RESEARCH & REFLECTION IN DERMATOLOGY

First edition. February 3, 2024.

ISBN: 979-8224195114

Written by Ram Malkani.

Table of Contents

Dr.   RAM MALKANI

RESEARCH & REFLECTIONS IN DERMATOLOGY

4 Decades of Clinical and Consultation Experience in India

DEDICATED TO MY SON
KABIR MALKANI

4 Decades of Clinical and Consultation Practice in India

A clinician has a certain limitations during his life time, though as years pass by, he may gloat over the popularity and reverence he enjoys from the patients. He may also enjoy the fact of his erudition, at times exaggerated, as part of a self aggrandisement tendency. His initial years, after becoming a Consultant, are spent in reinforcing his knowledge, testing it, and trying to get feed back of his skills through the therapeutic management of his patients. He cleverly learns the art of clinical acumen, which could take many long years. He learns the art and importance of eliciting good history from the patients. He has to network and become a self styled marketing person. He has to learn to win over the hearts of his patients by humouring them with his bed side mannerisms.

Over a period of time he learns to rise above contemptuous feelings he might have experienced towards his patients, staff, associates and colleagues. During the journey he may come across opportunities to excel in arriving at somewhat admirable diagnoses, have a collection of case reports, studies, drug trials and original articles. He by virtue of his seniority can help others around him grow, may be to greater heights than himself. He has the opportunity to set hemsilf as an example of a crusader in the alleviation of suffering of his patients. He can dedicate his life in empathizing and counseling his patients. If he is lucky to have an inquisitive mind he can make inroads into genuine research, avoiding duplication under the guise of research.

Completed Research

Preventive corticosteroid therapy prevents nerve damage in multibacillary leprosy patients, an assessment by NCV studies and clinical neurological examination: a study of 40 patients

To study the etiology, risk factors, skin changes of chronic venous insufficiency and existence of preceding or present deep venous thrombosis as an etiology, and association of thrombophilia -2014

Chronic Urticaria and Metabolic Syndrome: Markers of Systemic Inflammation

ETHICAL COMMITTEE OF DRSKINPIMPLES PVT LTD

Ethical Committee

HIV

Drug Resistance Mutations to Protease and Reverse Transcriptase Inhibitors in Treatment Naive HIV-1 Clade C Infected Individuals from Mumbai, India

A study of antiretroviral resistance patterns in treatment experienced and naive human immunodeficiency virus infected-patients

ONGOING RESEARCH

Hair morphology in heat damaged hair in females: A case-control study

Melasma and Metabolic Syndrome: More than meets the eye?

Studies

Assessment of Complete Hormonal Status in Female Acne Patients – A Study

Acanthosis nigricans: a marker of polycystic ovarian disease, insulin resistance, obesity, A Jaslok Hospital & Reseach Centre Study

Baseline CD4 T cell counts in HIV infected individuals who were diagnosed during voluntary counselling and testing in a resource poor setting

Subclinical DVT as an etiology of CVI- a study of 50 cases

Ongoing Studies

To study the prevalence of HIV, HBV, and HCV and trends of prevalence from 2009 through 2013;

Drug trials

Use of Buspirone (Buscalm), a psychotropic drug for treatment of atopic dermatitis in 20 patients – conducted a double blind controlled trial, at the Jaslok Hospital & Research Centre, 1995

Evaluation of Azithromycin for the treatment of acute non-gonococcal urethritis in males (Protocol AZM-II-92-003C) Trial conducted at the Jaslok Hospital & Research Centre

Efficacy and safety assessment of a new Ayurvedic antifungal Herbal cream - A study conducted at the Jaslok Hospital & Research Centre

Efficacy and Safety of Moxifloxacin (MXF) vs Cephalexin (with or without Metronidazole) in the Treatment of Mild to Moderate Uncomplicated Skin and Skin Structures Infections (USSSI)

Evaluation of clinical efficacy and tolerance of Tazarotene 0.05% gel in the treatment of Acne vulgaris & Psoriasis-March 2003 to June 2003.

Evaluation of azithromycin in the treatment of acute pyogenic skin infections

International Publications

Evaluation of Azithromycin / Zithromax for the treatment of skin infections

Anonymous Counselling & Testing Centre, Bombay - an intervention strategy

Medico-politics and HIV related responses in India - impact, as a product of historicization with the epidemic

IADVL Maharashtra Branch's anonymous testing centre (ATC) at Bombay.

Why is the Indian Dermatologist reluctant to acknowledge the magnitude of psychodermatology?

Acquired Zinc Deficiency in a Renal Transplant Recipient with Gastro-intestinal Tuberculosis Responding Promptly to Oral Correction

Leprosy or sarcoidosis? A diagnostic dilemma!

Psychodermatology

Institute of Psychosomatic Dermatology

Conceptualising Institute For Psychosomatic Dermatology

A study of stress in patients with acne excoriée, lichen and macular amyloidosis, and lichen planus

A study of DEPRESSION in patients with acne excoriée, lichen and macular amyloidosis, and lichen planus

Genodermatosis

Congenital Lip Pits

Kindler Weary Syndrome

Skin and Systemic Disease

A Rare Overlap of Epidermolysis Bullosa Acquisita and Seronegative Rheumatoid Arthritis

Infections

Erythema Necroticans

Chromomycosis

Pseudo elephantiasis of the vulva of tubercular etiology-An unusual presentation

Disseminated Mycofoacterium Bovis Infection from BCG Vaccination of a patient with Combined Immunodeficiency

Cutaneous presentation of atypical mycobacterial infection – An interesting case

Cutaneous Malakoplakia - A Rare Entity!

Cutaneous Myiasis

A Rare Case of Actinomycetoma

Malignancy

Follicular Mucinosis

Recalcitrant pruritus as primary manifestation of synchronous Hodgkins lymphoma and Langerhans cell histiocytosis

Skin - a mirror of internal disease

Neutrophilic Eccrine Hidradenitis in a patient of Chronic Lymphoid Leukemia

Drug Reactions

Management of pemphigus with gold compounds

Drug hypersensitivity syndrome to leflunomide

Dapsone induced Hemolysis in Glucose-6-Phosphate Dehydrogenase (G6PD) deficient individual

Dapsone syndrome : A case study

Toxic Epidermal Necrolysis

Lymphomatoid drug eruption due to levofloxacin

Myocarditis: A rare complication in DRESS syndrome

A rare complication of Rituximab therapy in Pemphigus vulgaris

Mononucleosis-Like Drug Rash: An Interesting Case Presentation

Review Articles

Oral Retinoids in Dermatology

IgE

Induction of contact dermatitis as a therapeutic measure in Alopecia Areata and Warts

Essential fatty acids and the skin

Cetirizine in urticaria and atopic dermatitis

Keloids and Hypertrophic Scars A Therapeutic Enigma

Lasers in Dermatology

Psychogenic Pruritus - an overview

Bifonazole: Focus on a Topical Azole

Epidemiological study of serum IgE levels in patients with atopic dermatitis.

In the process of completion for publication

Completed Research

Preventive corticosteroid therapy prevents nerve damage in multibacillary leprosy patients, an assessment by NCV studies and clinical neurological examination: a study of 40 patients

Phiroza Wadia, Sunil Ghate, Ram Malkani

Presented at the Jaslok Hospital & Research Centre, Founder`s day deliberation 2013

Presented at the National conference of the IADVL DERMOCON held at Hyderabad

Reflections

In Leprosy wasting of muscles, neuropathy and deformities have been a challenge. The nerve damage is more on a late diagnosis, reactions and mostly in Multibacillary Leprosy. Preventing motor deficit is what prompted the study. Conventionally administering cortisone helps in minimising damage. Hence it was proposed to see if prescribing cortisone from the day of initiation of anti leprosy treatment would prevent nerve damage as compared to prescribing as and when during reactions in leprosy.

One arm of 20 patients received cortisone from the beginning of treatment, second arm of 20 received as and when. For objective assessment clinical exam and NCV studies were done at regular intervals. It was a surprise to conclude at the end of the study, that the nerve damage was inevitable! By and large the experience was that, there was hardly any dropouts amongst the patients during follow up.

Introduction

Leprosy would have been a benign disease if it did not cause deformities. Reactions/neuritis lead to majority of deformities. Steroids have been used to treat reactions/neuritis for decades together. Newer studies demonstrated utility of prophylactic steroids in preventing reactions/neuritis & silent neuritis.

We undertook this study to analyse the effects of prophylactic steroids in comparison with Multidrug therapy (MDT). It was decided to enroll 40 cases divided into 2 groups of 20 each. The study group received prednisolone in addition to MDT from day 1. Prednisolone was tapered off in 4`th month.

Objectives

- To study utility of prophylactic steroids in preventing reactions/neuritis

- To study whether there is reversal of nerve function impairment after steroids

- To study incidence of silent neuritis

Material & Methods

Forty cases with one or more skin & or nerve lesions were included in the study. Baseline clinical assessment, slit skin smears, touch sensibility test (TST) & voluntary muscle test (VMT) were done. A punch skin biopsy was done to confirm the diagnosis. In cases presenting without skin lesions, a cutaneous nerve biopsy was done. Nerve conduction velocity (NCV) was done at baseline & at 3 monthly intervals. Clinical evaluation was carried out at monthly intervals. TST/VMT was repeated at 3 monthly intervals.

All cases received WHO MDT MB for 2 years.

Cases without reaction/neuritis were alternately assigned to prophylactic prednisolone (20 mg daily for 3 months, tapered off in the 4th month). This group was called Group A. The other Group (Group B) received only MDT.

Those presenting with reaction/neuritis were given therapeutic prednisolone (40 mg, 30 mg, 20mg, 15 mg, 10mg, 5 mg each for 14 days). This Group was also added to Gr A.

Observations

- Study group (Gr A) consisted of 18/40 cases of which 15/18 males & 3/18 females

- Out of 18 cases receiving prednisolone, 14/18 received prophylactic & 4/18 therapeutic steroid.

- Age of the patients varied between 17- 60 yrs. There was one child aged 8 years.

- Control Gr B had 22 cases, of them 13 were males & 9 females.

- Age of these patients ranged between 7- 60 yrs. There was no child in this group

- Reactions seen in two groups during follow up

- Gr A = 2/18 had neuritis. Both had baseline neuritis also

- Gr B = 3/22 had type I reaction & neuritis

- No case of silent neuritis recorded in our study by clinical means.

Clinical features

As is evident in this table,

LESIONS	Gr A	Gr B	Total
HPP`s	4	9	13
Erythematous	8	10	18
Icthyotic	2	1	3
Pure Neural	4	2	6
Total	18	22	40

Erythematous patches were the commonest presentation followed by hypo-pigmented patches in both the groups. Six cases of pure neural leprosy found of them, 4 belonged to Gr A & 2 to Gr B.

HISTOPATHOLOGY

The commonest histopathological finding was Borderline tuberculoid leprosy (BT). Midborderline (BB), Borderline lepromatous (BL) & Inderterminate (I) were the other classes seen. Two patients each in both the groups were no biopsied.

H/P	Gr A	Gr B	Total
BT	12	15	27
BB	2	1	3
BL	1	1	2
Indeterminate	1	3	4
Not done	2	2	4
Total	18	22	40

Baseline abnormal TST was recorded in 8 cases in Gr A & 3 cases in Gr B.

TST	Gr A	Gr B	Total
Normal	10	19	29
Abnormal	8	3	11
Total	18	22	40

Baseline abnormal VMT was recorded in 8 cases in Gr A & 2 cases in Gr B

VMT	Gr A	Gr B	Total
Normal	10	20	30
Abnormal	8	2	10
Total	18	22	40

NCV Baseline

NCV	Gr A	Gr B	Total
Normal	3	11	14
Mononeuritis Multiplex	6	5	11
One nerve	4	3	7
Two nerves	2	1	3
Not done	3	2	5
Total	18	22	40

Final abnormal TST was recorded in 7 in Gr A & 5 cases in Gr B

TST	Gr A	Gr B	Total
Normal	11	17	28
Abnormal	7	5	12
Total	18	22	40

Final abnormal VMT was recorded in 7 in Gr A & 2 in Gr B

VMT	Gr A	Gr B	Total
Normal	11	20	31
Abnormal	7	2	9
Total	18	22	40

NCV Final

NCV	Gr A	Gr B	Total
Normal	4	8	12
Mononeuritis Multiplex	6	5	11
One nerve	4	3	7
Two nerves	1	2	3
Not done	3	4	7
Total	18	22	40

Observations

Gr A & Gr B did not show significant difference with respect to occurrence of reactions/neuritis.

Sensory component was involved more commonly than motor component, by TST, VMT as well as NCV in both groups.

As the number of cases in Gr A involved cases with baseline reactional episodes, TST, VMT & NCV abnormality is seen more in that group.

TST & VMT improved in one case in Gr A, while TST deteriorated in 2 cases in Gr B which possibly explains the prophylactic effect of steroids.

NCV improved in one case in Gr A while it deteriorated in 3 cases in Gr B. That also possibly explains the utility of prophylactic steroids.

Conclusions

Prophylactic steroids do show a positive effect on nerve function improvement in this small study.

Those cases not receiving prophylactic steroids show deterioration in nerve function.

Steroids don`t have prophylactic role in preventing reactions/neuritis. As preservation ofnerve function is a priority to prevent deformities, prophylactic steroids may be considered in management of leprosy.

To study the etiology, risk factors, skin changes of chronic venous insufficiency and existence of preceding or present deep venous thrombosis as an etiology, and association of thrombophilia -2014

Sneh Thadani, Ram Malkani

Presented as a poster at the National conference of the IADVL at Mangalore DERMACON 2015

Reflections

On coming across the fact that, one third of patients attending a hospital OPD have Venous insufficiency in the legs, it was decided to underst and the pathology of Chronic venous insufficiency (CVI) in greater detail, as Stasis Dermatitis and Venous Ulcers are presentation seen not so infrequently by the Dermatologist in clinical practise. The exact etiology not known, the Dermatologist isill equipped to comprehend the therapy to be recommended. When going through the literature it was realised that venous hypertension was the common pathology for the skin changes. That venous hypertension was because of pooling of blood in the veins because of incompetent perforators. The incompetent perforators were hypothesised in the thesis as a result of an evanescent Deep Vein Thrombosis, which caused temporary pooling in the Deep vein, subsequently *leading to pooling in the superficial vein. The superficial veins draining into the Deep veins would have to dilate, to accommodate the pooled blood, which would result in the valves to be stretched away from each other, resulting in incompetent perforators and permanent venous hypertension.*

The hypothesis suggests the cause responsible is thrombosis, which resolves spontaneously in the Deep Veins. The cause of thrombosis is probably thrombophilia in the patient, which was responsible for the obstruction of the Deep vein temporarily. The Gold standard for diagnosis of resolving DVT requires expertise of the sonologist and the special more sensitive probes of Colour Doppler to identify the very fine images defining a resolving DVT. The thesis did not bring out the correct incidence of thrombosis because of the Limitations of the sonologist and the equipment used.

Background:

Venous disorders are clinically important; they range from telangiectasis to fatal events such as pulmonary embolism. The main objectives of the study were to evaluate the clinical presentation of chronic venous insufficiency (CVI) and assess the factors associated with it.

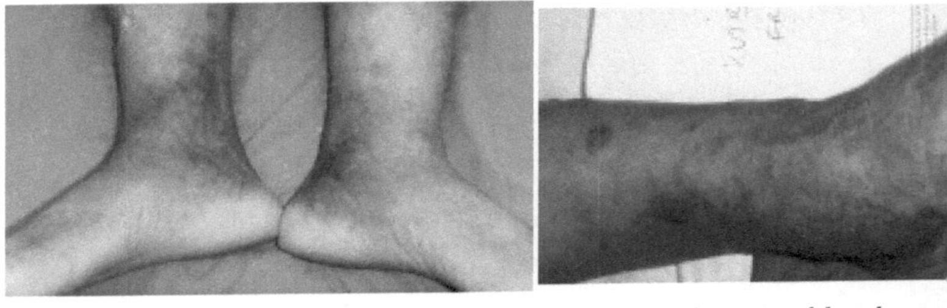

Image 1: showing hyper pigmentation on the medial aspect of both lower limbs and ankle flare due to chronic venous insufficiency

Image 2: showing dilated tort varicose veins on medial side of t associated hyper pigmentation

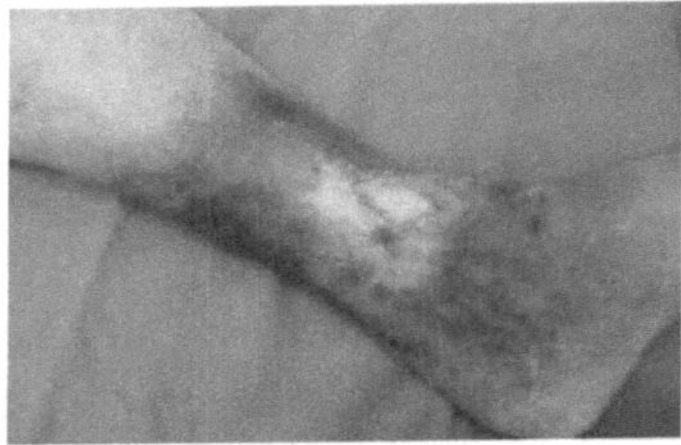

Image 3: venous ulcer measuring 1 cm,with irregular but well defin floor showing yellowish necrotic ba hyper pigmentation, lipoderma evidence of dilated tortuous varicos

Methods:

The present study is a cross-sectional analysis of 50 patients presenting with features of deep vein thrombosis (DVT). We collected demographic and clinical information (features of CVI, body mass index), used scales to measure the severity of CVI (Venous Severity Clinical Score [VSCS] and CEAP classification). We also did a colour Doppler duplex scanning and haematological investigations (Factor-V, D-DIMER, Lipid profile, and Serum Homocysteine).

Results:

We presented the results from 32 males and 18 females; there were no significant differences in mean ages (SD) of the males and female (43.1 (12.1) vs 47.6 (9.8) years; p=0.19).The most common symptoms were oedema (88%), pigmentation (78%), and distended veins (76%). Factor-V was significantly higher in patients who were classified as severe on VSCS (4% vs 0%, p=0.03). Furthermore, patients who were diagnosed with perforators (95% vs 55%, p=0.002), great saphenous vein incompetence (62% vs 21%, p=0.003), and with varicosities (71% vs 28%, p=0.002) on ultrasonography were significantly more likely be severe on clinical classification compared with those who were not. Patients with thrombosis on sonography had significantly higher serum homocysteine (100% vs 29%, p=0.04), Factor-V (100% vs 4%, p<0.0001) and altered lipid profile compared with those who did not.

Conclusion:

Haematological markers are useful to identify venous thrombosis as a cause of CVI, as this may be difficult to detect on ultrasonography.

Chronic Urticaria and Metabolic Syndrome: Markers of Systemic Inflammation

Dr. Ram Malkani, Dr. Anshu Agarwal, Dr. Maninder Singh Setia

Presented as a Free paper at the National Conference of theIADVL DERMACON 2016 conference held at Coimbatore

Reflections

Urticaria is a commonsymptom encountered in Dermatology. Yet no known definite etiology in Chronic spontaneous Urticaria is established. Urticaria is considered to be a systemic inflammation and so isMetabolic syndrome. Hence the need to see if Urticaria has a greater incidence of Mets than in Controls. Severe Urticaria does have higher CRP and at times even D Dimer is raised. In our study the sample was small and in the criteria of Mets, Only three parameters were chosen out of 5. Two left out were, Blood pressure and Fasting blood sugar, which in hind sight probably could be responsible for lesser number of Mets associated with urticaria in our study.

Introduction:

Metabolic syndrome (MetS) and chronic urticaria patients are considered to be markers of systematic inflammation.

We assessed prevalence of MetS in patients with chronic urticaria and their association with systemic inflammation.

Methods: We assessed MetS in 40 patients with chronic urticaria (cases) and 38 patients without chronic dermatological conditions (controls), using the National Cholesterol Education Program–III Adult treatment Panel. We assessed the severity of urticaria by Urticaria Severity System Score and measured C-Reactive protein (marker of systemic inflammation). We used logistic regression models for multivariate analysis.

Results: The mean (SD) age of cases was (37.6 [10.4]) and of controls was (36.1 [13.4]); p=0.56. The mean (SD) of waist circumference (WC) and low density liproproteins (LDL) was significantly higher in cases compared with controls (WC: 94.2 [10.4] vs 86.8 [9.1], p=0.001; LDL: 124.9 [21.5] vs 110.9 [31.7], p=0.02). High levels of CRP was similar in cases and controls (55% vs 45%, p=0.70). MetS was significantly higher in cases compared with controls (35% vs 10%, p=0.01). After adjusting for age, sex, and CRP, we found cases were significantly more likely to have MetS compared with controls (odds ratio: 5.2, 95% confidence intervals: 1.3 – 19.9). High levels of CRP was not associated with MetS. There was no significant association between the severity of chronic urticaria and presence of MetS.

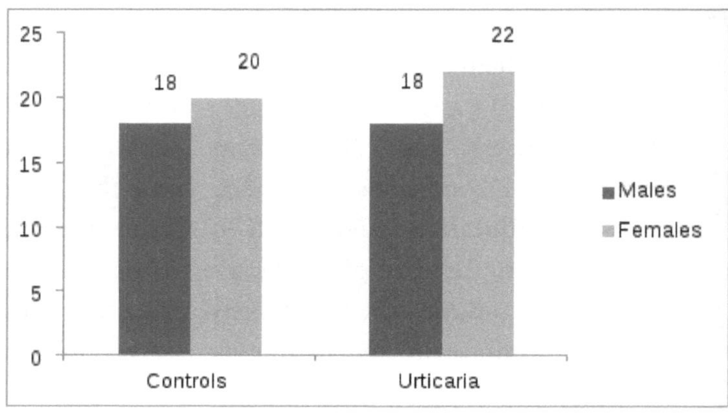

p= 0.83

Controls: 45% Males and 55% Females, Urticaria Patients: 47% Males and 53% Females

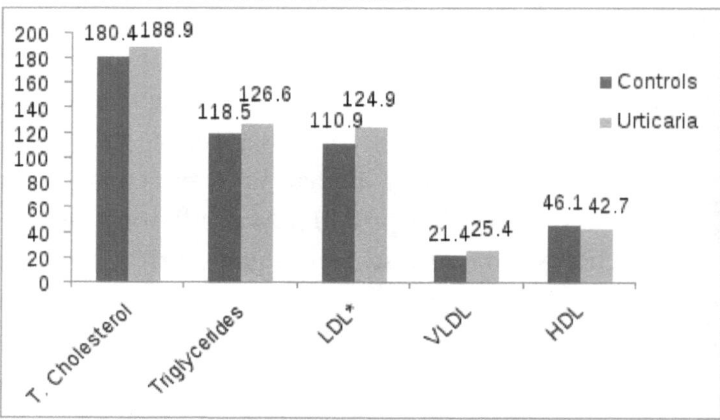

The mean (SD) LDL levels were significantly higher in urticaria patients compared with controls [124.9 (21.5) vs 110.9 (31.7), p=0.02]

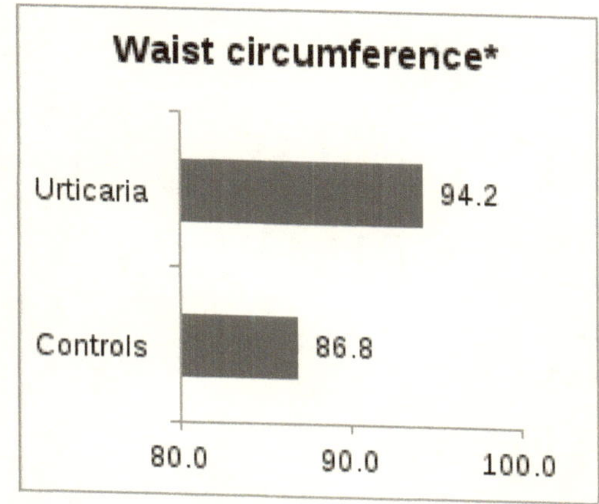

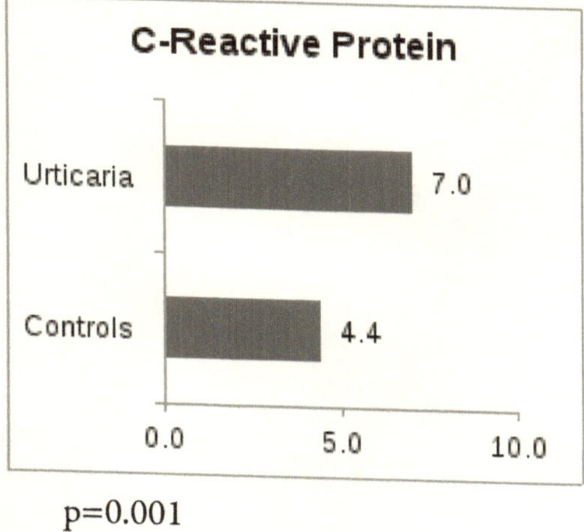

p=0.001

Conclusions

All patients with chronic urticaria should be evaluated for MetS and clinical treatment should focus on management of both conditions. Systemic inflammation was not associated with both conditions in our population.

ETHICAL COMMITTEE OF DRSKINPIMPLES PVT LTD

Ethical Committee

INTRODUCTION

One of the possibly only single clinic which is conducting an Ethical committee affiliated to Drskinpimples pvt ltd. In May 2017,which has its registered office at the private clinic of Dr Ram Malkani, a Consultant Dermatologist in practice for the last 45 years,at 305 Doctor House,opp Jaslok Hospital and Research Centre, 14,Dr G Deshmukh Rd , Mumbai 400 026.

ABOUT DRSKINPIMPLES PVT LTD

Drskinpimples Pvt Ltd is an organisation, with two Directors, Dr Ram Malkani and his elder sister Mrs Chandra Malkani. Drskinpimples Pvt Ltd has Memorandum of Association. The private ltd company has a PANCARD and submits its accounts to IT and pays income tax.

REGULATORY AUTHORITY REQIUSITES

For any research project, or a publication, it is mandatory for it to be scrutinised by an Ethical Committee, which is affiliated to DCGI,CDSCO, New Delhi. Drskinpimples Pvt Ltd has been registered with the DCGI, CDSCO, New Delhi, the National agency, authorised by the Central Government Ministry of Health.Essentially this Ethical Committee can scrutinise, only the research projects or the publications, where Dr Ram Malkani, who has to be is the Principal Investigator.

CONSTITUENT MEMBERS OF THE ETHICAL COMMITTEE

The Ethical committee consists of Chairperson, Member Secretary , two Clinicians, one Theologist, one lawyer, one from Applied Science, one lawyer, Two non medical representatives, one of them with Science background One of Non Science background. Every member has to acquire the certificate of having passed the examination of eligibility of becoming a member on an an Ethical committee, which is available online on the NIH website.

PROCESS OF REGISTRATION OF THE ETHICAL COMMITTEE

Most or all of the Ethical Committees existing in the country are affiliated to a teaching College, University or an Institution

The application is then made to DCGI, New Delhi for approval. The process of application requires a dedicated team to compile the documentation. After carefully going through the documents/dossier submitted, the approval is granted. The DCGI grants its approval for the next three years.

TIME TABLE OF THE FUNCTIONING OF THE ETHICAL COMMITTEE

A meeting of the committee must be held every 3 months with required quorum present. All members receive an honorarium for attending the meeting. The meeting is held in an austere place with basic minimum refreshments.

The Agenda and the Project to be discussed is/are circulated to all EC members a month before. Before deciding on the date, availability of all Members of the EC, is checked by the Member Secretary. The Member Secretary maintains the minutes and accounts. Minutes, once ready have to be signed by the Chairperson. A box file is maintained of the hard copies of the Agenda and the minutes. The EC must have an office and the Member Secretary must be present at least for 5 hrs daily for 6 days a week. At the end of the tenure of 3 years ,the existing EC has to apply for renewal. Each application involves many documents, CV of all members etc amounting Loads of A4 size papers.

MEMBER SECRETARY

A Research Secretary is mandatory who should be full time, atleast 5 hours per day. Finding a member secretary not easy for a single clinic. The Member Secretary must have some understanding of Research, documentation, coordination with committee members in organising the Ethical committee meeting. In an institute, on the other hand, faculty, dedicated staff available, who will carry out the responsibility of maintaining minutes, filing the protocols of the projects submitted, the comments of the members of the Ethical Committee, to the investigator/s, during the meeting, added to that the the responsibility of compiling their response to the queries of the EC members, then communicating to the members within a month online. The Member Secretary, can also be assigned the responsibility of reviewing the literature, of the Research projects planned by Drkinpimples' investigators and to prepare summaries.

FINANCIAL IMPLICATIONS

Each EC meeting is held every 3 months. It could cost Rs 15000 or more for each meeting as each member is given a token honorarium towards travel. In a year there are 4 meetings. Meeting cost itself amounting to Rs 60,000. The other miscellaneous expenses include Stationery, making copies, courier services expenses for getting a Signature of the Chairman. All together expenses could total upto an amount of Rs 70 to 80,000 a year. If in any Research project, if a grant is received, then it can probably help covers a part of the cost of the the expenses involved in maintaining the Ethical committee.

PURPOSE OF STARTING AN ETHICAL COMMITTEE IN A PRIVATE CLINIC

FOUR ARMS OF RESEARCH

1) Conceptualising the research hypothesis
2) Writing the protocol as per the guidelines of the DCGI

3) Approval of the Ethical Committee

4) Conducting the research project to its end point

THE PROTYPE OF AN AGENDA

- Reading the minutes of the last meeting
- Reviewing the comments` response of the last meeting
- Any new proposal
- Reviewing completion of the old Proposal/s

Dr. Malkani proposes to conduct epidemiological, cross-sectional, cohort, case-control, and other clinical studies in skin, hair, sexually transmitted infections (including HIV/AIDS), and leprosy.

Academically, as more unique patients come to the clinic, which may not happen in an institute. A patient of clinic, in a research in an institute, has to be shared and similarly authorship needs to be shared. In an institute bureaucratic procedures are time consuming, at times, colleagues / In the institute may show some animosity out of a professional competitiveness. With one`s own Ethical Committee, one can have the liberty of rolling out many publications, research projects to be reviewed by the EC.

SOME IMPORTANT ISSUES

One of the members in the initial first meeting which was held in a club, before the committee was formally formed said, that the meetings should be held in austere venue, it should not appear that the organisers are trying to influence the members ,influencing a favourable response. One of the initial chosen was a Chartered Accountant and a Fraud Auditor consultant, expressed his apprehensions, that he would not like to be a member as, there might be some litigation on EC members, which would disturb his piece of mind. One of the lady members consulted the Director of DrSkinpimples pvt ltd for a Dermatological consultation for her son, insisted on paying fees, as otherwise, it would amount To quid pro quo.

THE BOTTOM LINE

Existence of an Ethical committee, raises the bar of of ethics in routine day to day practice. It can offer colleagues,Pharma,who do not have access to an institution Ethical Committee, to get an approval of EC , which can have a common theme or partnership with drskinpimples Pvt Ltd.

HIV

Drug Resistance Mutations to Protease and Reverse Transcriptase Inhibitors in Treatment Naive HIV-1 Clade C Infected Individuals from Mumbai, India

P.D. Potdar, B.S. Daswani and N.J. Rane, Dr Ram Malkani, Dr Raj Harjani

International Journal of Virology
7(1),13-23 2011

INTRODUCTION

According to the AIDS Epidemic Update by the WHO (2008) it was estimated that an enormous 2.4 million people have been affected with HIV in India at the end of 2008 i.e., probably one in every eight people (Steinbrook, 2007). Of these, only an estimated 10-20% of infected people in India know that they have HIV infection (Steinbrook, 2007) and even fewer are those who have the privilege of well-timed drug resistance treatment and monitoring. The same is true in other developing countries like Nigeria (Olowosegun et al., 2008), Cameroon (Alemnji et al., 2006), Bangladesh (Khandoker et al., 2006) wherein the very lack of knowledge of HIV status poses a big challenge to control this disease. Fortunately, the easy accessibility and low cost of Highly Active Antiretroviral Therapy (HAART) since the year 2000 has dramatically decreased the AIDS (Acquired

Immunodeficiency Syndrome) related mortality and improved survival of HIV patients who are aware of the disease (Palella et al., 1998; Kumarasamy et al., 2005). However, the emergence of drug resistant viruses has been an undesired outcome which requires timely monitoring. Especially, the first line therapy is of paramount importance in controlling viral replication and thus the primary mutations should be taken into consideration before prescribing first line regimen (O'Neil et al., 2002). Several prospective controlled studies have shown that patients whose physicians have access to drug resistance data, particularly genotypic resistance data, respond better to therapy than control patients whose physicians do not have access to these assays (O'Neil et al., 2002). This assists the physicians in the initial choice of treatment (Weidle et al., 2003) and helps identify the genetic causes of treatment failure as a prerequisite in deciding the subsequent clinical course for better patient management (Kantor et al., 2010).

HIV pathogenesis is influenced by various factors such as route of exposure, dose of the inoculum, genetic predisposition, age, environment, other opportunistic infections, virus variants etc (Oguntibeju et al., 2007). Further, HIV-1 clade C infected persons comprise more than 56% of the infections worldwide and more than 98% of the infections in the Indian subcontinent (Robertson et al., 2000). Surprisingly, existing sequence data and interpretation algorithms are instead focused on HIV-1 clade B. Compared to the extensive information available on the B subtypes, there is hardly enough statistics on the predominant non-B subtypes to identify significant correlations and develop a sequence database. Therefore, extensive surveillance efforts are necessary to control the widespread dissemination of the clade C viruses.

The assay for antiretroviral response has become an indispensable diagnostic tool to increase the overall efficiency of treatment and management of HIV affected patients. The genotypic technique by gene sequencing remains the 'gold standard' for resistance testing due to the ability to detect mutations in variants that are present in low quantities as that can potentially cause resistance and also detect mutations that are responsible for selective drug pressure (Shafer, 2002). However, in India the laboratories having the facilities for genotyping are very few (Robertson et al., 2000). Moreover, the enormous cost of this assay makes patients shy away from it. Drug resistance testing has not been an integral part of routine treatment monitoring of patients receiving ARV drugs or as a prerequisite to initiate ARV treatment. Furthermore, there is a paucity of information regarding the presence of primary drug resistance to protease inhibitors in Indian literature (Shankarkumar et al., 2009). Especially, the studies on primary drug resistance mutations reported from Mumbai have mainly focused only on the reverse transcriptase region of the pol gene. Therefore, this study has analyzed primary drug resistance mutations in both protease and reverse transcriptase regions, in treatment naive HIV seropositive individuals from Mumbai, India. This is a report on the preliminary findings on drug resistance mutations in clade C individuals which may contribute to the HIV mutations data at a global level.

MATERIALS AND METHODS

Sample collection: The patients attending the clinics of Jaslok Hospital and Research Centre and other hospitals in Mumbai from the year 2008-2010 were enrolled for this study. The Scientific Advisory committee and Ethics committee of Jaslok Hospital and Research Centre had approved this study. Fifty naive HIV seropositive patients and 10 control individuals were enrolled with their informed consent. Five ml of blood was collected in EDTA BD Vacutainer® tubes and RNA isolation was immediately carried out using the Trizol® reagent (Invitrogen, USA).

HIV RNA PCR: HIV RT-PCR was performed using the QIAGEN ® OneStep RT-PCR Kit (QIAGEN, Hilden, Germany). The upstream primer SK462 (5'-TGC TAT GTC AGT TCC CCT TGG TTC TCT-3') and downstream primer SK438 (5'- AGT TGG AGG ACA TCA AGC AGC CAT GCA AAT-3') were utilized to amplify the HIV gag region. The cycling conditions were as follows: 50°C for 30 min, 94°C for 2 min, 40 cycles of 94°C for 15 sec, 55°C for 30 sec, 72°C for 1 min and final extension at 72°C for 5 min. The 142 bp amplicons obtained were loaded an 8% polyacrylamide gel and electrophoresis was carried out under non-denaturing conditions and visualized by silver staining.

HIV real time PCR: HIV RNA real time PCR was performed using RoboGene Human Immunodeficiency Virus (HIV-1) quantification kit (aj ROBOSCREEN, Germany). The 200 ng of Trizol® extracted RNA was added to the Master mix containing 2 x universal master mix+primer (200 nM) + probe (200 nM) + 1x RT enzyme

(SuperScriptTM III Platinum). For each experiment, a non template control (NTC) and a negative control (HIV seronegative individual's RNA confirmed by PCR) was run. The external control RNA was HIV-1 RNA (aj ROBOSCREEN, Germany) at various dilutions. The samples were transferred into a 96 well real time PCR plate and the plate was kept into the real-time PCR instrument (ABI 7700, Foster City, USA). The thermal conditions were set at 60°C for 45 min for initial incubation of reverse transcription, hold on 95°C for 2 min and then proceeding with 45 cycles of melting at 95°C for 15 sec and annealing at 57°C for 1 min. Viral copies were calculated from the Ct value using a proper standard graph and quality control measures were taken at every step.

Genotypic assay for detection of HIV drug resistance: The sequencing of the protease and reverse transcriptase genes was performed as described in the past by Balakrishnan et al. (2005) with a few modifications.

First round PCR: The RNA extracted was used in a Reverse transcriptase PCR using the QIAGEN ® OneStep RT-PCR Kit (QIAGEN, Hilden, Germany). The primers used were upstream PR1 (5' - ACC AGA GCC AAC AGC CCC ACC A-3') and downstream PR2 (5'- CTT TTG GGC CAT CCA TTC CTG GC-3') for protease and upstream RT1 (5'-TAG GAC CTA CAC CTG TCA ACA TA-3') and downstream RT6 (5'-TAG GCT GTA CTG TCC ATT TAT CAG G-3') for reverse transcriptase genes. The same cycling conditions for both protease and reverse transcriptase were used in the first round PCR which was set up at 50°C for 30 min, 94°C for 2 min, 40 cycles of 94°C for 15 sec, 55°C for 30 sec, 72°C for 1 min and 72°C for 5 min.

Second round PCR: The 2 μL of the first PCR products was used as template for the second round PCR. For the protease gene, the primers used were upstream PR3 (5' -GAA GCA GGA GCC GAT AGA CAA GG-3') and downstream PR2 (5'- CTT TTG GGC CAT CCA TTC CTG GC-3') and the PCR conditions were initial denaturation at 95°C for 1 min, 25 cycles of denaturation at 95°C for 15 sec, annealing at 55°C for 30 sec, extension 72°C for 45 sec and final extension at 72°C for 7 min. For the reverse transcriptase gene, the primers used were upstream R3 (5'- TAG GCT GTA CTG TCC ATT TAT CAG G-3') and downstream RT6 (5'-TAG GCT GTA CTG TCC ATT TAT CAG G-3') with the PCR conditions set up at initial denaturation at 95°C for 1 min with 25 cycles of denaturation at 95°C for 15 sec, annealing 55°C for 30 sec, extension at 72°C for 1 min and final extension at 72°C for 7 min.

The amplicons obtained for both protease and reverse transcriptase genes were analyzed on a 2% agarose gels stained with ethidium bromide (20 mg mL-1) and observed under UV light. The purified PCR product was subjected to DNA sequencing using Big Dye Terminator (Applied Biosystems, USA) in an ABI PRISM 3100 Genetic Analyzer (Applied Biosystems).

Analysis using HIV stanford database: The sequences obtained were analyzed for homology with HIV protease and reverse transcriptase genes using NCBI BLAST search and HIV clade detection was done using the online NCBI

Viral Genotyping tool. Further, the online HIV Stanford Database (http://hivdb.stanford.edu) was utilized for genotypic drug resistance analysis and all sequences were defined as compared with clade B as per the database rules.

RESULTS

Preliminary observations (Table 1) of the HIV seropositive naive patients enrolled for the study regarding gender and age revealed that 76% were males and their ages ranged from 7 to 55 years with a median age of 30 years. HIV seropositivity was confirmed by RT-PCR of gag gene expression for all fifty samples. Out of the 50 HIV seropositive patients, 18 samples had an undetectable viral load i.e. plasma HIV-1 RNA viral load = 1000 copies mL-1 and thus could not be sequenced. The remaining samples were within a range of 1.4x103 to 2.8x106 viral copies mL-1 and had a median value of 3.6x105 viral copies mL-1.

HIV Protease and reverse transcriptase regions of the pol gene were successfully amplified and sequenced in fifteen samples. RT-PCR for the reverse transcriptase and protease regions have been shown in Fig. 1 and 2, respectively. Further, clade identification was done using the NCBI viral mutations (Table 2) at the following positions: V32I (1 out of 15); M46L (5 out of 15); I47M (8 out of 15); I50V (1 out of 15); V82A/D/G (6 out of 15); N88S (3 out of 15). This study further showed that M46L, I47M and V82A/D/G were most prominent mutations found in almost more than 30% of patients analysed for this study and this needs further investigation with more number of samples. These PR mutations impart resistance to drugs like Indinavir

(IDV), Lopinavir (LPV), Nelfinavir (NFV) etc. Also, minor protease mutations/polymorphisms in ten of the fifteen samples studied were seen at the following positions: L10I (1 out of 15); V11F (1 out of 15); L23H (2 out of 15); K43I/R (2 out of 15); A71D (1 out of 15); G73A (2 out of 15); T74A/P/S (8 out of 15); N83D (8 out of 15). As far as Reverse transcriptase gene mutations are concerned, Nucleotide Reverse Transcriptase Inhibitors (NRTIs) mutations at positions M41L (1 out of 15); D67N (1 out of 15); M184V (2 out of 15); T215A/G/R (5 out of 15); K219E/R (3 out of 15), L210V (1 out of 15) were seen as shown in Table 3.

Table 1: Preliminary observations of HIV-1 infected individuals enrolled for the study

Preliminary observations	Patients (n = 50)
Gender	
Males (%)	76
Females (%)	24
Age	
Range (years)	7-55
Median (years)	30
Viral load	
Number of detectable samples i.e., >1000 copies mL^{-1}	32*
Number of undetectable samples i.e., <1000 copies mL^{-1}	18
Range of viral load of detectable samples (copies mL^{-1})	1.4×10^3 to 2.8×10^6
Median of viral load of detectable samples (copies mL^{-1})	3.0×10^5

*Out of 32 samples which had detectable HIV viral loads, 15 samples were successfully sequenced

Fig. 1: A region in the HIV reverse transcriptase obtained by 1 step RT-PCR and subsequent nested PCR (above) and the amplification of beta-Actin gene (below), respectively

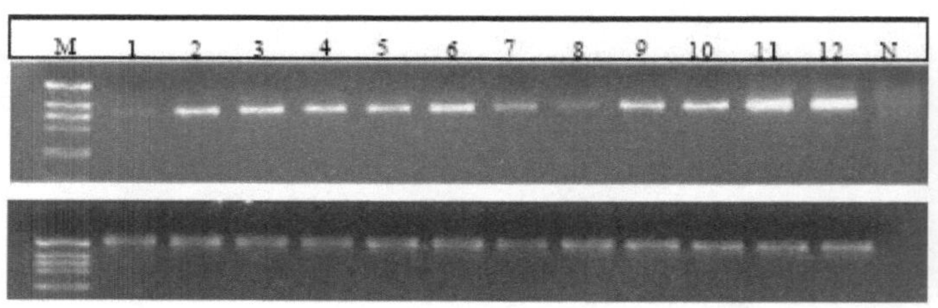

Fig. 2: A region in the HIV protease obtained by 1 step RT-PCR and subsequent nested PCR (above) and the amplification of beta-Actin gene (below), respectively

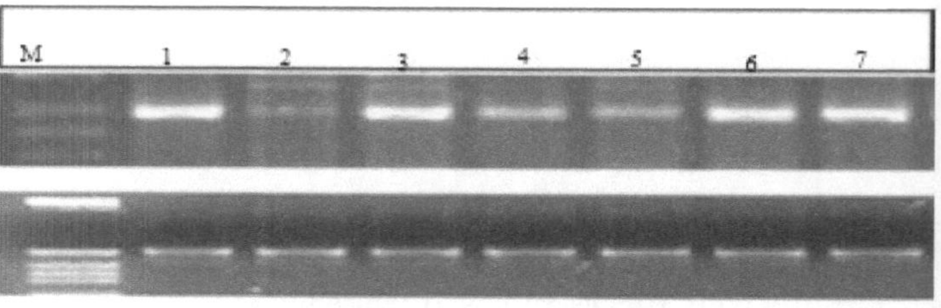

Table 2: Major protease drug resistance mutations obtained in indian HIV seropositive naive patients

Mutation	No. of patients	%	Reduced sensitivity to drugs
V32I	1/15	7	All PI, except Saquinavir (SQV)
I47M	8/15	53	Reduced susceptibility to FPV, IDV, LPV, TPV, DRV. Highly unusual mutation
V82A/D/G	6/15	40	Reduce susceptibility to IDV, LPV with other mutations NFV ATV, FPV. V82DG highly unusual mutation.
N88S	3/15	22	High resistance to NFV, ATV, increased susceptibility to FPV
I50V	1/15	7	Causes intermediate resistance to FPV
M46L	5/15	33.35	Resistance to IDV, NFV, FPV, LPV, ATV

FPV: Fosamprenavir, ATV: Atazanavir, IDN: Indinavir, LPV: Lopinavir, TPV: Tiprinavir, DRV: Duranavir, NFV: Nelfinavir, SQU: Saquinavir

The most prominent among these was T215A/G/R as seen in 33.3% of the study cohort. Mutations associated with Non Nucleoside Reverse Transcriptase Inhibitors (NNRTIs) were also observed in this study at positions: Y181C (5 out of 15); Y188L (1 out of 15); G190A (1 out of 15); H221F/P (4 out of 15); P225H (3 out of 15). Therefore, Y181C (33.3%), H221F/P (26.6%) and P225H (20%) were the prominent mutations seen in the study cohort as shown in Table 4. Overall, many of the patients whose samples were sequenced for RT were resistant to Stavudine (D4T) and Efavirenz (EFV).

Table 3: NRTI mutations found in present study in Indian HIV seropositive naive patients

Mutation	No. of patients	%	Resistant to drug
T215A/R/G	5/15	33.3	AZT, D4T, ABC, DDI and TDF and is highly unusual.
M41L	1/15	7	Usually occurs with T215G High level resistance to AZT, D4T, ABC and TDF
M184V	2/15	14	High resistance to 3TC, FTC, increased susceptibility to AZT, TDF and D4T
D67N	1/15	7	Low resistance to NRTIs, susceptible to 3TC, FTC.
K219E/R	3/15	20	Decreased susceptibility to AZT and D4T
L210V	1/15	7	Usually occurs with the mutations M41L and T215Y and is highly unusual

AZT: Zidovudine, D4T: Stavudine, ABC: Abacavir, DDI: Didanosine, TDF: Tenafovir, FTC: Emtricitabine, 3TC: Lamivudine

Table 4: NNRTI Mutations found in our study in Indian HIV seropositive naive patients

Mutation	No. of patients	%	Resistant to drug
Y181L	1/15	7	High level resistance to NVP and EFV Low resistance to ETR
Y181C	5/15	33.3	Cause high level resistance to ETR, NVP/PLV, Low resistance to EFV
H221F/P	4/15	26.6	It is uncommon NNRTI associated mutation
P225H	3/15	20	Increased EFV resistant when in presence of P225LQR
G190A	1/15	7	Causes high level resistance to NVP and EFV and increased DLV susceptibility

NVP: Nevirapine, ETR: Etravivine, DLV: Delavidine, EFV: Efavirenz

This information is particularly useful in a country wherein resource limited settings and financial constraints limit the access to genotypic drug resistance data, thereby further investigations on the prevalence of these mutations in theIndian HIV gene pool can lead to the avoidance of these drugs for the treatment of HIV clade C patients of Indian origin.

DISCUSSION

According to the UNAIDS (2010) findings HIV in India is more prevalent in males than females which is concordant with the current findings. The same was true in a research study conducted in Malaysia consisting of 693 newly diagnosed HIV patients (Nissapatorn et al., 2007). Conversely, HIV seems to be equally prevalent in males and females in other developing countries such as Nigeria (Akhigbe et al., 2010) and more prevalent in females in other Nigerian studies (Nwachukwu and Orji, 2008;

Amegor et al., 2009). Further, the accurate diagnosis of this disease largely relies on PCR techniques rather than serological assays (Jamehdar et al., 2007), hence we confirmed the HIV seropositive status of all the patients using RT-PCR. Furthermore, HIV drug resistance assays are inseparable components of effective clinical management of individuals commencing or undergoing ART. The events of early HIV infection, mainly the saturation of the target cells, influences the transmitted drug resistant viruses to become well established in reservoirs that maintain long term resistance (Brenner et al., 2002; Delaugerre et al., 2004; Ghosn et al., 2006). Also, the replicative fitness of the viruses can be reduced with the correct ART combination (Gandhi et al., 2003). Therefore, the initial knowledge of the resistance status in an HIV seropositive individual commencing antiretroviral therapy is extremely vital. The International AIDS Society (IAS), USA, also recommends genotypic testing before commencing ART as this will detect mutations that may not be revealed in phenotypic assays and identify the subtype (Hirsch et al., 2008). In the present investigations, 15 samples could be screened for protease inhibitor resistance mutations of which many major and minor mutations were detected. It is noteworthy that although it is rare to observe major mutations in the PR region in treatment naive HIV patient samples, we came across many major mutations in the samples analyzed. Confirmation of the homology of these sequences with HIV wild type sequence was done using NCBI blast. The plausible explanation for observing many PR mutations is that the infrequent occurrence of major PR mutations makes many researchers overlook PR mutation analysis, which is also a tricky task. It was observed that I47M (substrate cleft position), a rare mutation, was present in more than 50% of samples analyzed. Interestingly, Mousavi et al. (2010), have recently reported I47M in a study from Iran. Isoleucine (I) at position 47 is typically mutated to valine(V) or Alanine(A) leading to decreased susceptibility to Fosamprenavir (FPV), Atazanavir (ATV), Indinavir (IDV), Lopinavir (LPV), Tipranavir (TPV) and Darunavir (DRV). Additionally, two most common mutations detected were M46L (flap position) and V82A/D/G (substrate cleft position). The former mutation is responsible for reducing susceptibility to almost all the protease inhibitors namely IDV, Nelfinavir(NFV), FPV, LPV, ATV, TPV and possibly Saquinavir (SQV) and DRV. The latter mutation has been reported as 10% of all primary mutations in a recent study from western India by Sachdeva et al. (2005) and results in contraindication to IDV and LPV. Further, mutation at position 88 (interior enzyme position) was observed in 22% of samples analyzed causing high level resistance to ATV and NFV. Mutations at position 82 and 88 are generally co-existent and result in contraindication to many PIs particularly NFV. Other major mutations in the protease gene were seen in low frequency (6%) at positions V32I and I50V which result in high level resistance to FPV. Besides, minor mutations/polymorphisms in the protease region were also observed in high frequencies the most common being at positions 74 (53%) and 83 (53%). These polymorphisms may have a negligible contribution to drug resistance. Nevertheless, physicians have to take into account these accessory mutations before making treatment decisions as they may be play a role in increasing viral fitness in association with major mutations (Alexander et al., 2001; Cane et al., 2001; Cerquerira et al., 2004; Escoto-Degadillo et al., 2005; Han et al., 2007; Paraschiv et al., 2007)

Studies from Southern India on ART naive individuals show absence of any primary NRTI and NNRTI drug resistance mutations (Balakrishnan et al., 2005; Soundararajan et al., 2007). In contrast, 6 NRTI and 5 NNRTI mutations were noticed in most samples that were screened for reverse transcriptase region. This is in agreement with earlier studies from Mumbai, India, which report prevalence of primary drug resistance (Deshpande et al., 2004). The resistance to Nucleotide Reverse Transcriptase Inhibitors were most frequent (33.3%) at position 215 known as Thymidine Analog Mutation (TAMs) which was seen alone or in combination with K219E. Moreover, TAMs are common in low-income countries and decrease susceptibility to Nevirapine (NVP) and Stavudine (D4T). The next most prevalent mutation was M184V seen in 14% of the samples analyzed. This is the most commonly occurring NRTI mutation and confers high level resistance to lamivudine (3TC) and emtricitabine (FTC). Thus, a higher prevalence of T215Y than M184V was seen while a study from Northern India among ART naive individuals have reported higher prevalence of M184V (Hira et al., 2004). This may be due to several factors such as differences in sample size, geographical distribution, mode of transmission etc. Further, a single case of 4 NRTIs namely M41L, D67N, T215A, M184V along with M46V protease inhibitor mutation was observed which may result in high/ intermediate level resistance to many drugs except for NVP. Although, these are isolated cases among ART naive individuals, they highlight the fact that genotyping for drug resistance mutations may be a crucial factor in commencing antiretroviral therapy. Other NRTIs include L210V (7%) and K219E (15%). L210V which was recently reported in naive subjects from Italy (Monno et al., 2009) and its more common form, L210W confers resistance to each of the NRTIs except for 3TC and FTC.

Regarding the NNRTIs, the most common mutation observed was Y181C (33.3%). The same has been true for HIV-1 infected pregnant women from south India after single dose NVP (Rajesh et al., 2010). Y181C is primarily responsible for resistance to NVP and DLV and low-level resistance to EFV. Additionally, Y was substituted by L at position 181 in one case which is an unusual mutation at this position. Subsequently, the next most prominent mutation was as position 221(26.6%) which is concordant with a recent study in patients from Mumbai undergoing NRTI plus NNRTI (Deshpande et al., 2007). Besides, P225H was detected in 20% of the cases. This being a secondary mutation confers resistance to EFV when in combination with other mutations like K103N, Y188L or G190A (Bacheler et al., 2001). Likewise, G190A was seen in one individual in combination with P225H. Substitution of A instead of G has also been recently observed by Kandathil et al. (2009) in clade C infected individuals in India. By and large, the NNRTIs observed generally impart EFV resistance.

Overall, despite some limitations in this study like small sample size, unknown routes of transmission etc., the findings well correlate with the fact that clade C viruses predominate in India (Robertson et al., 2000). Furthermore, the prevalence of drug resistance mutations in HIV-1 infected untreated patients in India was hitherto thought to be low (Pachamuthu et al., 2006; Chaturbhuj et al., 2010). Most notably, the present results suggest that these primary drug resistance mutations need to be thoroughly investigated and large-scale studies are required to evaluate the transmission of HIV drug resistance in Mumbai and other parts of India. Genotypic drug resistance data can give clinicians a true picture of drug resistance and susceptibility and ensure the commencement of the most suitable ART combination for the management of this disease.

CONCLUSIONS

The current findings draw attention to the fact that there may be high levels of primary HIV drug resistance in Mumbai. Further, from the HIV drug resistance mutations analyzed in our cohort, the most prominent resistant drugs were: Indinavir (IDV), Lopinavir (LPV), Nelfinavir(NFV), Stavudine (D4T) and Efavirenz (EFV). Simply put, the genotypic assay for HIV drug resistance is imperative to initiate and monitor the progress of ART. Further, continued efforts in HIV molecular epidemiology is essential which will not only aid in effective patient management but also enhance our understanding on the clade C mutations prevalent in the Indian HIV gene pool.

ACKNOWLEDGMENTS

We are very thankful to the Scientific Advisory committee and Management of Jaslok Hospital and Research Centre for sanctioning and funding this project on HIV infection. We highly appreciate the co-operation of the clinicians Dr.R. Harjani, Dr. Ram Malkani and Jaslok consultants for providing HIV patient samples.

REFERENCES

1. Akhigbe, R.E., J.O. Bamidele and O.L. Abodunrin, 2010. Seroprevalence of HIV infection in kwara, Nigeria. Int. J. Virol., 6: 158-163.

2. Alemnji, G., J. Mbuagbaw, G. Afetane and M. Nkam, 2006. Associations between CD4 Cell counts and clinical presentations among HIV/ AIDS patients in Cameroon. J. Med. Sci., 6: 843-847.

3. Alexander, C.S., W. Dong, K. Chan, N. Jahnke and M.V. O'Shaughnessy et al., 2001. HIV protease and reverse transcriptase variation and therapy outcome in antiretroviral naive individuals from a large North American cohort. AIDS., 15: 601-607.

4. Amegor, O.F., D.A. Bigila, O.A. Oyesola, T.O. Oyesola and S.T. Buseni, 2009. Hematological changes in HIV patients placed on anti retroviral

therapy in markurdi, Benue State of Nigeria. Asian J. Epidemiol., 2: 97-103.

5. Bacheler, L., S. Jeffrey, G. Hanna, R. D'Aquila and L. Wallace et al., 2001. Genotypic correlates of phenotypic resistance to efavirenz in virus isolates from patients failing nonnucleoside reverse transcriptase inhibitor therapy. J. Virol., 75: 4999-5008.

6. Balakrishnan, P., N. Kumarasamy, R. Kantor, S. Solomon and S. Vidya et al., 2005. HIV Type 1 Genotypic Variation in an Antiretroviral Treatment-Naive Population in Southern India. AIDS Res. Hum. Retroviruses., 21: 301-305.

7. Brenner, B.G., J.P. Routy, M. Petrella, D. Moisi and M. Oliveira et al., 2002. Persistance and fitness of multidrug-resistant of human immunodeficiency virus type 1 acquired in primary HIV infection. J. Virol., 76: 1753-1761.

8. Cane, P.A., A. De Ruiter, P. Rice, M. Wiselka, R. Fox and D. Pillay, 2001. Resistance-associated mutations in the human immunodeficiency virus type 1 subtype C protease gene from treated and untreated patients in the United Kingdom. J. Clin. Microbiol., 39: 2652-2654.

9. Cerquerira, D.M., E.D. Ramalho, C.P. Oliveira, R.R. Silva and M. Franchini et al., 2004.

HIV-1 subtypes and mutations associated to antiretroviral drug resistance in human isolates from central Brazil. Braz. J. Microbiol., 35: 187-192.

10. Chaturbhuj, D.N., N.K. Hingankar, P. Srikantiah, R. Garg and S. Kabra et al., 2010. Transmitted HIV drug resistance among HIV-infected voluntary counseling and testing centers (VCTC) clients in Mumbai, India. AIDS Res. Hum. Retroviruses., 26: 927-932.

11. Delaugerre, C., L. Morand-Joubert, M.L. Chaix, O. Picard and A.G. Marcelin et al., 2004. Persistence of multidrug-resistant HIV-1 without antiretroviral treatment 2 years after sexual transmission. Antivir. Ther., 9: 415-421.

12. Deshpande, A., P. Recordon-Pinson, R. Deshmukh, M. Faure and Jauvin et al., 2004. Molecular characterization of HIV type 1 isolates from unrelated patients of Mumbai (Bombay) India and detection of rare resistance mutations. AIDS. Res. Hum. Retroviruses., 20: 1032-1035.

13. Deshpande, A., V. Jauvin, N. Magnin, P. Pinson and M. Faure et al., 2007. Resistance mutations in subtype C HIV type 1 isolates from Indian patients of Mumbai receiving NRTIs plus NNRTIs and experiencing a treatment failure:

Resistance to AR. AIDS. Res. Hum. Retroviruses., 23: 335-340.

14. Escoto-Degadillo, M., E. Vazquez-Valls, M. Ramirez-Rodriguez, A. Corona-Nakamura and G. Amaya-Tapia et al., 2005. Drug resistance mutations in antiretroviral-naive patients with established HIV-1 infection in Mexico. HIV Med., 6: 403-409.

15. Gandhi, R.T., A. Wurcel, E.S. Rosenberg, M.N. Johnston, N. Hellmann et al., 2003. Progressive reversion of human immunodeficiency virus type 1 resistance mutations in vivo after transmission of a multiply drug-resistant virus. Clin. Infect. Dis., 37: 1693-1698.

16. Ghosn, J., I. Pellegrin, C. Goujard, C. Deveau and J.P. Viard et al., 2006. HIV-1 resistant strains acquired at the time of primary infection massively fuel the cellular reservoir and persist for lengthy periods of time. AIDS, 20: 159-170.

17. Han, X., M. Zhang, D. Dai, Y. Wang and Z. Zhang et al., 2007. Genotyping resistance mutations to antiretroviral drugs in treatment-naive HIV/AIDS patients living in Liaoning province, China: Baseline prevalence and subtype-specific difference. AIDS. Res. Hum. Retroviruses, 23: 357-364.

18. Hira, S.K., K. Panchal, P.A. Parmar and V.P. Bhatia, 2004. High resistance to antiretroviral drugs the Indian experience. Int. J. STD. AIDS., 15: 173-177.

19. Hirsch, M.S., H.F. Gunthard, J.M. Schapiro, F. Brun-Vezinet and B. Clotet et al., 2008. Antiretroviral drug resistance testing in adult HIV-1 infection: 2008 recommendations of an international AIDS society-USA panel. Clin. Infect. Dis., 47: 266-285.

20. Jamehdar, S.A., F. Sabahi, M. Forouzandeh, M. Haji, M.H. Abdolbaghi, M. Kazemnejad and F. Mahboudi, 2007. Evaluation of a new, highly sensitive and specific primer set for Reverse-transcriptase PCR detection of HIV-1 infected patients: Comparison with standard primers. J. Boil. Sci., 7: 954-958.

21. Kandathil, A.J., R. Kannangai, V.P. Verghese, S.A. Pulimood and P. Rupali et al., 2009. Drug resistant mutations detected by genotypic drug resistance testing in patients failing therapy in clade C HIV-1 infected individuals from India. Indian J. Med. Microbiol., 27: 231-236.

22. Kantor, R., D. Katzenstein, R. Camacho, P.R. Harrigan and A. Tanuri et al., 2010. Genotypic analyses of RT and protease sequences from persons infected with non-subtype B HIV-1.

http://gateway.nlm.nih.gov/MeetingAbstracts/
ma?f=102261251.html

23. Khandoker, A., M.M.H. Khan, N. Ahsan, M. Fazley Elahi Chowdhury, M. Kabir and M. Mori, 2006. Association between decision making autonomy and knowledge of HIV/AIDS prevention among ever married women in Bangladesh. J. Medical Sci., 6: 155-163.

24. Kumarasamy, N., S. Solomon, S.K. Chaguturu, A.J. Cecelia and S. Vallabhaneni et al., 2005. The changing natural history of HIV disease: Before and after the introduction of generic antiretroviral therapy in Southern India. Clin. Infect. Dis., 41: 1525-1528.

25. Monno, L., L. Scudeller, G. Brindicci, A. Saracino and G. Punzi et al., 2009. Genotypic analysis of the protease and reverse transcriptase of non-B HIV type 1 clinical isolates from naive and treated subjects. Antiviral Res., 83: 118-126.

26. Mousavi, S.M., R. Hamkar, M.M. Gouya A. Safaie and S.M. Zahraei et al., 2010. Surveillance of HIV drug resistance transmission in Iran: Experience gained from a pilot study. Arch. Virol., 155: 329-334.

27. Nissapatorn, V., C.K.C. Lee, Y.A.L. Lim, K.S. Tan and I. Jamaiah et al., 2007. Toxoplasmosis:

A silent opportunistic disease in HIV/AIDS patients. Res. J. Parasitol., 2: 23-31.

28. Nwachukwu, N.C. and A. Orji, 2008. Sero prevalence of human immunodeficiency virus among some fresh Nigerian graduates. Res. J. Immunol., 1: 51-55.

29. O'Neil, P.K., G. Sun, H. Yu, Y. Ron, J.P. Dougherty and B.D. Preston, 2002. Mutational analysis of HIV-1 long terminal repeats to explore the relative contribution of reverse transcriptase and RNA polymerase II to viral mutagenesis. J. Biol. Chem., 277: 38053-38061.

30. Oguntibeju, O.O., W.M.J. van den Heever and F.E. van Schalkwyk, 2007. A review of the epidemiology, biology and Pathogenesis of HIV. J. Biol. Sci., 7: 1296-1304.

31. Olowosegun, T., A.M. Sule, O.A. Sanni, H.U. Onimisi and O.M. Olowosegun, 2008. Awareness of HIV/AIDS pandemic in selected fishing communities in North Central Nigeria. Asian J. Epidemiol., 1: 17-23.

32. Pachamuthu, B., S. Shanmugam, K. Nagalingeswaran, S.S. Solomon and S. Solomon et al., 2006. HIV-1 drug resistance among untreated patients in India: Current status. J. Postgrad. Med., 52: 183-186.

33. Palella Jr. F.J., K.M. Delaney, A.C. Moorman, M.O. Loveless and J. Fuhrer et al., 1998. Declining morbidity and mortality among patients with advanced human immunodeficiency virus infection. N. Engl. J. Med., 338: 853-860.

34. Paraschiv, S., D. Otelea, M. Dinu, D. Maxim and M. Tinischi, 2007. Polymorphism and resistance mutations in the protease and reverse transcriptase genes of HIV-1 F subtype Romanian strains. Int. J. Infect. Dis., 11: 123-128.

35. Rajesh, L., K. Ramesh, L.E. Hanna, P.R. Narayanan and S. Swaminathan, 2010. Emergence of drug resistant mutations after single dose nevirapine exposure in HIV-1 infected pregnant women in South India. Indian J. Med. Res., 132: 509-512.

36. Robertson, D.L., J.P. Anderson, J.A. Bradac, J.K. Carr and B. Foley et al., 2000. HIV-1 nomenclature proposal. Science, 288: 55-56.

37. Sachdeva, N., S. Sehgal and S.K. Arora, 2005. Frequency of drug resistant variants of HIV-1 coexistent with wild-type in treatment naive Patients of India. Med. Gen. Med., 7: 68-68.

38. Shafer, R.W., 2002. Genotypic testing for human immunodeficiency virus type 1 drug resistance. Clin. Microbiol. Rev., 15: 247-277.

39. Shankarkumar, U., A. Pawar and K. Ghosh, 2009. HIV-1 evolution, drug resistance and host genetics: The Indian scenario. Virus Adaption Treat., 1: 1-4.

40. Soundararajan, L., R. Karunajanandham, V. Jauvin, M.H. Schrive and R. Ramachandran et al., 2007. Characterization of HIV-1 isolates from antiretroviral drug naive children in southern India. AIDS. Res. Hum. Retroviruses, 23: 1119-1126.

41. Steinbrook, R., 2007. HIV in India: A complex epidemic. N. Engl. J. Med., 356: 1089-1093.

42. UNAIDS, 2010. UNAIDS report on the global AIDS epidemic. http://www.unaids.org/globalreport/Global_report.htm.

43. WHO, 2008. Epidemiological fact sheet on HIV and AIDS: Core data on epidemiology and response. AIDS epidemic update, 2008. http://www.who.int/hiv/pub/epidemiology/pubfacts/en/.

44. Weidle, P.J., R. Downing, C. Sozi, R. Mwebaze and G. Rukundo et al., 2003. Development of phenotypic and genotypic resistance to antiretroviral therapy in the UNAIDS HIV drug access initiative-uganda. AIDS, Suppl., 3: S39-S48.

A study of antiretroviral resistance patterns in treatment experienced and naive human immunodeficiency virus infected-patients

Raj Harjani, Ram Malkani

Indian Journal of Sexually Transmitted Diseases and AIDS. 2016;37:167-72

INTRODUCTION

India currently has about 2.1 million people living with human immunodeficiency virus/acquired immunodeficiency syndrome (HIV/AIDS) and an adult HIV prevalence of 0.27%.[1] The most common routes of transmission are sexual (89%), parent to child (5%), and injecting drug use.[2] Even though antiretroviral therapy (ART) was available to those who could afford it for about two decades in India and was regularly used by physicians, the National AIDS Control Organisation (NACO) Department of AIDS Control initiated free ART in 2004. From a modest start of 25 ART centers and 6845 patients on ART in 2005; currently, NACO has about 425 ART centers and 768,000 people on ART. Thus, there has been an increase the number of people on ART.[1]

One major concern while administering ART is the presence of resistance to these drugs.[3] Apart from clinical implications of ART resistance, the cost of management increases with the presence of resistance mutations.[4] Given, the elaborate laboratory set up required for antiretroviral (ARV) resistance testing, it is expensive and not easily available to a large proportion of HIV-infected individuals in resource-limited countries such as India.

However, with increased use of ART in the Indian population, it is important to document the resistance patterns and the clinical implications, if any, of these in the Indian population. Thus, this study was undertaken to assess the resistance to protease inhibitors (PIs), nucleoside reverse transcriptase inhibitors (NRTIs), and non-NRTIs (NNRTIs) in treatment experienced and naive HIV-infected patients in Mumbai, Maharashtra, India.

METHODS

This study was a cross-sectional assessment of consecutive consenting 21 HIV-infected individuals attending an HIV care center in a tertiary care center in Mumbai, Maharashtra, India.

The study was conducted at a private tertiary care center in South Mumbai, Maharashtra, India. Data were collected from consecutive HIV-infected patients in whom resistance patterns could be assessed. All HIV-infected individuals included in the present analysis were tested for CD4 count, viral load, and resistance to ARVs. We tested them for the following drugs: (1) PIs: Atazanavir (ATV), darunavir (DRV), fosamprenavir (FPV), indinavir (IDV), lopinavir (LPV), nelfinavir (NFV), saquinavir (SQV), and tipranavir (TPV); (2) NRTIs: Lamivudine (3TC), abacavir (ABC), azidothymidine (AZT), stavudine (D4T), didanosine (DDI), emtricitabine (FTC), and tenofovir (TDF); and (3) NNRTIs: Efavirenz (EFV), etravirine (ETR), nevirapine (NVP), and rilpivirine (RPV). The HIV RNA PCR was done using QIAGEN OneStep RT-PCR Kit (QIAGEN, Hilden, Germany) and HIV RNA real-time PCR was done using RoboGene HIV-1 Quantification Kit (ROBOSCREEN, Germany). A detailed explanation of the molecular diagnostic methods has been published elsewhere.[5] HIV Stanford Database was used for genotypic drug resistance analysis.[6] The resistance patterns were classified as: Susceptible (resistance mutation score [RMS] 0 and 5), potential low-level resistance (RMS 10), low-level resistance (RMS 15–25), intermediate resistance (RMS 30–55), and high-level resistance (HLR) (RMS 60 and above). We also calculated the overall prevalence HLR in all the resistance tests conducted among PIs, NRTIs, and NNRTIs.

Demographic data (age, sex), date of HIV testing, and treatment (regimen and duration) were also collected. All the data were entered in MS Excel (©Microsoft Corp., USA) and converted to Stata Version 13 (©StataCorp, College Station, TX, USA). We calculated the means and standard deviations (SDs) for the linear variables, and proportions for categorical variables. We compared the means using t-test and the differences in proportions were compared using the Fisher's exact test for low cell counts. We also calculated the correlations for resistance patters in these drugs.

The study was approved by the Ethics Committee of the hospital in which the study was conducted.

RESULTS

A total of 13 male and 8 female were included in the present analysis. The mean (SD) age of the participants was 38.9 (8.1) years; there was no significant difference between the ages of males (38.5 [5.8]) and females (39.5 [11.3]) (P = 0.78). Only three participants were on treatment currently. The median duration from the time of diagnosis was 71 days (range 0 days to 2496 days). The median CD4 count before drug resistance testing was 146 (range 12–674) and the median CD4 counts after drug resistance 246 (range 10–659); this change was significantly significant (P = 0.003). The mean (SD) log viral load of the subjects before resistance testing was 5.06 (0.74); this was significantly higher in those on treatment compared with those who were not (5.20 [0.68] vs. 4.23 [0.56], P = 0.03).

Treatment-naive patients

Among PIs, high susceptibility was observed for DRV (89%) followed by LPV (72%) and FPV (67%). HLR was observed only in NFV, ATV, and IDV. In general, susceptibility was high for most of the NRTIs: 3TC (94%), FTC (94%), and TDF (89%). HLR was also found only in FTC (6%) and 3TC (6%). The susceptibility was similar for all the NNRTI tested; it was 61% for EFV, ETV, NVP, and RPV. We recorded HLR for NVP.

A total of 144 resistance tests were conducted for PIs (we tested eight PIs for each of 18 treatment-naive patients); of these, we found seven cases of HLR (5%). Similarly, the prevalence of HLR among NRTIs was 2% and among

NNRTIs was 11%; the proportion of HLR was significantly different across these three groups (P = 0.01).

Treatment experienced patients

In treatment-experienced patients, HLR was found for IDV, NFV, TPV, ATV, FPV, and SQV. Similarly, it was also found for 3TC, ABC, AZT, D4T, and FTC. However, HLR was only found for NVP. Resistance patterns were significantly different in treatment naive and experienced patients for FPV, LPV, TPV, and AZT.

We have presented a detailed analysis of the resistance patterns for each drug in Tables 1-4.

Table 1: Levels of resistance among protease inhibitor in those who were exposed to treatment (yes) and those who were not exposed to treatment (no), Mumbai, Maharashtra, India

Drugs	Susceptible, n (%)	Potential low-level, n (%)	Low-level, n (%)	Intermediate, n (%)	High-level resistance, n (%)	P
ATV						
Yes	0 (0)	0 (0)	0 (0)	2 (67)	1 (33)	0.1
No	10 (56)	3 (17)	1 (6)	2 (11)	2 (11)	
DRV						
Yes	2 (67)	0 (0)	0 (0)	1 (33)	0 (0)	0.3
No	16 (89)	1 (6)	1 (6)	0 (0)	0 (0)	
FPV						
Yes	0 (0)	0 (0)	1 (33)	1 (33)	1 (33)	0.0
No	12 (67)	2 (11)	1 (6)	3 (17)	0 (0)	
IDV						
Yes	0 (0)	0 (0)	0 (0)	1 (33)	2 (67)	0.0
No	10 (56)	3 (17)	1 (6)	3 (17)	1 (6)	
LPV						
Yes	0 (0)	0 (0)	1 (33)	2 (67)	0 (0)	0.0
No	13 (72)	1 (6)	1 (6)	3 (17)	0 (0)	
NFV						
Yes	0 (0)	0 (0)	0 (0)	1 (33)	2 (67)	0.0
No	10 (56)	2 (11)	2 (11)	0 (0)	4 (22)	
SQV						
Yes	0 (0)	0 (0)	1 (33)	1 (33)	1 (33)	0.0
No	11 (61)	2 (11)	2 (11)	3 (17)	0 (0)	
TPV						
Yes	0 (0)	0 (0)	0 (0)	1 (33)	2 (67)	0.0
No	11 (61)	1 (6)	2 (11)	4 (22)	0 (0)	

TPV=Tipranavir; SQV=Saquinavir; NFV=Nelfinavir; LPV=Lopinavir; IDV=Indinavir; FPV=Fosamprenavir; DRV=Darunavir; ATV=Atazanavir

Table 2: Levels of resistance among nucleoside reverse transcriptase inhibitors in those who were exposed to treatment (yes) and those who were not exposed to treatment (no), Mumbai, Maharashtra, India

Drugs	Susceptible, n (%)	Potential low-level, n (%)	Low-level, n (%)	Intermediate, n (%)	High-level resistance, n (%)	P
3TC						
Yes	2 (67)	0 (0)	0 (0)	0 (0)	1 (33)	0.27
No	17 (94)	0 (0)	0 (0)	0 (0)	1 (6)	
ABC						
Yes	2 (67)	0 (0)	0 (0)	0 (0)	1 (33)	0.26
No	11 (61)	4 (22)	3 (17)	0 (0)	0 (0)	
AZT						
Yes	1 (33)	1 (33)	0 (0)	0 (0)	1 (33)	0.05
No	13 (72)	0 (0)	3 (17)	2 (11)	0 (0)	
D4T						
Yes	1 (33)	1 (33)	0 (0)	0 (0)	1 (33)	0.06
No	12 (67)	0 (0)	4 (22)	2 (11)	0 (0)	
DDI						
Yes	2 (67)	0 (0)	0 (0)	1 (33)	0 (0)	0.18
No	11 (61)	5 (28)	2 (11)	0 (0)	0 (0)	
FTC						
Yes	2 (67)	0 (0)	0 (0)	0 (0)	1 (33)	0.27
No	17 (94)	0 (0)	0 (0)	0 (0)	1 (6)	
TDF						
Yes	2 (67)	0 (0)	0 (0)	1 (33)	0 (0)	0.16
No	16 (89)	2 (11)	0 (0)	0 (0)	0 (0)	

TDF=Tenofovir; FTC=Emtricitabine; DDI=Didanosine; D4T=Stavudine; AZT=Azidothymidine; ABC=Abacavir; 3TC=Lamivudine

Table 3: Levels of resistance among nonnucleoside reverse transcriptase inhibitors in those who were exposed to treatment (yes) and those who were not exposed to treatment (no), Mumbai, Maharashtra, India

Drugs	Susceptible, n (%)	Potential low-level, n (%)	Low-level, n (%)	Intermediate, n (%)	High-level resistance, n (%)	Susceptible
EFV						
Yes	1 (33)	0 (0)	0 (0)	2 (67)	0 (0)	0.65
No	11 (61)	0 (0)	1 (6)	5 (28)	1 (6)	
ETV						
Yes	1 (33)	0 (0)	0 (0)	2 (67)	0 (0)	0.54
No	11 (61)	1 (6)	2 (11)	4 (22)	0 (0)	
NVP						
Yes	1 (33)	0 (0)	0 (0)	0 (0)	2 (67)	0.55
No	11 (61)	0 (0)	0 (0)	0 (0)	7 (39)	
RPV						
Yes	1 (33)	0 (0)	0 (0)	2 (67)	0 (0)	0.23
No	11 (61)	0 (0)	3 (17)	4 (22)	0 (0)	

RPV=Rilpivirine; NVP=Nevirapine; ETV=Etravirine; EFV=Efavirenz

Table 4: Levels of resistance and resistance mutation scores among protease inhibitors, nucleoside reverse transcriptase inhibitors, and nonnucleoside reverse transcriptase inhibitors in all tests conducted among 18 treatment-naive patients, Mumbai, Maharashtra, India

Anti-retrovirals	Total tests	Susceptible	Potential low-level	Low-level	Intermediate	High-level resistance
PIs	144	93 (65)	15 (10)	11 (8)	18 (13)	7 (5)
NRTIs	126	97 (77)	11 (9)	12 (10)	4 (3)	2 (2)
NNRTIs	72	44 (61)	1 (1)	6 (8)	13 (18)	8 (11)

*P=0.001. PIs=Protease inhibitors; NRTIs=Nucleoside reverse transcriptase inhibitors; NNRTIs=Nonnucleoside reverse transcriptase inhibitors

As seen in Table 5, among the correlation of resistance patterns of PI, we found that ATV correlated highly with DRV, FPV, NFV, IDV, LPV, SQV, and TPV. We also found a high correlation in the resistance patterns of FPV and LPV (0.92), FPV and NFV (0.92), and NFV and IDV (0.99). In NRTIs, we found very high correlation in the resistance patterns of ABC and DDI, DDI and D4T, and D4T and AZT. Among NNRTIs, we found a high correlation in the resistance patterns of NVP and the other three NNRTIs (RPV [0.97], ETR [0.97], and EFV [0.98]). In general, the resistance patterns were similar within the same class of medications. Additional correlation values have been presented in Table 2.

Table 5: Correlation matrix of resistance patters of drugs (protease inhibitors, nucleoside reverse transcriptase inhibitors, nonnucleoside reverse transcriptase inhibitors) among 18 treatment-naive patients, Mumbai, Maharashtra, India*

ARVs/ ARVs	ATV	DRV	FPV	IDV	LPV	NFV	SQV	TPV	3TC	ABC	AZT	D4T	DDI	FTC	TDF	RPV	EFV	ETR	NVP
ATV	1.00																		
DRV	0.53	1.00																	
FPV	0.89	0.61	1.00																
IDV	0.99	0.49	0.90	1.00															
LPV	0.83	0.57	0.92	0.82	1.00														
NFV	0.99	0.53	0.92	0.99	0.85	1.00													
SQV	0.93	0.48	0.80	0.94	0.71	0.91	1.00												
TPV	0.81	0.55	0.73	0.85	0.54	0.83	0.77	1.00											
3TC	-0.21	-0.09	-0.17	-0.21	-0.15	-0.21	-0.19	-0.19	1.00										
ABC	0.16	-0.27	0.12	0.20	0.08	0.15	0.26	0.08	0.40	1.00									
AZT	0.13	-0.22	0.10	0.21	-0.03	0.14	0.23	0.29	-0.15	0.76	1.00								
D4T	0.30	-0.25	0.23	0.34	0.17	0.29	0.40	0.20	-0.17	0.83	0.91	1.00							
DDI	0.21	-0.28	0.16	0.25	0.11	0.20	0.31	0.12	0.24	0.99	0.84	0.92	1.00						
FTC	-0.21	-0.09	-0.17	-0.21	-0.15	-0.21	-0.19	-0.19	1.00	0.40	-0.15	-0.17	0.24	1.00					
TDF	0.08	-0.13	0.18	0.17	0.22	0.11	0.16	0.14	-0.09	0.59	0.69	0.66	0.63	-0.09	1.00				
RPV	0.12	0.16	0.09	0.15	0.16	0.11	0.14	0.21	0.19	0.28	0.25	0.17	0.25	0.19	0.41	1.00			
EFV	0.01	0.10	0.00	0.04	0.07	0.00	0.04	0.10	0.30	0.42	0.34	0.26	0.39	0.30	0.55	0.95	1.00		
ETR	0.12	0.16	0.09	0.15	0.16	0.11	0.14	0.21	0.21	0.27	0.23	0.15	0.24	0.21	0.37	0.99	0.93	1.00	
NVP	0.01	0.10	0.00	0.04	0.07	0.00	0.04	0.10	0.30	0.40	0.32	0.24	0.37	0.30	0.44	0.97	0.98	0.97	1.00

*The correlation values in bold indicate a P<0.05 and values in bold and italics indicate P<0.01. TPV=Tipranavir; SQV=Saquinavir; NFV=Nelfinavir; LPV=Lopinavir; IDV=Indinavir; FPV=Fosamprenavir; DRV=Darunavir; ATV=Atazanavir; TDF=Tenofovir; FTC=Emtricitabine; DDI=Didanosine; D4T=Stavudine; AZT=Azidothymidine; ABC=Abacavir; 3TC=Lamivudine; RPV=Rilpivirine; NVP=Nevirapine; ETV=Etravirine; EFV=Efavirenz; ARVs Anti-retrovirals

DISCUSSION

HLR was relatively low for PIs and NRTIs. However, the highest proportion of HLR was found among NRTIs in treatment-naive patients. Furthermore, in these patients, susceptibility was highest for DRV among PIs, for 3TC and

FTC among NRTIs, and similar for all NNRTIs tested. Interestingly, resistance patterns were correlated among the same groups of drugs, whereas the correlation was in general not significant across three groups of ARVs.

Although ARVs have been used in India for nearly two decades, there was limited literature on ARV resistance patterns.[7] However, there has been an increase in the number of reports highlighting the presence of ARV resistance in the Indian population. The pattern and proportion of resistance patterns vary in these studies. For instance, Deshpande et al. reported surveillance drug-related mutations for NNRTIs and PIs in about 10% of the patients.[8] However, Gupta et al. reported that about 96% had resistance to at least one ARV and the resistance was maximum for NRTIs and minimum for PIs.[9] Both these studies were from the same geographic location (Mumbai, Maharashtra, India). Interestingly, other authors have also reported high resistance patterns for NRTIs and NNRTIs and low to none for PIs.[10,11] We found resistance patterns to be high in treatment-experienced patients – particularly for PIs and NRTIs. Saravanan et al. also reported a relatively high proportion of resistance mutations for PIs, even though this was lower than that found for NRTIs.[12] A study by Richman et al. reported 76% resistance to any ARV drug, 71% resistance to NRTIs, 41% resistance to PIs, and 25% resistance to NNRTIs in the United States.[13] As reported elsewhere[5] some of the common mutations we found were M46 L, I47M, V82A/D/G, in addition to minor protease mutations or polymorphisms of L10I, V11F, L23H, K43I/R, A71D, G73A, T74A/P/S, and N83D.

The presence of resistance to various ARVs is important for clinical management of patients. Furthermore, the presence of resistance to ARVs even in treatment-naive patients is an important marker to suggest transmission of resistant viruses in the population. Interestingly, Sen et al., and Azam et al. did not find any mutations in treatment-naive patients.[14,15] The current NACO guidelines have suggested nevirapine-based regimens as first line of therapy in adults.[16] As per our findings, a high proportion of treatment experienced and a substantial proportion of treatment-naive patients have HLR to NVP. It has been well documented that single-dose NVP may result in a relatively high proportion of resistance mutations.[17-19] Lockman et al. found that LPV/ritonavir combination with TDF-FTC was superior compared with NVP-TDF-FTC combination in women who were exposed to single-dose NVP in pregnancy.[20] Since single-dose NVP was being used in the Prevention of Parent to Child Treatment Programme in India,[21] it is quite likely that there is the presence of resistance mutations to NVP in the population. Furthermore, as observed in our data resistance patterns in NVP and other NNRTIs may be highly correlated. Similar cross-resistance and class resistance in NNRTIs have also been reported by others.[19,22] The WHO also recommends the use of TDF + 3TC (or FTC) + EFV as the first line management for adult patients.[23] Given, the Cross-resistance among NNRTIs, it may be useful to assess the resistance before starting NNRTI-based therapies in patients. The NACO guidelines suggest ATV-based regimens to be second-line treatment.[24] As observed in our data, susceptibility was relatively low to ATV even in treatment-naive patients. Furthermore, there was a high correlation of resistance patterns with other PIs. Thus, it may be worthwhile conducting a detailed ARV resistance testing before initiating second-line therapy. The PI which showed best susceptibility was DRV; thus, DRV may be a useful alternative for management of patients. Indeed, other authors have also reported high susceptibility to DRV and that it should be the preferred choice of drug for third-line management.[12,25] It may be worthwhile to consider DRV as a drug of choice for second-line treatment. In addition, LPV, TPV, and SQV may be useful alternatives for clinical management of patients.

We included data from 21 patients in our analysis; the sample was relatively small. Thus, the generalizability of these data may be limited nonetheless we have presented a detailed analysis of all three groups of ARVs. Furthermore, we have also presented correlation between resistance patterns of various ARVs. Although we have not included detailed information on resistance mutations in our manuscript, this has been presented elsewhere.[5]

In spite of the above limitations, this is an important contribution to the literature and has important treatment implications. We found a high proportion of HLR for many PIs in treatment-experienced patients; however, HLR was not observed in treatment-naive patients for most of the PIs. Similarly, HLR was not observed in for NRTIs in treatment-naive patients. HLR in treatment-naïve patients was however relatively high for NNRTIs. Furthermore, there was a high correlation in general among drugs belonging to the same group. Thus, it may be useful to conduct ARV resistance even in newly infected HIV patients and those receiving medications for the first time.

Acknowledgments

We would like to acknowledge Dr. P. D. Potdar and Department of Molecular Biology, Jaslok for help with microbiological assessment and We would like to acknowledge Dr. Prasita Kshirsagar, Associate Professor of Medicine (Rajiv Gandhi Medical College) for support. We would also like to acknowledge Dr. Maninder S. Setia, Consultant Epidemiologist for feedback on the manuscript.

References

1. National AIDS Control Organization. Annual Report 2013-14. New Delhi, India: Department of AIDS Control, Ministry of Health & Family Welfare, Government of India; 2014.

2. National AIDS Control Organization. Annual Report 2010-11. New Delhi, India: Department of AIDS Control, Ministry of Health & Family Welfare, Government of India; 2012.

3. Frentz D, Van de Vijver DA, Abecasis AB, Albert J, Hamouda O, Jørgensen LB, et al. Increase in transmitted resistance to

non-nucleoside reverse transcriptase inhibitors among newly diagnosed HIV-1 infections in Europe. BMC Infect Dis 2014;14:407.

4. Krentz HB, Ko K, Beckthold B, Gill MJ. The cost of antiretroviral drug resistance in HIV-positive patients. Antivir Ther 2014;19:341-8.

5. Potdar PD, Daswani BS, Rane NJ. Drug resistance mutations to protease and reverse transcriptase inhibitors in treatment naive HIV-1 clade C infected individuals from Mumbai, India. Int J Virol 2011;7:13-23.

6. Stanford University HIV Drug Resistance Database. Available from: http://www.hivdb.stanford.edu/. [Last accessed on 2016 Mar 15].

7. Lakhashe S, Thakar M, Godbole S, Tripathy S, Paranjape R. HIV infection in India: Epidemiology, molecular epidemiology and pathogenesis. J Biosci 2008;33:515-25.

8. Deshpande A, Karki S, Recordon-Pinson P, Fleury HJ. Drug resistance mutations in HIV type 1 isolates from naive patients eligible for first line antiretroviral therapy in JJ Hospital, Mumbai, India. AIDS Res Hum Retroviruses 2011;27:1345-7.

9. Gupta A, Saple DG, Nadkarni G, Shah B, Vaidya S, Hingankar N, et al. One-, two-, and three-class resistance among HIV-infected patients on antiretroviral therapy in private care clinics: Mumbai, India. AIDS Res Hum Retroviruses 2010;26:25-31.

10. Saini S, Bhalla P, Gautam H, Baveja UK, Pasha ST, Dewan R. Resistance-associated mutations in HIV-1 among patients failing first-line antiretroviral therapy. J Int Assoc Physicians AIDS Care (Chic) 2012;11:203-9.

11. Sinha S, Shekhar RC, Ahmad H, Kumar N, Samantaray JC, Sreenivas V, et al. Prevalence of HIV drug resistance mutation in the Northern Indian population after failure of the first line antiretroviral therapy. Curr HIV Res 2012;10:532-8.

12. Saravanan S, Vidya M, Balakrishnan P, Kantor R, Solomon SS, Katzenstein D, et al. Viremia and HIV-1 drug resistance mutations among patients receiving second-line highly active antiretroviral therapy in Chennai, Southern India. Clin Infect Dis 2012;54:995-1000.

13. Richman DD, Morton SC, Wrin T, Hellmann N, Berry S, Shapiro MF, et al. The prevalence of antiretroviral drug resistance in the United States. AIDS 2004;18:1393-401.

14. Azam M, Malik A, Rizvi M, Rai A. Zero prevalence of primary drug resistance-associated mutations to protease inhibitors in HIV-1 drug-naive patients in and around Aligarh, India. J Infect Dev Ctries 2014;8:79-85.

15. Sen S, Tripathy SP, Patil AA, Chimanpure VM, Paranjape RS. High prevalence of human immunodeficiency virus type 1 drug resistance mutations in antiretroviral treatment-experienced patients from Pune, India. AIDS Res Hum Retroviruses 2007;23:1303-8.

16. National AIDS Control Organization. Antiretroviral therapy guidelines for HIV-infected adults and adolescents – May 2013. New Delhi, India: Department of AIDS Control, Ministry of Health & Family Welfare, Government of India; 2013.

17. Johnson JA, Li JF, Morris L, Martinson N, Gray G, McIntyre J, et al. Emergence of drug-resistant HIV-1 after intrapartum administration of single-dose nevirapine is substantially underestimated. J Infect Dis 2005;192:16-23.

18. Palmer S, Boltz V, Martinson N, Maldarelli F, Gray G, McIntyre J, et al. Persistence of nevirapine-resistant HIV-1 in women after single-dose nevirapine therapy for prevention of

maternal-to-fetal HIV-1 transmission. Proc Natl Acad Sci U S A 2006;103:7094-9.

19. Rajesh L, Ramesh K, Hanna LE, Narayanan PR, Swaminathan S. Emergence of drug resistant mutations after single dose nevirapine exposure in HIV-1 infected pregnant women in South India. Indian J Med Res 2010;132:509-12.

20. Lockman S, Hughes MD, McIntyre J, Zheng Y, Chipato T, Conradie F, et al. Antiretroviral therapies in women after single-dose nevirapine exposure. N Engl J Med 2010;363:1499-509.

21. National AIDS Control Organization. Updated guidelines for prevention of parent to child transmission (PPTCT) of HIV using multi drug anti-retroviral regimen in India. New Delhi, India: Department of AIDS Control Basic Services Division, Ministry of Health & Female Welfare, Government of India; 2013.

22. Sluis-Cremer N. The emerging profile of cross-resistance among the nonnucleoside HIV-1 reverse transcriptase inhibitors. Viruses 2014;6:2960-73.

23. World Health Organization. Consolidated guidelines on the use of antiretroviral drugs for treating and preventing HIV infection: Recommendations for a public health approach

June 2013. Switzerland, Geneva: World Health Organization; 2013.

24. National AIDS Control Organization. National guidelines on second-line and alternative first-line ART for adults and adolescents – May 2013. New Delhi, India: Department of AIDS Control, Ministry of Health & Family Welfare, Government of India; 2013.

25. Saravanan S, Madhavan V, Balakrishnan P, Smith DM, Solomon SS, Sivamalar S, et al. Darunavir is a good third-line antiretroviral agent for HIV type 1-infected patients failing second-line protease inhibitor-based regimens in South India. AIDS Res Hum Retroviruses 2013;29:630-2.

ONGOING RESEARCH

Hair morphology in heat damaged hair in females: A case-control study

Ram H Malkani, Consultant Dermatologist, Jaslok Hospital

Maninder Singh Setia, Consultant Epidemiologist, Jaslok Hospital

Ms. Priyanka Mithbawkar, Research Secretary, Dr Skinpimples Pvt Ltd.

ABSTRACT

Hair loss is one of the most common presenting complaints in the Dermatology Clinics. There has been an increase in the use of hair styling in India in the past few years. With the advent of new saloons and changing life styles, hair grooming is common among women and men, even at younger ages. Some of the changes associated with the use of these styling and grooming procedures have not been extensively studied in the Indian population. In this study, we propose to compare the hair morphology in female patients who have used any heat application to their hair in the past six months with those who have not used any heat application ever to their hair.

The comparison will include gross features, various hair indices, microscopic features (including light and electron microscopy). We propose to recruit 100 subjects (50 cases – those exposed to heat damage, and 50 controls those not exposed to heat damage) for the present study. After consent, a detailed socio-demographic history, details of hair loss, treatment taken for hair loss, applications of hair products, detailed use of hair straightening procedures in cases were taken (type of procedure, detailed history of the procedures, frequency of treatment, first use, any complaints associated with it). We will then evaluate the hair morphology in cases and controls. The evaluation will include: naked examination of hair, hair pull test, hair density, hair breakage index, light microscopy, and transmission electron microscopy. We will be able to study the association between morphological changes in hair damage and heat application. We will also be able to define heat related changes in hair in the Indian female population. A detailed examination of light and TEM will be a useful contribution to the Indian literature.

BACKGROUND

Hair loss is one of the most common presenting complaints in the Dermatology Clinics. Though, a common cause of hair loss in men is androgenetic alopecia, the common causes of hair loss in women often discussed are acute or chronic telogen effluvium, and female pattern baldness. However, there are other causes of hair damage such as physical friction or use of chemical and/or cosmetic products (such as bleaching or hair colouring) and other causes such as exposure to ultraviolet light, excessive grooming, use of hair straightening agents, hair irons, and small electric warmers may damage hair. One of the common features of hair damage due to excessive heat is the presence of 'bubble hair'. This may also lead to weakening and breakage of hair. A microscopic evaluation of hair may show uneven breakages on light microscopy. In addition some other features may be gas like or bubble appearance in electron microscopy. Thus, this may be an important cause of hair loss in women; an issue that needs to explored in detail in the Indian population. (1-8)

There has been an increase in the use of hair styling in India in the past few years. With the advent of new saloons and changing life styles, hair grooming is common among women and men, even at younger ages. Some of the changes associated with the use of these styling and grooming procedures have not been extensively studied in the Indian population. There are few electron microscopy studies of hair changes associated with use of heat styling hair products in India. The present study will be an important contribution to the literature on hair research in India, and eventually may help add new dimension to diagnosis and care of hair loss among women in India.

AIMS AND OBJECTIVES

To compare the hair morphology in female patients who have used any heat application to their hair in the past six months with those who have not used any heat application ever to their hair.

The comparison will include gross features, various hair indices, microscopic features (including light and electron microscopy).

METHODS

The present study will be a prospective case-control study.

Study site: The study will be conducted in the Department of Dermatology, Jaslok Hospital.

Definition of a case: All females 18-40 years who present to the Dermatology clinic and report any of the following in the past six months: blow drying of hair, hair straightening, use of hair iron.

We will exclude females with an evidence of cicatricial alopecia, alopecia areata, and infections of the scalp.

Definition of a control: Females (age matched + 2 years, only females > 18 years) who do not report any of the above mentioned procedures, and have not used hair colour or hair bleach ever in their life time.

Procedure

After consent, a detailed socio-demographic history, details of hair loss, treatment taken for hair loss, applications of hair products, detailed use of hair straightening procedures in cases (type of procedure, detailed history of the procedures, frequency of treatment, first use, any complaints associated with it).

Evaluation of hair

Naked eye examination of scalp and hair: Record the texture and type of hair loss.

Hair pull test: A hair-pull test will be performed in all the four quadrants of the scalp.

Hair Density and Hair Breakage Index: (9, 10)

Hair mass index (HMI) is a measure of hair density and hair diameter. HMI=(cross-sectional area of hair (mm2)/sample scalp area)x100.

Hair Breakage Index (HBI) is another important measurement of hair weathering. It is a measurement of the diameter of hair in the proximal region of the scalp to the distal region of the scalp. A higher HBI indicates higher level of hair damage.

Light microscopy: The hair collected from the cases and controls will be examined under light microscopy. We will look for changes in the hair structure – any uneven breakages or even the presence of bubbles.8

Transmission Electron Microscopy: we will also perform a TEM of the hair collected from cases and controls. The TEM will evaluate the cortex and cuticle of the hair samples. We will evaluate all the cortical components (including melanin granules and cortical cells).(7)

SAMPLE SIZE

Assuming that about 80% of the cases will have heat changes (such as changes in cortex/cuticle or presence of bubbles) and 50% of the controls will have these changes, with an alpha of 0.05 and power of 80% we will require 45 cases and controls each. To account for data loss, we will inflate the sample size of 10%. Thus, we will recruit 50 cases and 50 controls for the present study.

STATISTICAL ANALYSIS

We will calculate the proportion for categorical variables and prevalence proportion for categorical outcomes (such as proportion of women with hair damage). We will calculate the means and standard deviations for continuous variables. The proportions will be compared using the chi square tests and the means will be compared using the t-test. We will also estimate the odds ratios and their 95% confidence intervals as a measure of association using the logistic regression models.

EXPECTED OUTCOMES

We will be able to demonstrate the proportion of women with heat related damage to hair in the population who have not used any hair heating products.

We will be able to demonstrate the proportion of women with heat related damage to hair in the population who used any hair heating products.

We will be able to study the association between morphological changes in hair damage and heat application. We will also be able to define heat related changes in hair in the Indian female population. A detailed examination of light and TEM will be a useful contribution to the Indian literature

TIMELINE

It will be a one year project

3 months: Administrative Approval (Ethics Committee approval, designing the data collection sheet & piloting the

data collection sheet, standardisation of light microscopy and TEM procedures)

6 months: Data collection from cases and controls

3 months: Data analysis and manuscript preparation

REFERENCES

1. Ahn HJ, Lee WS. An ultrastuctural study of hair fiber damage and restoration following treatment with permanent hair dye. Int J Dermatol 2002;41(2):88-92.

2. Bolduc C, Shapiro J. Hair care products: waving, straightening, conditioning, and coloring. Clin Dermatol 2001;19(4):431-6.

3. Hearle JW. A critical review of the structural mechanics of wool and hair fibres. Int J Biol Macromol 2000;27(2):123-38.

4. Jeon SY, Pi LQ, Lee WS. Comparison of hair shaft damage after UVA and UVB irradiation. J Cosmet Sci 2008;59(2):151-6.

5. Kon R, Nakamura A, Takeuchi K. Artificially damaged hairs: preparation and application for the study of preventive ingredients. Int J Cosmet Sci 1998;20(6):369-80.

6. Lee WS, Oh TH, Chun SH, Jeon SY, Lee EY, Lee S, et al. Integral lipid in human hair follicle. J Investig Dermatol Symp Proc 2005;10(3):234-7.

7. Lee Y, Kim YD, Hyun HJ, Pi LQ, Jin X, Lee WS. Hair shaft damage from heat and drying time of hair dryer. Ann Dermatol 2011;23(4):455-62.

8. McMichael AJ. Hair breakage in normal and weathered hair: focus on the Black patient. J Investig Dermatol Symp Proc 2007;12(2):6-9.

9. Mhaskar S, Kalghatgi B, Chavan M, Rout S, Gode V. Hair breakage index: an alternative tool for damage assessment of human hair. J Cosmet Sci 2011;62(2):203-7.

10. Wikramanayake TC, Mauro LM, Tabas IA, Chen AL, Llanes IC, Jimenez JJ. Cross-section Trichometry: A Clinical Tool for Assessing the Progression and Treatment Response of Alopecia. Int J Trichology 2012;4(4):259-64.

Melasma and Metabolic Syndrome: More than meets the eye?

Ram H Malkani, Harish Ahuja, Namrata Shindekar

A Jaslok Hospital & Research Centre Study

SPECIFIC AIMS:

Melasma, a common condition seen in the dermatology clinics. It has been estimated that women outnumber male patients attending the clinic for melasma in a ratio of 9:1; thus it being an important dermatological and cosmetic condition. Another important issue that has received a lot of attention in the dermatological arena recently is the Metabolic Syndrome (MetS). The overall prevalence of metabolic syndrome in India is 34%, the prevalence being higher in females compared with males (42% vs 25%). We propose to conduct a case-control study of 160 women (80 cases of melasma and 80 controls) attending the Department of Dermatology at Jaslok Hospital. We will assess metabolic syndrome, exposure to sunlight, family history, menstrual irregularities, and radiological features of polycystic ovarian syndrome in these patients. Data will be analysed to estimate the odds ratio as a measure of association.

In the last two decades, there is a growing concern regarding the negative impact of diseases on the quality of life of patients. Dermatological conditions are distinguished by certain peculiarities. Despite the small mortality rates for skin diseases, the aesthetic appearance could negatively influence the daily activities of patients. And hence a clinical condition of primary aesthetic significance could have a far greater clinical significance on emotional health of patients. The attending physician needs to take into consideration this aspect and deliver necessary amount of empathy while treating such aesthetic skin concerns.

Specific questionnaires on quality of life in diseases have been developed for various medical fields such as psychiatry (schizophrenia and depression), endocrinology (diabetes), rheumatology (rheumatoid arthritis), gynaecology (menopause) and oncology. There are validated instruments in dermatology for psoriasis, atopic dermatitis, acne, hives, onychomycosis, lower limb ulcers, pemphigus, vitiligo, alopecia, Hidradenitis suppurativa, photodamage, ichthyosis and, more recently, for melasma.

The present study will be a case-control study to evaluate the association between metabolic syndrome and melasma among Indian population. More specifically, we will:

1) Estimate the prevalence of metabolic syndrome in patients with and without melasma.

2) Evaluate the association between melasma and metabolic syndrome by conducting a case-control study.

3) As a first secondary objective in this study, we will assess the Quality of Life index in Indian melasma patients.

4) As a second secondary objective, we will perform a comparative study of IDF criteria of metabolic syndrome with other tests like High Molecular Weight Adiponectin andProinsulin Insulin ratio in the diagnosis of metabolic syndrome.

Objective and scope of the project:

1. To estimate prevalence of metabolic syndrome in persons with and without melasma.

2. To evaluate the association between melasma and metabolic syndrome.

3. To compare between IDF criteriawithother tests like HMW Adiponectin and insulin proinsulin/insulin ratio in the diagnosis of metabolic syndrome

4. To assess the emotional burden of melasma in Indian male and female patients.

5. To assess the Quality of Life in melasma patients.

6. To correlate the MASI score with MELASQOL score.

BACKGROUND AND SIGNIFICANCE:

Melasma is one common condition seen in the dermatology clinics. It has been estimated that women outnumber male patients attending the clinic for melasma in a ratio of 9:1; thus it being an important dermatological and cosmetic condition. Indeed, an epidemiological study in India reported that the prevalence of melasma is as high as 50% in pregnant women. Even though it is an important dermatological condition, the factors that influence pathogenesis of pigmentation in melasma are complex; in fact, a range of factors have been suggested as the potential etiological factors. Some of these factors are as follows pregnancy, ultraviolet lights, oral contraceptive use. Though, it has been demonstrated that melasma skin had higher oestrogen receptor levels compared with normal skin; however, authors have also concluded that the evidence for hormonal role in etiopathogenesis provided conflicting results.

Another important issue that has received a lot of attention in the dermatological arena recently is the Metabolic Syndrome (MetS). It is a syndrome associated with obesity, insulin resistance, and a high blood pressure. The overall prevalence of metabolic syndrome in India is 34%, the prevalence being higher in females compared with males (42% vs 25%). The same study also found that metabolic syndrome was also associated with being older, being female, and general obesity. It has also been argued that MetS is involved with an inflammatory response in the body. Plonka and colleagues have suggested that, hypothetically, melanin synthesis may occur in the adipocytes as a counter to oxidative damage in obese individuals.

Melasma, an acquired pigmentary disorderis quite prevalent, chronic and relapsingin nature which provides numerous medical expenses and medications and procedures.Being primarily a skin of the face, even small, discrete patches may provide considerable harm to the welfare of affected patients.

In 2003, Balkrishnan and colleagues developed and validated the Melasma Quality of Life Scale (MELASQOL), a questionnaire with ten specific items for measuring the quality of life of patients with melasma.This instrument was made from seven issues of scale SKINDEX-16 (questionnaire on quality of life of patients with skin diseases in general) and threequestions in Skin Discoloration Questionnaire. The final score of MELASQOL can vary between 7 and 70, with higher scores indicating worse quality of life.

Rationale of the research:

As discussed earlier, we propose to study the association of metabolic syndrome and melasma. Though, currently, we did not find sufficient evidence to understand the association between these two clinical entities few studies have prompted us to propose the hypothesis. We have stated that melanin synthesis may be higher as an anti-oxidant mechanism in obese individuals. Furthermore, it has also been suggested that Adiponectin may modulate the production of Proopiomelanocortin (based on the colocalisation of receptors seen in the animal models).

Alpha-MSH one of the products from POMC is known to stimulate melanogenesis. Thus, the above mentioned studies have made us hypothesise that potentially; metabolic syndrome is one of the associations of melasma in female patients.

There is evidence of association between metabolic syndrome and psoriasis in literature; thus, metabolic syndrome has been discussed in dermatology. Furthermore, studies have also shown that women who have Polycystic Ovarian Syndrome and Insulin Resistance are also more likely to have upper body adiposity and acanthosis nigricans. However, there are no studies that evaluate the association between metabolic syndrome and melasma.

Studies in several populations have shown that even a small amount of melasma can cause significant emotional and psychological distressed Patients with lower levels of education or underlying psychiatric disorders may be at greater risk of emotional impairment.

Melasma is often psychologically distressing in affected patients. The most commonly used tool for assessment of quality of life in patients with melasma is MELASQOL.

Interestingly, the effect of melasma on quality of life was not correlated with the severity of melasma, suggesting that even a small amount of pigmentation can take a significant emotional toll.

It is clear that melasma significantly affects quality of life, and its effect on a particular patient may be profound. Given the impact that this condition has on patients' quality of life and the lack of highly effective treatment options, additional research into understanding the biologic basis of this disease will be crucial to developing more effective treatment options.

MELASQOL has been shown to have discriminatory power and high consistency; social life, recreation and leisure, and emotional well-being are the most affected domains of quality of life.

Since colour of skin varies with different geographies and so does social settings and thereby the emotional ramifications, it is worthwhile studying the Quality of Life in Indian female melasma patients objectively.

The MELASQOL scores can also be used as useful tool in guiding treatment methods as well as tracking the improvement of patients QOL.

RESEARCH DESIGN AND METHODS:

Detailed research plan:

The present study will be a clinic based case-control study.

Study Site: The study will be conducted at the Department of Dermatology, Jaslok Hospital. It is a private hospital in South Mumbai. The average out-patient attendance of the Department of Dermatology is 30-50 patients per day.

Study Design: As discussed above it will be a case control study among patients:

Cases will be all patients who currently have melasma.

Controls will all patients who have never had melasma. Though for current melasma, we will be able to evaluate the patients clinically for past melasma, patients will be shown clinical photographs. They will be classified as controls only after they confirm that they have never had the pigmentary condition in the past.

Inclusion criteria:

1) All consenting women aged 18-45 years.

Exclusion criteria:

1) Pregnant women (currently) and six months post-partum/post-abortion/post-delivery (any form).

2) Women who are on oral contraceptive pills (currently) or have been on pills in the past six months.

Data collection:

All consecutive consenting melasma patients and controls will be eligible for the current study.

Examination for both cases and controls:

A) Questionnaire (For both Cases and Controls):We will collect information on socio-demographics, body mass index detailed history of pregnancy, menstrual history, past OC pill use, daily activities (exposure to sunlight), application on face, and family history of melasma in these women. All the women will also undergo an ultrasonography to evaluate for

PCOS, since central obesity is associated with PCOS and we can adjust for this condition during analysis.

B) Evaluation for Metabolic Syndrome (For both Cases and Controls): 1) Waist circumference measurement at the approximate midpoint between the lower margin of the last palpable rib and the top of the iliac crest; 2) Triglycerides; 3) High density lipoproteins; 4) Serum glucose (or a history of type 2 diabetes mellitus); 5) blood pressure; 6) Serum insulin; 7) Serum pro-insulin; 8) Serum High Molecular Weight Adiponectin. (According IDF criteria, clinically Metabolic Syndrome is defined if there is positive finding in any three or more of the above five risk factors).

C) Evaluation for Melasma (For cases only): In addition, the cases will be clinically evaluated for melasma (Wood's lamp examination), MASI scores, and detailed history and treatment taken for melasma will also be recorded.

D) Evaluation for Quality Of Life in patients suffering from Melasma (For cases only): We propose to include 80 male and female patients with melasma in the study. Every patient will be will be administered the 10 point MELASQOL.

All the data will be collected in a pre-designed data collection sheet.

TOTAL MASI SCORE:

A numerical value for area of involvement, ranging from 1 (<10% of the area involved) to 6 (90-100% of the area involved) is assigned. The total score is calculated as follows:

MASI = 0.3 A (D+H) + 0.3 A (D+H) + 0.3 A (D+H) + 0.1 A (D+H)

Forehead Rt. Malar Lt. Malar Chin

The range of scores is 0 to 48

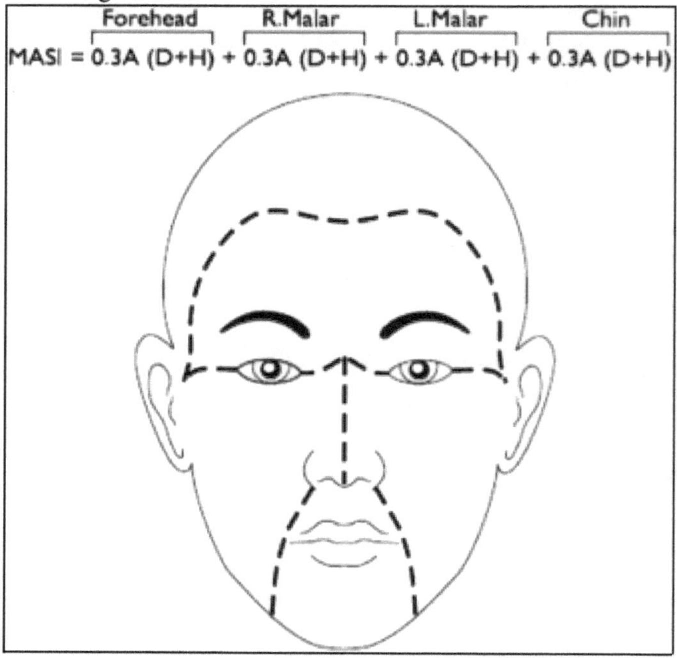

Timeline:

	6 months	6 months	6 months	6 months
Administrative	XXXX			
Data collection	XXXXX XXXXXXXXX	XXXXXXXXX	XX	
Data analysis		XXXX	XXXXXXXX	XXX
Manuscript Preparation/ Report submission				XXXXX

Sample size:

The baseline prevalence of metabolic syndrome is 42% (Prasad and co-workers, 2012). If we assume an alpha error of 0.05 and power of 80%, with 73 patients in each group (case and control), we will be able to show a significant association at an estimate of 65% (Power Analysis Figure). This sample will also cover one direction alternate hypothesis. To account for 10% data loss, we will recruit 80 participants in each group. Thus, our total sample size will be 160 participants.

Data analysis: All the clinical and laboratory data will be entered in EpiInfo and converted to Stata for further analysis. We will calculate the means and standard deviations for continuous variables (such as triglyceride levels, HDL, and BMI). The difference in means between the cases and controls will be assessed using the t-test. We will estimate the proportions for categorical variables and differences in the proportions will be assessed using the chi square test. We will then use logistic regression models to estimate the Odds ratios and multivariate analysis.

Expected Outcome and its utility to Indian dermatology:

Though, there is some evidence for this hypothesis (as discussed in rationale), a case-control study to estimate the association has not been conducted. Since melasma and metabolic syndromes are two common conditions in India, this will be a useful and an ideal contribution to literature. In addition, detection of metabolic syndrome and prompt diagnosis may potentially also be useful in therapeutic care of melasma patients – a possible future study area. Advantage of performing the tests like High Molecular Weight Adiponectin and Insulin and pro-insulin ratio in future is that these tests can be done commercially for patients visiting Jaslok Hospital, once these tests are standardized.

1. Title of the Project:

Melasma and Metabolic Syndrome: More than meets the eye?

2. Name and Designation of

a) Principal investigator: Dr. Ram H Malkani, Consultant Dermatologist, Jaslok Hospital

b) Co-investigators: NA

3.   Sponsoring   Collaborating   Institution (Address): NA

4. Duration of the Project

a) Period (No. of year): Two Years.

b) Tentative starting date: April, 2016. (After getting approval)

c) Period of collecting data:

3 months: Administrative Approval (Ethics Committee approval, designing the data collection sheet & piloting the data collection sheet, standardization of procedures) –April, 2016 to June, 2016.

6 months: Data collection from cases and controls: July, 2016 to December, 2017.

d) Period for complete analysis of data.

3 months: Data analysis and manuscript preparation: January, 2018 to March, 2018.

To be filled in by the Principal investigator
Name: Dr. Ram H.Malkani.
Address: Room No 200, Dermatology Clinic,
Jaslok Hospital,
Dr. G. B.Deshmukh Road,
Mumbai – 400 026.

Start Date: February, 2016.

Sponsor/Funding/Agency: NA.

Conflict of Interest:

Project Title: Melasma and Metabolic Syndrome: More than meets the eye?

Please answer the following questions in the covering letter attached with the proposal submitted to the Ethics Committee.

1. Please provide a precise description of how human subjects will be involved in the research, including a clear of all activities and responsibilities of the subjects.

We propose to recruit 160 study participants for the study. After consent, we will collect information on socio-demographics, body mass index detailed history of pregnancy, menstrual history, past OC pill use, daily activities (exposure to sunlight), application on face, and family history of melasma in these women. All the women will also undergo an ultrasonography to evaluate for PCOS, since central obesity is associated with PCOS and we can adjust for this condition during analysis. As a subpart of this study, we will be assessing the quality of life in the patients having melasma.

Examination for both cases and controls:

Evaluation for metabolic syndrome: 1) Waist circumference; 2) Triglycerides; 3) High density lipoproteins; 4) Serum glucose (or a history of type 2 diabetes mellitus); 5) blood pressure.

Evaluation for Cases only

Evaluation for melasma:

In addition, the cases will be clinically evaluated for melasma (Wood's lamp examination), MASI scores, and detailed history and treatment taken for melasma will also be recorded.

Evaluation for Quality of Life:

The cases will be asked a questionnaire.Patients will be asked to determine both their quality of life with melasma and also what their quality of life would have been, hypothetically, if they did not have melasma.

All the data will be collected in a pre-designed data collection sheet.

References

1. Cornier, M. A., D. Dabelea, et al. (2008). "The metabolic syndrome." Endocrine Rev29(7): 777-822.

2. Guillod-Maximin, E., A. F. Roy, et al. (2009). "Adiponectin receptors are expressed in hypothalamus and colocalized with proopiomelanocortin and neuropeptide Y in

rodent arcuate neurons." J Endocrinol200(1): 93-105.

3. Khanna, N. and S. Rasool (2011). "Facial melanoses: Indian perspective." Indian J DermatolVenereolLeprol77(5): 552-563; quiz 564.

4. Lieberman, R. and L. Moy (2008). "Estrogen receptor expression in melasma: results from facial skin of affected patients." J Drugs Dermatol7(5): 463-465.2

5. Perez, M., J. L. Sanchez, et al. (1983). "Endocrinologic profile of patients with idiopathic melasma." J Invest Dermatol81(6): 543-545.

6. Plonka, P. M., T. Passeron, et al. (2009). "What are melanocytes really doing all day long...?" ExpDermatol18(9): 799-819.

7. Salmenniemi, U., E. Ruotsalainen, et al. (2004). "Multiple abnormalities in glucose and energy metabolism and coordinated changes in levels of adiponectin, cytokines, and adhesion molecules in subjects with metabolic syndrome." Circulation110(25): 3842-3848.3

8. Sheth, V. M. and A. G. Pandya (2011). "Melasma: a comprehensive update: part I." J Am AcadDermatol65(4): 689-697; quiz 698.1

9. Rathore, S.P., S. Gupta, and V. Gupta, Pattern and prevalence of physiological cutaneous changes in pregnancy: a study of 2000 antenatal women. Indian J DermatolVenereolLeprol, 2011. 77(3): p. 402.

10. Prasad, D.S., et al., Prevalence and risk factors for metabolic syndrome in Asian Indians: A community study from urban Eastern India. J Cardiovasc Dis Res, 2012. 3(3): p. 204-11.

11. Passeron, T., Melasma pathogenesis and influencing factors - an overview of the latest research. J EurAcadDermatolVenereol, 2013. 27 Suppl 1: p. 5-6.

12. The IDF consensus worldwide definition of the metabolic syndrome; http://www.idf.org/webdata/docs/MetS_def_update2006.pdf [Accessed on 13 March 2014].

13. Balkrishnan R, McMichael AJ, Camacho FT, Saltzberg F, Housman TS, GrummerS, et al. Development and validation of a health-related quality of life instrument for women with melasma. Br J Dermatol 2003; 149: 572–577.

14. Dominguez AR, Balkrishnan R, Elizey AR, Pandya AG.Melasma in Latina patients: cross-cultural adaptation andvalidation of a quality-of-life questionnaire in Spanish language.J Am AcadDermatol 2006; 55: 59–66.

15. Cestari TF, Hexsel D, Viegas ML, Azulay L, Hassun K, Almeida AR, et al. Validation of a melasma quality of life questionnaire for Brazilian Portuguese language: theMelasQol-BP study and improvement of QoL of melasma patients after triple combination therapy. Br J Dermatol 2006; 156: 13–20.

16. Dogramaci AC, Havlucu DY, Inandi T, Balkrishnan R. Validation of a melasma quality of life questionnaire for the Turkish language: theMelasQoL-TR study. J Dermatology Treat 2009; 20: 95–99.

17. Melasma: Measure of the Impact on Quality of Life Using the French Version of MELASQOL after Cross-cultural Adaptation Laurent Misery, Anne-Marie Schmitt, Sami Boussetta, Nora Rahhali and Charles Taieb. Journal Compilation © 2010 ActaDermato-Venereologica. ISSN 0001-5555.

Studies

Assessment of Complete Hormonal Status in Female Acne Patients – A Study

Ram Malkani, Vandana Punjabi nee Budhraja

Received CT Bannerjee award at the National Conference, IADVL Bangalore

Reflections

The study was carried out in women with acne, as the hormonal status in women with Acne is misunderstood even in 2017, while writing this. Women with acne are considered by many as having hormonal imbalance and also taken for granted that they have PCOD. Both parts of the statement are not entirely true. Some do have significantly higher levels of androgens, but very few in numbers. Similarly about only 30 to 40 percent of females with acne have PCOD. What can be concluded is that most probably have a higher end organ sensitivity or they have increased conversion of testosterone to more potent Dihydrotestoster one peripherally, probably because of overactive 5 alpha reductase enzyme. Minor elevations of Testosterone, Free testosterone, DHEA-S, Andostanedione were considered normal, as it happens as an accompaniment of PCOD. No patients had higher levels of 17 –OH Progesterone, suggesting Congenital adrenal hyperplasia or Late onset adrenal hyperplasia not so common.

AIMS

To assess the androgen environment of female acne patients using RIA technique and compare the same with healthy female controls.

To determine the prevalence of ultrasonically defined polycystic ovaries in women with acne.

Materials & Methods

Patients   92 with Acne Vulgaris
             Aged 12-37 years (mean 23.07 yrs)

Controls   28 healthy women
             Aged 16-36 years (mean 23.04 yrs)

             Pregnant Women
             H/O delivery, OCPs, Hormones-6 months
Excluded S/S of Virilism
             -Hirsutism (Feriman – Gallwey score > 8)
             -androgenetic Alopecia

Results

1. History, Physical Examination

2. RIA Tests : S. Prolactin

Total & Free Testosterone

DHEA-S

Androstenedione

In some pts: 17-OH Progesterone

Post ACTH 17-OH Progesterone

FSH, LH

TSH, T3, T4

S. Cortisol

3. Pelvic USG : Follicular Phase

4. Statistical Analysis

Total No. of Patients	92
Duration of Acne	2 months – 25 years Mean : 5.97 years
Age of Onset of Acne	Mean 17 years
Menstrual Abnormalities	28.57%
Family H/O Acne	58%
Severity of Acne - Mild	19.57%
Moderate	63.04%
Severe	17.39%

Mean Values of RIA

Test Normal Range		Patients	Controls	Significance (P Value)
Total testosterone	N	90	26	S*
(0.3 – 0.9 ng/ml)	mean	0.61	0.49	(P = 0.05)
Free testosterone	N	54	27	NS
(0.2 – 3.2 pg/ml)	mean	2.35	2.29	(P = 0.69)
S. Prolactin	N	62	20	NS
(1.1 – 23.8 ng/ml)	mean	15.87	13.91	(P = 0.86)
DHEA-S	N	64	28	NS
(0.82 – 3.38 l g/ml)	mean	2.96	2.48	(P= 0.13)
Androstenedione	N	92	28	NS
0.9 – 2.8 ng/ml)	mean	3.03	2.72	(P = 0.44)

N = No. of Subjects in whom test was done

S* = Significant (P < 0.05) NS = Not significant (P > 0.05)

No. of Patients & Controls with Values above the Normal Range

Test	Patients N	% above N range	Controls N	% above N range	Significance (P Value)
Total testosterone	90	14.4	26	0	S* (P = 0.03)
Free testosterone	54	16.7	27	25.9	NS (P = 0.27)
S Prolactin	62	19.4	20	15	NS (P = 0.98)
DHEA – S	64	32.8	28	21.4	NS (P = 0.23)
Androstenedione	92	42.4	28	46.4	NS (P = 0.81)

S* = Significant (P < 0.05) NS = Not significant (P . 0.05)

Clinical Features & Abnormal Test Results

Variable	% of Pts	% of Pts showing abnormal Results
H/O Menstrual AbN+	28.57%	92.86% NS
H/O menstrual AbN-	-	80.00%

Test Used: Sign Test

Clinical Features & Abnormal Test Results (contd.)

Variable	% of Pts	% of Pts showing Abnormal Results
Family H/ O Acne +	58.00%	81.25% NS
Family H/ O Acne -		86.36%
Duration <= 2 yrs	27.51%	75.00% NS
>2 yrs upto 10 yrs	60.34%	91.00%
> 10 yrs	12.07%	71.40%
Severity - Mild	19.57%	72.22% NS
Moderate	63.04%	68.96%
Severe	17.39%	75.00%

Test Used: Sign Test

Results

1 Abnormal Biochemical Results

1 Abnormal Biochemical Results or PCOD

Pelvic Ultrasound

Pelvic USG	Patients N %	Controls N %	Significance (P Value)
PCOD	30 38%	5 21.70%	NS
No. PCOD	49 62%	18 78.30%	(P = 0.23)
Total	79 100%	23 100%	

N = No. of Patients in whom test was done

Test Used : Chi – Square Test

Conclusions

- 3/4th of female acne patients studied showed disturbed endocrine environment

- Significant increase in Total Testosterone values

- No correlation between Abnormal test results and menstrual abnormality, family history, duration & severity of acne

Polycystic ovaries were present in 38% of patients

Acanthosis nigricans: a marker of polycystic ovarian disease, insulin resistance, obesity, A Jaslok Hospital & Reseach Centre Study

Meenakshi Verma, Ram Malkani

Presented at the National IADVL conference, Mumbai

Reflections

It is common knowledge now, that Acanthosis nigricans is a marker of hyperinsulemia. It is an enigma if Acanthosis Nigricans can be reversed. One of our female case, of course the study was only on females, took metformin for one year, lost 10 kg and her Acanthosison the neck disappeared. At times slim females also were found to have clinically acanthosis on the neck. Occassionally, a female who was slim and had no clinical evidence of Acanthosis on the neck, on biopsy, showed, evidence of Acanthosis Nigricans.

AIMS AND OBJECTIVES

The study was conducted to evaluate the demographic pattern and establish Acanthosis nigricans as a cutaneous marker of systemic conditions such as polycystic ovarian disease, insulin resistance, elevated body mass index.

METHODS AND MATERIALS

Study design

This is a prospective study in which 25 cases of acanthosis nigricans and 20 age and sex matched controls were evaluated over a period of two years.

Inclusion Criteria for cases:

1. Presence of Acanthosis nigricans diagnosed clinically and histopathologically

2. Female

3. Age group 13 to 45 yrs

4. No underlying malignancy

5. Healthy individuals

Inclusion Criteria for controls:

1. Absence of acanthosis nigricans
2. Female
3. Age group 13 to 45 yrs
4. Healthy individuals

Insulin resistance was computed using the formula : fasting glucose/ fasting insulin < 4.5

Body mass index : weight in kgs/ height in mt^2
Polycystic ovarian disease was diagnosed on basis of ultrasonography of pelvis

Assessment

Written informed consent/Parental consent
    Demography noted
    Medical history noted
    Clinical examination

Investigations

lipid profile status
    serum glucose[fasting] levels
    serum insulin[fasting] levels
    Skin biopsy to confirm presence of acanthosis nigricans
from involved areas
    Radiological   studies   included   an
ultrasonography[pelvis] to study ovarian disease
    Family history of diabetes – 40%of cases had a family
history of daibetes mellitus
    Family history of acanthosis nigricans - 28% of cases had
a family history ofacanthosis nigricans

Age distribution

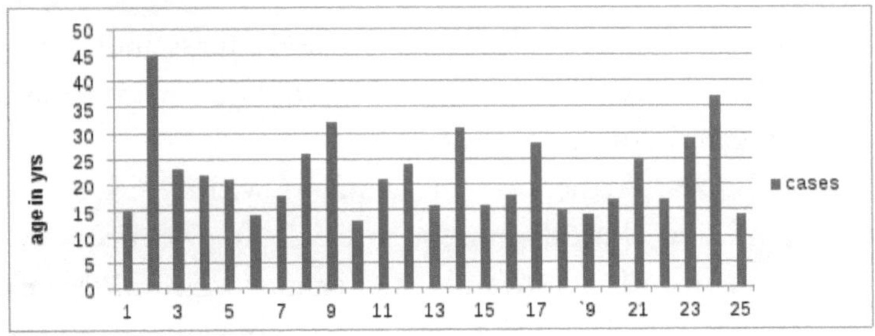

The mean age among cases was 22 yrs

RESULTS

80% of cases Vs 11% of controls had a high body mass index [P<0.001] The relative risk{RR} was 3.82 [1.76<RR<8.30]

64% cases Vs 35% controls had polycystic ovarian disease [P=0.05] The relative risk was 1.70 [0.96<RR<3.01]

68% cases Vs 26%controls had insulin resistance [P<0.01]The relative risk was 2.13[1.17<RR<3.86]

CASES VS CONTROLS

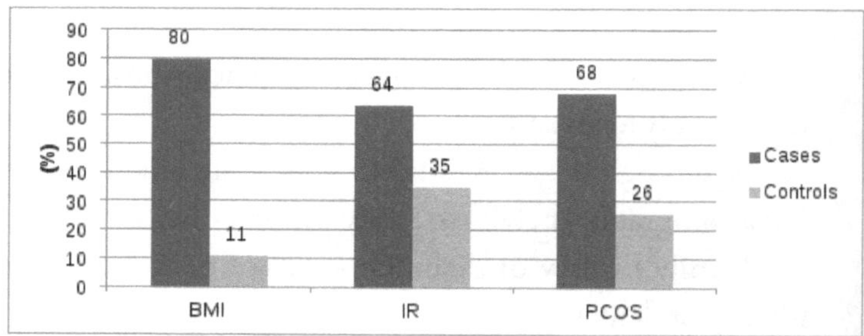

BMI= Body mass index, IR = Insulin resistance, PCOS = Polycystic ovarian syndrome.

Conclusion

Polycystic ovarian disease, high body mass index, insulin resistance are factors positively correlated with acanthosis nigricans in our population.

Insulin resistance in women with PCOS entails significant clinical consequences. It is evidenced by the prevalence of significantly higher glucose intolerance and a risk which is seven times greater for developing type 2 diabetes.

Acanthosis nigricans is a valuable cutaneous marker of hyperinsulinemia in obese individuals, PCOS.

Baseline CD4 T cell counts in HIV infected individuals who were diagnosed during voluntary counselling and testing in a resource poor setting

Namrata Sippy, Meenakshi Verma & Ram Malkani

Won the first prize on the Best Poster award at the XXIVth National Conference of the IADVL held at Ahmedabad Jan 25-28 1996 on the paper

Ladymeade Reference Unit, Ministry of Health, Barbados; Jaslok Hospital and Research Centre, Mumbai, India; IADVL HIV anonymous testing centre, Mumbai, India

ABSTRACT:

Background: Measurement of CD4 cells are required for staging HIV disease and making decisions regarding the initiation of antiretroviral therapy.Baseline determinations help to predict the impact of therapy and plan management strategies.Baseline measurements were evaluated in an Indian cohort who participated in voluntary HIV counselling and testing.

Methods: CD4 cell counts were determined for 71 adults (57M/14F) between January and December 2004 after being confirmed HIV+ve by ELISA and Western

Blot.Samples were processed at the MGM Hospital, Panvel, India.Statistical analyses were conducted using VassarStats (Richard Lowry, USA). T cell counts were assessed for differences in gender and age.

Results: Age of studied persons varied between 22 – 64 years (Median age- 38 years).CD4 counts ranged from 130-1772 cells/microliter (Overall Median -728; Median (Males) – 742 (95%CI=697-925), Median (Females) – 832 (95% CI=671-1142).No significant difference in CD4 cell counts were observed between males and females of different ages (P > 0.05).

1 person had a CD4 cell count of <200; 9 had CD4 cell counts between 200 and 350 cells/microlitre.

Conclusions: Over one-half of adults and baseline CD4 counts consistent with normal ranges of CD4 established in Indian adults; indicating that persons participating in VCT are presenting at an earlier stage of the disease process.Although not significant, females had a higher CD4 cell count than males.Gender and age had no affect on CD4 cell counts.

INTRODUCTION:

The HIV epidemic in India has increased at an alarming rate with over 5 million people being positive at the end of 2003.India's population being over 1 billion people, this epidemic has a major impact for spread of disease in Asia, the Pacific and worldwide. The mode of transmission is primarily through heterosexual behaviour.Effective surveillance activities are necessary for resource requirement planning, care and management of people living with HIV/

AIDS (PLWHA) and devising strategies for HIV prevention. HIV voluntary counselling and testing (VCT) is an extremely useful surveillance tool and furthermore serves as an entry point for access to care, support, treatment and laboratory monitoring of PLWHA's. The Indian Association of Dermatologists Venereologists and Leprologists (IADVL) runs a VCT centrein Mumbai, a city which is severely affected by the HIV epidemic. CD4 T cell count are determined on all persons diagnosed HIV positive after VCT. The CD4 T cell count is a marker of disease progression and required by clinicians when staging HIV disease and to make decisions when to initiate antiretroviral therapy or opportunistic infection prophylaxis. In India there are not many published studies on CD4 T cell counts at presentation . It isessential to determine at what stage are person presenting in their HIV disease to plan effective management strategies and in order to maximise treatment access in line with the WHO 3x5 initiative. This study was conducted to assess baseline CD4 T cell counts of all HIV positive persons diagnosed after VCT.

METHODS:

Blood samples collected duringVCT were tested by ELISA and confirmed by Western blot.All persons who were diagnosed HIV+ between January and December 2004 were included in the study.Laboratory analyses were conductedat the MGM Medical college and Hospital, Panvel India.CD4 T cell counts and viral load (available only for 25 patients) were determined.CD4 T cell counts in peripheral blood samples were determined using the Whole

Blood Capcellia immunoenzymatic method.The HIV viral load was measured by Quantitative RT-PCR.Statistical analyses of data was performed using Vassarstats, a web-based software for statistical computation (Richard Lowry, Vassar College, USA)

RESULTS:

The study cohort comprised of 57 Males and 17 Females (Total – 71 persons).44% of persons were age of persons diagnosed was 38 years.13% of persons had CD4+ T cell counts above the clinically relevant WHO described threshold (<200 cells/microliter) for defining AIDS condition, but below 350 cells/microliter.Majority (86%) of persons had CD4 T cell counts above 350 cells/ microliter.Overall MedianCD T4 cell count – 728 cells/ microliter; Median (Males) – 742 (95% CI=697-925), Median (Females) – 832 (95% CI=671-1142).There was no significant difference in CD4 cell counts between males and females of different ages (P>0.05).All but one person were asymptomatic.Median viral load (n=25) was 14,200 HIV RNA copies/ml.Viral loads for 24/25 persons was <30,000 copies/ml.

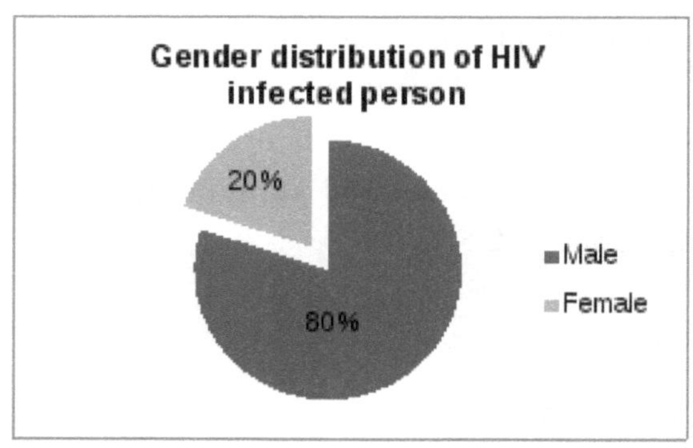

Gender distribution of HIV infected person
20%
80%
Male
Female

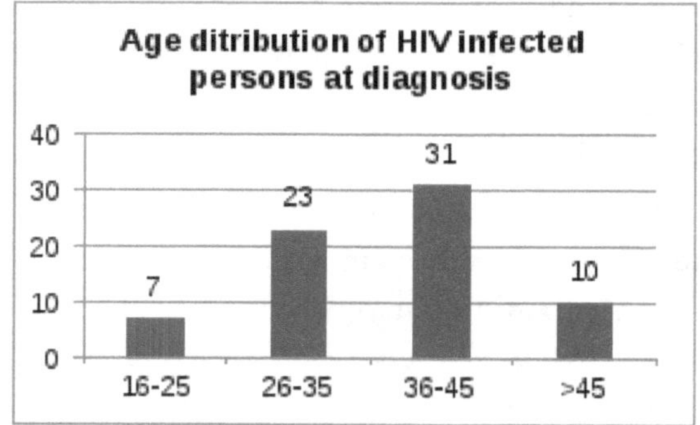

Age ditribution of HIV infected persons at diagnosis
40
30
20
10
0
7
23
31
10
16-25
26-35
36-45
>45

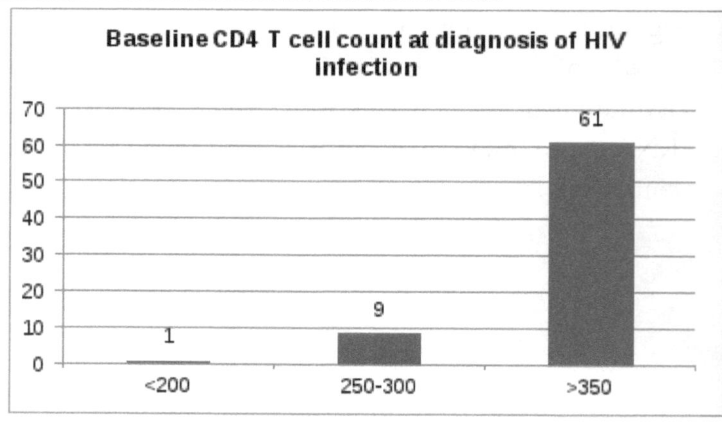

Baseline CD4 T cell count at diagnosis of HIV infection
70
60
50
40
30
20
10
0
1
9
61
<200
250-300
>350

CONCLUSION:

Majorityof persons diagnosed HIV positive after VCT presented at a very early stage in their disease as indicated by their high CD4 T cell counts.Early presentation and early access to care positively impacts treatment success and overall clinical outcome, when therapy will be required by these persons.The results indicate that persons who other wise may feel healthy are readily participating in VCT programmes.This tool has shown to be effective in this cohort of infected persons and is strongly advocated.

Subclinical DVT as an etiology of CVI- a study of 50 cases

Sneh Thadani, Rusina Karia, Ram Malkani

INTRODUCTION:

Various studies have been done to establish risk factors of chronic venous insufficiency. Studies suggest that it can occur due to congenital valve or vessel abnormalities, but it most commonly occurs when the valves of the deep veins are damaged as a result of DVT (1) (2) Valves maintain the hydrostatic venous pressure in the lower extremities by preventing the reflux of venous blood when its being pumped against gravity towards the heart. With no valves to prevent deep system reflux, the hydrostatic venous pressure in the lower extremity increases dramatically. Even after the DVT resolves the damage to the valves remains permanent, later culminating in CVI. But prior DVT can be clinical or subclinical and often not diagnosed on ultrasound after resolution. The hypothesis that prior (clinical/subclinical) DVT is the main cause of CVI and it is not diagnosed after resolution on ultrasound is the basis of our study to find markers of thrombosis even if DVT has resolved and other ultrasound features suggestive of CVI so that physicians can start patients on treatment on the basis of these markers and non-thrombotic ultrasound findings to control the future CVI

MATERIALS AND METHODS

We carried out the study on patients visiting the dermatology outpatient department at JASLOK HOSPITAL AND RESEARCH CENTRE which is a tertiary care hospital in a Mumbai, India catering to middle class and higher upper class patients. It was an observational study and consecutive consent was taken from 50 patients between 18 -65 years of age of both gender presenting with symptoms of pain, edema , pigmentation, distended veins , ulcers of the lower limbs and/or with a history of past or preceding symptoms or sign of deep venous thrombosis.

We collected a detailed history of presenting symptoms (onset, progression and duration) and associated history of aggravating factors. Local cutaneous examination and the BMI of the patient was taken and noted. Patients were classified using two scoring systems- Venous severity clinical score (VSCS) (3) and CEAP - Clinical signs (C0-C6); Etiology (primary venous etiology present or not); anatomic distribution (superficial/deep/perforator or none); and pathophysiology (reflux/obstruction/both or none) (4)(5)(6). In VSCS using the seven classes of the C classification (pain , varicose veins, venous edema, skin pigmentation, inflammation, induration, ulcers, compression therapy) a 0 to 3 grading scheme is assigned to clinical manifestations of each class 0=absent, 1=mild,2=moderate,3=severe. Then the score is added and patients with VSCS score = 1-4 are classified as non-severe and VSCS score ≥5 are classified as severe.

After classifying the patients color doppler investigation for deep venous thrombosis (DVT) and venous incompetence and blood investigations like factor V, d-Dimer, T.cholesterol, T.triglycerides, homocysteine, High density lipoproteins (HDL) , low density lipoproteins (LDL), very low density lipoproteins (VLDL) were carried out to to evaluate their levels in severe and non-severe patients and their significance as proxy markers for DVT.

All the data collected on a pre determined clinical perfroma was entered in a Microsoft office Excel sheet which were further converted to Stata. (copyrights stata, corp , college , station , texas USA) . we calculated the means and the standard deviation (SD) for continuous variables with difference between the means assessed using the T- test calculated the proportions for the categorical variable and the difference in proportion was assessed using the chi square test. P value of less than 0.05 was considered statistically significant.

	Total	Males	Females	P value
Occupational category	50 (100)	32 (100)	18 (100)	
Desk job	15 (30)	13 (41)	2 (11)	
Labour	6 (12)	4 (13)	2 (11)	
Housewives	13 (26)	0 (0)	13 (100)	<0.001
Others(ward boys/ kitchen managers/ sales executive)	16 (32)	15 (47)	1 (6)	
Associated history and symptoms				
A] SYMPTOMS				
Pain	34 (68)	21 (65)	13 (72)	0.63
Oedema	44 (88)	27 (84)	17 (94)	0.29
Distended veins	38 (76	22 (69)	16 (89)	0.11
Pigmentation	39 (78)	27 (84)	12 (67)	0.15
Ulcers	12 (24)	9 (28)	3 (17)	0.36
B] HISTORY				
Prolonged standing	38 (76)	23 (72)	15 (83)	0.36
Trauma	6	4	2 (11)	0.89

	(12)	(13)		
Surgery	7 (14)	6 (19)	1 (6)	0.20
Immobilisation (> 2 weeks)	2 (4)	1 (3)	1 (6)	0.67
OC pills	3 (6)	0 (0)	3 (17)	**0.02**
Altered bowel habits	24 (48)	15 (47)	1 (50)	0.83
Episode of DVT	2 (4)	2 (6)	0 (0)	0.28
Blood in stools	5 (10)	3 (9)	2 (11)	0.84
Family history of Varicose	19 (38)	11 (34)	8 (44)	0.48

Investigations	VSCS			CLINICAL CLASSIFICATION			ETIOLOGICAL CLASSIFICATION		
	VSCS (≥5) 24 (100)	VSCS (1-4) 26 (100)	p value	C4a to C6 21 (100)	C0 to C3 29 (100)	P value	Primay venous etioloy 36 (100)	No venous etioloy 14 (100)	P v
A. Blood investigations									
Homocysteine (high)	10 (42)	6 (23)	0.16	7 (33)	9 (31)	0.86	12 (33)	4 (29)	0.7
D-Dimer (high)	6 (26)	4 (15)	0.35	5 (25)	5 (17)	0.51	8 (23)	2 (14)	0.5
Factor V (+)	4 (17)	0 (0)	**0.03**	4 (19)	0 (0)	**0.01**	4 (11)	0 (0)	0.1
T. Cholesterol (high)	5 (21)	7 (21)	0.61	5 (24)	7 (24)	0.98	8 (22)	4 (29)	0.6
T. Triglycerides (high)	10 (42)	8 (31)	0.42	8 (38)	10 (35)	0.79	14 (39)	4 (29)	0.5
HDL (low)	8 (33)	7 (27)	0.62	6 (29)	9 (31)	0.85	9 (25)	6 (43)	0.2
VLDL (high)	3 (13)	1 (4)	0.26	1 (5)	3 (10)	0.47)	3 (8)	1 (7)	0.8
LDL (high)	5 (12)	5 (19)	0.89	4 (19)	6 (21)	0.89	6 (17)	4 (29)	0.3
TG/HDL ratio (high)	11 (46)	9 (35)	0.42	10 (48)	10 (34)	0.35	16 (44)	4 (29)	0.3
B. Doppler findings									
Perforators (+)	21 (88)	15 (58)	**0.02**	20 (95)	16 (55)	**0.002**	35 (97)	1 (7)	<0

Great Saphenous Vein (+)	11 (46)	8 (31)	0.27	13 (62)	6 (21)	**0.003**	18 (50)
Varicosities (+)	16 (67)	7 (27)	**0.005**	15 (71)	8 (28)	**0.002**	23 (64)
Thrombosis (+)	2 (8)	0 (0)	0.13	2 (10)	0 (0)	0.09	2 (6)

Number of perforators	Total 50 (100)	Males 32 (100)	Females 18 (100)	P value
A. Above knee				
0	49 (98)	31 (97)	18 (100)	0.45
2	1 (2)	1 (3)	0 (0)	
B. Below knee				
0	41 (82)	26 (81)	15 (83)	0.88
1	4 (8)	3 (9)	1 (6)	
2	5 (10)	3 (9)	2 (11)	
C. Medical malleolus				
0	13 (26)	9 (28)	4 (22)	0.60
1	17 (34)	9 (28)	8 (44)	
2	14 928)	9 (28)	5 (28)	
3	3 (6)	3 (9)	0 (0)	
4	3 (6)	2 (6)	1 (6)	

RESULT

A total of 50 patients (32 males and 18 females) with chronic venous insufficiency were evaluated. There was no difference between the mean age of males and females (SD:

47.6 , 43.1 , p value=0.19). Patients having Occupations such as kitchen managers, ward boys, sales executive were highest (32%) followed closely by desk jobs (30%) and the commonest history was of prolonged standing among our patients (76%) without any significant difference between male and female. The most frequent symptoms found in our patients were oedema (88%), pigmentation (78%) and distended veins (76%). The symptom seen significantly less than others was ulcers (24%). BMI of our patients is high, 32% are obese (BMI $\geq$30) and 22% are overweight (BMI$\geq$25)

INVESTIGTIONS: A comparison between different classifications and their investigations is made. We found a raised Factor V significantly more in patients classified as severe under clinical classification compared with non severe (19% and 0%; p value=0.05) and in patients with a high VSCS score compared to those with a low VSCS score (17% and 0%; p value=0.03). No such significant difference was found when patients are classified according to etiology, anatomy and pathology. Similarly factors such as D-dimer , homocysteine, T.cholesterol and T.triglycerides are raised but no significant difference is found in the raised distribution between patients after classification according to VSCS and CEAP . VDRL is negative in our patients .On color doppler it was seen that perforators were found significantly more in patients with a high VSCS score compared to patients with low VSCS score (perforators: 88% and 58% ; p value=0.02) , in patients with a primary venous etiology compared to those without any venous etiology (97% and 1%; p value $\leq$0.0001), in patients with obstruction/reflux compared to those without any pathology(95% and 0%; p value≤0.0001) and in patients with severe clinical classification compared with non-severe patient(95% and 55%; p value=0.002). Similarly, varicosity and saphenous vein incompetence findings were seen . There were two patients with thrombosis and both had high homocysteine , Factor V , T. Cholesterol T. Triglycerides and low HDL. In table 3 we identified the perforators , most common perforators were medial malleolus (74%), followed by below knee (18%) and above knee (2%).

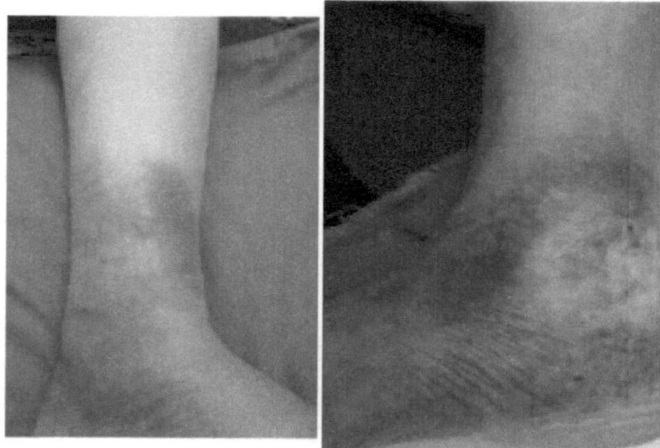
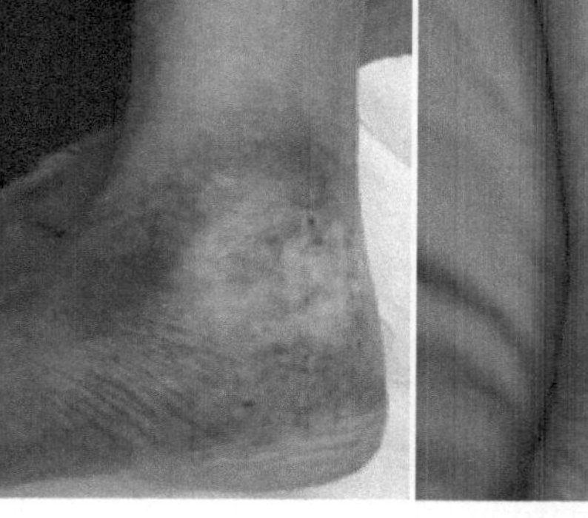

Dermatosclerosis   Stasis   Phlebitis

DISCUSSION:

Thus, we found patients with CVI had raised Factor V and homocysteine levels. However, none of our patients had features suggestive of active or resolved DVT on sonography. We also found that these patients had a high BMI (7)(8) and a history of standing for longer hours due to their occupation(9)(10)(11). Only those patients who were classified as severe cases of CVI had raised factor V.

However, both - severe and non-severe cases of patients with CVI had raised homocysteine & D-dimer. Despite these changes in the blood parameters, we did not find any signs of active DVT in any of our patients(12) .

Studies have suggested that high plasma levels of factor V might lead to an increased prothrombinase activity causing an increased risk of thrombosis (13) and implicate that hyperhomocysteinemia (HH) promotes thrombosis by an imbalanced redox status because its sulfhydryl group is a strong reductant (14) (15). Studies have shown that D-dimer has a sensitivity of 91% for DVT which means patients with raised d-dimer will have a higher likelihood of DVT and both our patients with thrombosis had raised D-dimer but other patients with raised D-dimer did not show a DVT on USG (16)(17). D-dimer has a low specificity because its raised in other conditions too like bleeding, aortic dissection, renal and liver diseases (18) thus raised D-dimer values should be interpreted in view of the history and the overall coagulation profile . We also found that all patients with CVI had high cholesterol and triglyceride levels. These parameters also have a role in thromboembolic events. Though the exact mechanism is unclear, it has been hypothesised that cholesterol and trigylcerides may cause an impairment in coagulation through changes in blood viscosity or mediation through tissue factor pathway inhibitor. (19) (20). Thus a raised factor V, Hyperhomocysteinemia, or altered lipid profile – proxy markers for DVT – may be used for diagnosis of CVI in patients without any evidence of any active thrombus on ultrasonography (21)(22)(23).Once the DVT resolves, usually it cannot be seen on ultrasound. However other features suggestive of valvular incompetence leading to CVI like incompetent perforators, saphenous vein incompetence, and varicosities can be noted on color doppler (24) (25). In our study even though evidence of active DVT was not found , our patients did show some features of CVI on color doppler (26)(27) Furthermore, all these patients were more likely to be classified as severe CVI and have a higher VSCS score. (28) Knowledge of these parameters is important in diagnosis of DVT in patients presenting with symptoms of CVI without any active thrombus (29)(30). It is quite likely that we may not find any feature suggestive of active or resolved thrombus on an ultrasound. However, even in the absence of these findings, it is essential to have a complete coagulation profile of these patients for effective diagnosis and management. It may be difficult to identify the subtle chronic changes in these veins like eccentric or diffuse thickening of the vein wall , calcification or partial recanalization of vein lumen with irregular channels , if the treating physician does not inform to sonologist to look for these changes due to a clinical suspicion of resolved DVT. Thus doppler findings such as perforator incompetence, saphenous vein incompetence and varicosities along with blood markers of previous DVT could be a good way of diagnosing CVI.

CONCLUSION:

An important limitation of our study is lack of a control group. In absence of this, we could not estimate the predictive values of these blood parameters. Nonetheless, our study presents some important findings. As highlighted clinical or subclinical DVT - an important cause of CVI, though its features may not always be seen on ultrasound, especially after resolution may have the presence of blood parameters suggestive of DVT such as raised factorV/Hyperhomocystenemia/raised T.triglycerides & T.cholesterol and which can be used as proxy markers for current or previous DVT. This needs further study to elucidate the role of Ultrasound,CT venogram and a complete thrombotic profile in the evaluation of a subclinical DVT in cases of CVI. Thus, it is imperative that all treating physicians become aware of USG findings as well as communicate with the sonologist to actively look for these changes. Even if these findings are missing (as was the case in our study), the blood profile should be examined to look for any alteration in the coagulation parameters suggestive of predeliction to thrombosis, and plan the treatment protocol accordingly. These patients should also be regularly followed for evidence of any recurrence of thrombotic episodes.

References

1] Robert Weiss, MD; Chief Editor: William D James, MD .Venous Insufficiency.

2] Thayer E. Scott, MPH, Wayne W. LaMorte, MD, PhD, MPH, Daniel R. Gorin, MD, and James O. Menzoian, MD, Boston, Mass. Risk factors for chronic venous insufficiency: A dual case control study. J VASC SURG 1995322:622-8.

3] Rutherford, R.B., et al., Venous severity scoring: An adjunct to venous outcome assessment. Journal of Vascular Surgery, 2000. 31(6): p. 1307-12)

4] Porter, J.M. and G.L. Moneta, Reporting standards in venous disease: an update. International Consensus Committee on Chronic Venous Disease.. Journal of Vascular Surgery, 1995. 21(4): p. 635-45.)

5] Porter, J.M., et al., Reporting standards in venous disease.Journal of Vascular Surgery, 1988. 8(2): p. 172-181)

6] Carpentier, P.H., et al., Appraisal of the information content of the C classes of CEAP clinical classification of chronic venous disorders: a multicenter evaluation of 872 patients. Journal of Vascular Surgery, 2003. 37(4): p. 827-33

7] Danielsson, G., et al., The influence of obesity on chronic venous disease. Vascular & Endovascular Surgery, 2002.36(4): p. 271-6.

8] Oganov RG, Savel'ev VS, Shal'nova SA, Kirienko AI, Zolotukhin IA. Risk factors of chronic venous insufficiency of the lower extremities and possibilities of its medication in therapeutic practice. Ter Arkh, 2006;78(4):68-72.

9] Stvrtinova, V., J. Kolesar, and G. Wimmer, Prevalence ofvaricose veins of the lower limbs in the women working at a department store. International Angiology, 1991. 10(1): p. 2-5.

10] Tuchsen, F., et al., Standing at work and varicose veins.Scandinavian Journal of Work, Environment & Health, 2000. 26(5): p. 414-20

11] Shai A1, Karakis I, Shemesh D. [Possible ramifications of prolonged standing at the workplace and its association with the development of chronic venous insufficiency]. Harefuah. 2007 Sep;146(9):677-85, 734.

12] Prandoni, P., et al., Vein abnormalities and the postthrombotic syndrome. 2005: Journal of Thrombosis & Haemostasis February 2005;3(2):401-402.)

13] P W Kamphuisen , Frits R Rosendaal Jeroen Eikenboom Rogier M Bertina. Factor V Antigen Levels and Venous Thrombosis : Risk Profile, Interaction With Factor V Leiden, and Relation With Factor VIII Antigen Levels Arteriosclerosis Thrombosis and Vascular Biology 20(5):1382-6 • June 2000 with 19 Reads DOI: 10.1161/ 01.ATV.20.5.1382

14] Coppola A , Davi G, De Stefano V et al. Homocysteine , coagulation, platelet function and thrombosis, Semin Thromb Haemost . 2000. 26: 243- 254

15] Yunyoung Chang, MDa Ganary Dabiri, MD, PhD,b Elizabeth Damstetter, MD,a Emily Baiyee Ebot, MD,c Jennifer Gloeckner Powers, MD,d and Tania Phillips, MDa Boston, Massachusetts; Providence, Rhode Island; and Nashville, Tennessee. Coagulation disorders and their cutaneous presentations: Pathophysiology

16] Turkstra F, Van Beek E , Buller H. Observer and biological variation of a rapid whole blood D-dimer test, Thromb Haemost 1998. 79:91-93.

17] Bounameaux H, Cirafici P, de Moerloose P et al. Measurment of D-dimer in plasma as diagnostic aid in suspected pulmonary embolism , Lancet . 1991. 337: 196-200

18] Goran pante K. MD,Phd. Pragmatic classification of causes of D-dimer. American Journal of Emergency Medicine (2009) 27, 1016.e5–1016.e7

19] Amparo Vayá,Yolanda Mira,Fernando Ferrando, MaTeresa Contreras. Hyperlipidaemia and venous thromboembolism in patients lacking thrombophilic risk factors. British Journal of Haematology 2002, 118 (1): 255-9.

20] Belaj K1, Hackl G, Rief P, Eller P, Brodmann M, Gary T. Changes in lipid metabolism and extension of venous thromboembolism. 2014;64(2):122-6. doi: 10.1159/000360484. Epub 2014 Jul 5.

21] Frederick A. Anderson, Jr., PhD; Frederick A. Spencer, MD. Risk Factors for Venous Thromboembolism © 2003 American Heart Association, Inc. Circulation. 2003;107:I-9.

22] Kane WH, Majerus PW. Purification and characterization of human coagulation factor V. J Biol Chem. 1981;256:1002–1007.

23] Monkovic DD, Tracy PB. Activation of human factor V by factor Xa and thrombin. Biochemistry. 1990;29:1118–1128

24] Vivek Choudhary Professor , Saurabh Patil Assistant Professor. Role of Doppler Ultrasound In Lower Limb Chronic Venous Insufficiency. Indian journal of applied research Volume : 6 | Issue : 3 | March 2016 | ISSN - 2249-555X | IF : 3.919 | IC Value : 74.50

25] Rajiv K Chander, Thomas S Monahan. Ultrasound assessment of great saphenous vein insufficiency. Journal of Vascular Diagnostics and Interventions 15 June 2015 Volume 2015:3 Pages 25—31 .

26] Folse, R. and R.H. Alexander, Directional flow detection for localizing venous valvular incompetency. Surgery, 1970. 67(1): p. 114-21.

27] Sarin, S., et al., Duplex ultrasonography for assessment of venous valvular function of the lower limb.British Journal of Surgery, 1994. 81(11): p. 1591-5.

28] Marc A. Passman, MDa, , , Robert B. McLafferty, MDb, Michelle F. Lentz, MASc, Shardul B. Nagre, MBBS, MS, MPHa, Mark D. Iafrati, MDd, W. Todd Bohannon, MDe, Colleen M. Moore, MDb. Validation of Venous Clinical Severity Score (VCSS) with other venous severity assessment tools from the American Venous Forum, National Venous Screening Program Journal of Vascular Surgery Volume 54, Issue 6, Supplement, December 2011, Pages 2S–9S.

29] Esmon CT, Owen WG, Jackson CM. A plausible mechanism for pro-thrombin activation by factor Xa, factor Va, phospholipid, and calcium ions. J Biol Chem. 1974;249:8045–8047.

30] Rosing J, Tans G, Govers-Riemslag JW, Zwaal RF, Hemker HC. The role of phospholipids and factor Va in the prothrombinase complex. J BioChem. 1980;255:274–283

Ongoing Studies

To study the prevalence of HIV, HBV, and HCV and trends of prevalence from 2009 through 2013;

Principal Invesigator: Dr Haresh Ahuja;

Co-investigators: Dr Ram Malkani, Dr Aditya Tare

SPECIFIC AIMS

India is the second most populous nation in the world. The Indian subcontinent is classified as intermediate HBV endemic (HBsAg carriage 2-7 %) zone and has the second largest global pool of chronic HBV infections.(1) India has a population of more than 1.2 billion with 5.7 (reduced to 2.5) million HIV positive, 43 million HBV positive and 15 million HCV positive persons.(2)

In light of these findings,x we propose to conduct a retrospective study of the prevalence of HIV, HBV and HCV infections in patients visiting the Jaslok Hospital from the years 2009 to 2013. We will conduct retrospective secondary data analysis. The present retrospective study is an endeavor to detect the current prevalence of HBV and/ or HCV co-infection in patients infected with HIV in the visiting patients.We will compare our findings with similar other studies. The study will thus help us to estimate the prevalence of these viruses in the community at large.

The specific objectives of the study are:

1) To study the prevalence of HIV, HBV, and HCV and trends of prevalence from 2009 through 2013;

2) To study the association between these three infections: HIV, HBV, and HCV; and

3) To study the association between demographic factors and these three infections.

BACKGROUND & SIGNIFICANCE

People at high risk for Human Immunodeficiency Virus (HIV) infection are also likely to be at increased risk for other pathogens like the Hepatitis B Virus (HBV) and the Hepatitis C Virus (HCV), which share the route of transmission with HIV. There is a high degree of epidemiological similarity between these viruses in terms of routes of transmission, associated risk factors and the presence of these viruses in various body fluids.(3-5)

The co-infection of HCV with HIV is associated with a loss of immunological control of HCV and more rapid progression of HCV disease.(4,6) In a multi-center AIDS cohort study (MACS) in 2002, it was observed that liver-related mortality rates per 1000 person-years of observation were 1.7 in HIV-seropositive patients, 0.8 in HBsAg positive patients and 14.25 in the co-infected patients (significantly higher as compared with monoinfected patients.(3)

Furthermore, co-infection with hepatitis viruses may complicate the delivery of anti retroviral therapy (ART) by increasing the risk of drug-related hepatotoxicity and may interfere with the selection of specific agents. Expert guidelines developed in the United Sates and Europe recommend screening of all individuals infected with HIV for infection with HCV and HBV to help in appropriate management of such patients. In developing countries like India, no such uniform guidelines are available.(7)

Globally, the studies conducted on the prevalence of hepatitis viruses in patients infected with HIV have shown the rate of HIV and HBV/HCV co-infection to be around 12 to 15%.(8-10)

Few studies conducted in India have shown the prevalence of co-infection of HBV with HIV to vary in different geographical areas from as low as 9% to as much as 30% and of HCV with HIV to vary from 2 to 8%. (11-14)

RATIONALE OF THE RESEARCH

Since there is increased availability of antibiotics and antifungals, majority of the secondary infections associated with HIV have been taken care of. But HBV and HCV infections are becoming a cause of concern for individuals infected with HIV. Also with the advent of HAART liver disease has emerged as a cause of morbidity and mortality in these patients at later stages. Preliminary screening of the associated hepatitis viruses in patients with HIV will help in proper management of the coinfection.This limited information on correlation between these three infections in India – particularly in private health care settings.

Furthermore, the five-year data will help us assess the trends in prevalence and changes in correlation patterns.

RESEARCH DESIGN & METHODS:

Detailed research plan:

The present study will be a retrospective study.It is a secondary data analysis of data collected as apart of laboratory records from 2009 through 2013.

Study Site:

The study will be conducted at Jaslok Hospital. It is a private hospital in South Mumbai. Data will accessed from the laboratory records of patients who have undergone the tests at Jaslok Hospital.Study Design:

As discussed earlier, the present study is a secondary data analysis of data collected as a part of the laboratory records. We will abstract the following data from the records: 1) Age; 2) Sex; 3) Indoor or Outdoor patient; 4) Results of HIV test; 5) Results of HBV test; and 3) Results of HCV test. We will abstract data from all consecutive records from 2009 through 2013.

Sample size: The total number of records for the

Inclusion criteria:

1) Records with individuals more than or equal to 18 years of age
2) Analysis of secondary data from the period 2009 to 2013.

Exclusion criteria:

1) If the results are missing for all the three infections, the records will be excluded from the analysis

Data Collection:

All consecutive cases will be screened for HIV, HBV and HCV. The hospital data of 2009 to 2013will be collected in pre-designed data collection sheet.

Data analysis

All the data will be entered in Ms Excel and converted to Stata for analysis. We will calculate the means and standard deviations for continuous variables and proportions for categorical variables. The means will be compared using the t-test (for two groups) or the Analysis of Variance test (for more than two groups). The proportions will be compared using the chi square test or the Fisher's exact test for low expected cell counts. We will use the chi square for trend to assess the trends of prevalence over a period of five years. We will We will also use a logistic regression model for multivariate analysis (to account for potential confounders such as age and sex). A p value of < 0.05 will be considered statistically significant.

References

1. Lavanchy D. Hepatitis B virus epidemiology, disease burden, treatment and current and

emerging prevention and control measures. A review. J Viral Hepat. 2004;11:97-107

2. Nancy Singh. NAT: Safe Blood, Safe India. Available from http://www.expresshealthcare.in

3. Sulkowski MS. Viral hepatitis and HIV coinfection. J Hepatol 2008;48:353-67.

4. Rustgi VK, Hoofnagle JH, Gerin JL, Gelmann EP, Reichert CM, Cooper JN, et al. Hepatitis B virus infection in the acquired immunodeficiency syndrome. Ann Intern Med 1984;101:795-7.

5. Brendon Mc Caroon, Thyagarajan SP. Human Immunodeficiency virus and hepatotropic viruses: Interaction and treatment. Indian J Med Microbiol 1998;16:4-11

6. Thio CL, Scaberg EC, Skolasky R Jr, Phair J, Visscher B, Muñoz A, et al. HIV-1, hepatitis B virus and risk of liver related mortality in the Multicenter cohort study (MACS). Lancet 2002;360:1921-6.

7. Jain, et al.: Seroprevalence of hepatitis viruses in patients infected with HIV

8. Rouet F, Chaix ML, Inwoley A, Anaky MF, Fassinou P, Kpozehouen A, et al. Frequent occurrence of chronic hepatitis B virus infection

among West African HIV type 1 infected children. Clin Infect Dis 2008;46:361-6.

9. Telatela SP, Matec MI, Munubhi EK. Seroprevalence of hepatitis B and C viral co infection with Human Immunodeficiency Virus attending the pediatric HIV care and treatment center at Muhimbili National Hospital in Dar-es-Salaam, Tanzania. BMC Public Health 2007;7:338.

10. Egah DZ, Banwat EB, Audu ES, Iya D, Mandong BM, Anele AA, et al. Hepatitis B surface antigen, hepatitis C and HIV antibodies in a low –risk donor group, Nigeria. East Mediterr Health J 2007;13:961-6.

11. Tankhiwale SS, Khadase RK, Jalgoanker SV. Seroprevalence of anti HCV and hepatitis B surface antigen in HIV infected patients. Indian J Med Microbiol 2003;21:268-70

12. Saravanan S, Velu V, Kumarasamy N, Nandakumar S, Murugavel KG, Balakrishnan P, et al. Coinfection of hepatitis B and hepatitis C virus in HIV infected patients in South India. World J Gastroenterol 2007;13:5015-20.

13. Kumarasamy N, Solomon S, Flanigan TP, Hemalatha R, Thyagarajan SP, Mayer KH. Natural history of human immunodeficiency

virus disease in southern India. Clin Infect Dis 2003;36:79-85.

14. Padmapriyadarsini C, Chandrabose J, Victor L, Hanna LE, Arunkumar N, Swaminathan S. Hepatitis B or hepatitis C co-infection in individuals infected with human immunodeficiency virus and effect of antituberculosis drugs on liver function. J Postgrad Med 2006;52:92-6.

Drug trials

Use of Buspirone (Buscalm), a psychotropic drug for treatment of atopic dermatitis in 20 patients – conducted a double blind controlled trial, at the Jaslok Hospital & Research Centre, 1995

VL Aswani, Ram Malkani

Merind India Ltd.

Atopic dermatitis (AD) is a chronic relapsing dermatitis which can be categorized into the extrinsic and intrinsic types.

The diagnostic Criteria for Atopic Dermatitis (AD) by Hanifin and Rajka (7) are as follows:-

Major criteria: Must have three or more of:

Pruritus

Typical morphology and distribution

Flexural lichenification or linearity in adults

Facial and extensor involvement in infants and children

Chronic or chronically-relapsing dermatitis

Personal or family history of atopy (asthma, allergic rhinitis, atopic dermatitis)

Minor criteria: Should have three or more of:

Xerosis

Ichthyosis, palmar

The criteria for the diagnosis of Atopic Dermatitisfor the Double blind Placebo control trial, were

1) Personal or family history of atopy (asthma, allergic rhinitis, atopic dermatitis)

2) Flexural lichenification

3) Chronic or chronically relapsing dermatitis

4) Pruritus

The inclusion criteria were

1) Adults above the age of18 either sex satisfying the criteria of Atopic Dermatitis

Exclusion Criteria

1) Already receiving treatment for Atopic Dermatitis

Patients were given medication in a blinded fashion, unknown to the therapist, as the tablets were identical.

Assessment of the severity as per SCORAD and a score for itching.

At the end of one year 15 patients were enrolled.

Patients were followed up for a minimum of 6 weeks.

RESULTS :

The study was abandoned after one year, as the pharma responsible for the study changed. When the decoding was done the placebo, the medication arms showed equal results.

A total no of 50 were expected to be enrolled.

Evaluation of Azithromycin for the treatment of acute non-gonococcal urethritis in males (Protocol AZM-II-92-003C) Trial conducted at the Jaslok Hospital & Research Centre

Ram H. Malkani

Papers presented at the XXVth National Conference of the IADVL Madras June 1995

Summary

20 adult male patients (mean age 30 ± 6 yr) with acute urethritis, without Gram (-) intracellular diplococci in the smear and > 5 PMNs/HPF, were treated with a single oral dose of azithromycin (ZITHROMAX, Pfizer) given as 4 x 250 mg capsules (1 g). Symptoms and signs, were monitored on days 0, 8, and if necessary 15. Urethral smear was examined for Gram (-) intracellular diplococci and PMNs/ HPF at baseline and when completing the clinical evaluation (day 8 or 15). Blood chemistry was done on days 0 and 8/15 for safety assessment. Of the 20 patients, 17 (85%) were clinically cured, 2 (10%) improved, and 1 (5%) was a failure. There were no side effects, either biochemical or clinical. Single-dose convenience, good clinical efficacy (95%), and excellent toleration should make azithromycin a drug of choice for acute non-gonococcal urethritis in males,

which is mostly due to *Chlamydia trachomatis* or Mycoplasma species.

Introduction

Azithromycin, an azalide antibiotic resembling macrolides, is highly active against many Gram (+) and Gram (-) organisms, both aerobic and anaerobic, including Chlamydia trachomaris, *Mycoplasma hominis* and Urea-plasma urealyticum (Peters et al, 1992). Its pharmacokinetic features of special interest are (i) a long half-life of about 50 hours, which makes once-daily dosage possible, and (ii) its propensity to be concentrated in tissues cells rather than serum and be released slowly, which permits a single, 1 g oral dose to produce effective concentrations in urogenital tissues for 10 days (Foulds and Johnson, 1993). Such a dose has been reported to be highly effective for non-gonococcal urethritis (NGU) in men (Nilsen et al, 1992; Lister er al, 1993) and for chlamydial cervicitis in women (Ossewaarde et al, 1992; Martin et al, 1992). In view of the convenience of this regimen, which permits completion of supervised treatment of these infections on the spot, we investigated its efficacy and tolerability in our patients.

Patients and Methods

Selection Criteria: Adult males, aged 18-60 years, with symptoms of acute urethritis^ were selected if microscopic examination of their urethral smear showed > 5 PMNs/ HPF and absence of Gram(-) intracellular diplococci, and if they gave written consent to participate in the study after being explained its nature and purpose.

Exclusion Criteria: Patients were excluded if (i) they had known allergy to macrolides, hepatic or renal impairment, malabsorption, history of antibiotic treatment during previous 3 days,or participationin another study during the previousmonth;and(ii) theyneeded concomitant treatment with ergotamine, carbamazepine or digoxin.

Dosage Regimen: Azithromycin was used as 250 mg capsules (ZITHROMAX,™ Pfuer). The dose was 4 capsules (1 g) administered once only. Patients were instructed to take the capsules either 1 hour before a meal or 2 hours after a meal. The dose was administered under observation if these conditions were satisfied. No other antibiotic was allowed concomitantly. Vitamin capsules (BECOSULES,™ Pfizer) were given from day 4 onwards, one daily, as incentive for follow-up.

Observations: Each patient was seen at least 3 times, on days 1, 4 and 8, and if necessary a fourth time, on day 15, for proper assessment of response symptoms and signs were recorded on days 1, 4 and 8/15; investigations for diagnosis and response (Gram's stain) and for safety (serum chemistry) were done on day 1 and 8/15. At each visit, inquiry was made about side effects or any concomitant illness using an open-ended question.

Assessment: First, nonevaluable patients, if any, were segregated into dropouts and exclusions, with cause for it as far as it could be determined. Each evaluable patient's response was classified as: cure, if the symptoms and signs were completely or almost completely relieved and investigations, if abnormal initially, had returned to normal; improvement, if the symptoms and signs were markedly relieved, investigations showed normalcy or near-normalcy, and no further treatment was needed; failure, if there was no change in or worsening of clinical condition, requiring change of treatment; relapse, if there was improvement on day 4/7 with worsening on day 8/15, requiring change of treatment.

Results

Patients: The 20 patients enrolled had a mean age of 30 years (range 22-45 years, SEM 1.4 years). All fulfilled the selection criteria, and in 5 the Giemsa stain result was positive, suggesting the presence of chlamydial inclusions.

Dropouts: There were no dropouts; all patients completed the trial.

Compliance: This was 100% as no patient defaulted.

Clinical Efficacy: As shown in Table 1, 19 patients (95%) showed a satisfactory clinical response, and one patient (5%) was a failure, his Giemsa stain test on urethral smear being positive on day 15. The symptomatic relief at successive follow-up visits is shown in Table 2. As can be seen, most of the symptoms were relieved in a majority of patients by day 8, while in a few they were relieved by day 14.

Table 1 Clinical Efficacy

Cure	17 (85 %)
Improvement	2 (10%)
Failure	1 (5%)
Total	20 (100%)

Table 2 Relief of Symptoms

Symptom	Day 1	Day 8	Day 15
Burning micturition	19	9	3
Urinary frequency	16	5	1
Purulent discharge	1	0	0
Mucoid discharge	19	2	2
Meatal erythema	1	1	0
Epididymitis	3	1	0
Orchitis	2	1	0
Prostatic tenderness	1	0	0
Inguinal lymph nodes +	3	1	0
Early morning gleet	10	4	1
Painful erection	5	0	0

Microscopically, only one patient who did not respond clinically showed > 5 PMNs/HPF on day 15. Of the 5 patients whose urethral smear was Giemsa-positive on day 1, 4 became negative by day 8 and remained so on day 15; one patient who failed clinically remained Giemsa-positive.

Side Effects: There were no side effects reported by any of the patients, so that tolerability was uniformly good. As shown in Table 3, there were also no adverse effects on serum chemistry variables pertaining to hepatic and renal function.

Table 3. Serum Chemistry

Test	Initial	Final
Hemoglobin, g/dl	14.0 ± 0.3	13.7 ± 0.3
Total WBC count/ul	6.7 ± 0.5	7.6 ± 0.4
ESR, mm at I h	6.5 ± 1.0	3.7 ± 0.6
Bilirubin, mg/dl	0.8 ± 0.1	0.7 ± 0.1
Alkaline Pbosphatase, U/ml	68.4 ± 4.3	71.4 ± 5.4
SGOT, U/ml	27.6 ± 1.8	25.4 ± 1.6
SGPT, U/ml	24.8 + 2.7	27.1 ± 2.4
BUN, mg/dl	11.0 ± 0.4	11.3 ± 0.5
Creatinine, mg/dl	1.0 ± 0.0	1.0 ± 0.1

Discussion

Our results show that a single, 1 g dose of azithromycin is highly effective for treating acute NGU in males and is very well tolerated. This efficacy of the drug, which has been shown to be comparable to the standard treatment with doxycycline (100 mg twice daily for 7 days), is due to its ability to provide sustained concentrations in urogenital tissues in excess of the MIC90, viz. 0.25 Mg/g> for *Chlamydia trachomatis*, the commonest cause of NGU. In this respect, azithromycin seems to fulfil Ehrlich's dream of a "magic bullet" for the treatment of a very common sexually transmitted infection.

Waugh (1993) has reported 93% cure rate in male and female patients with gonorrhea using the same dose of azithromycin, viz. 1 g once only, which is highly encouraging. Concomitant chlamydial infection was also cleared in 22 of his patients, indicating the value of this regimen in outdoor or supervised treatment of sexually transmitted urethritis.

In view of our own experience and the review of available literature, it can be said that azithromycin represents a landmark in the treatment of sexually transmitted infections due to Chlamydia trachomaris, Mycoplasma hominis, Ureaplasma urealyticum and Neisseria gonorrhoeae—all common causes of urethritis in males and cervicitis in females.

Acknowledgements

Capsules containing 250 mg of azithromycin as dihydrate (ZITHROMAX™) were supplied by Pfizer Ltd, Bombay, who also supported the study with a research grant.

References

1. Foulds G, Johnson RB. Selection of dose regimens of azithromycin. J Antimicrob Chemother 1993; 31(Suppl E):39-50.

2. Lister PJ, Balechandran T, Ridgway GL, et al. Comparison of azithromycin and doxycycline in the treatment of non-gonococcal urethritis in men. J Aruimicrob Chemother 1993; 31(Suppl E): 185-192.

3. MartinDH,MroczkowskiTF,DaluZA,et al. A controlledtrialof a single dose of azithromycin for

the treatment of chlamydiaJ urethritis and cervicitis. N Engl J Med 1992; 327(13):921-925.

4. Nilsen A, Halsos A, Johansen A, et al. A double blind study of single dose azithromycin and doxycycline in the treatment of chlamydial urethritis in males. Genitourin Med 1992; 68:325-327.

5. Ossewaarde JM, Plantema FHF, Rieffe M, et al. Efficacy of single-dose azithromycin versus doxycycline in the treatment of cervical infections caused by Chlamydia trachomatis. Eur J Microbiol Infect Dis 1992; 11 (8):693-697.

6. Peters DH, Friedel HA, McTavish D. Azithromycin: a review of its antimicrobial activity, pharmacokinetic properties and clinical efficacy. Drugs 1992; 44(5):750-799.

7. Waugh MA. Open study of the efficacy and safety of a single oral dose of azithromycin for the treatment of uncomplicated gonorrhoea in men and women. J Antimicrob Chemother 1993; 31(Suppl E): 193-198

Efficacy and safety assessment of a new Ayurvedic antifungal Herbal cream - A study conducted at the Jaslok Hospital & Research Centre

Ram Malkani

Presented Posterat the XXIVth National Conference held at Ahmedabad June 25-28 1996.

Reflections

Antifungal cream that too, an Ayurvedic cream, the idea then not appealing. In 2016 and 2017, now that fungous has become resistant, probably this Ayurvedic cream formula could bring relief to the harassed patients of Fungal infections and the beneficiary Pharma manufacturer along with the Dermatology community.

Merind India wished to introduce an Ayurvedic anti fungal cream. 25 cases were enrolled with clinically and mycologically conformed cases of fungal Infections of the skin, in men and women, above the age of 14. Ayurvedic cream was dispensed to them, which they applied sparingly judiciously to a selected areas only and were followed up every two weeks for 6 weeks. At the end of the trial the results showed that all of them had clinical and mycological cure.

Efficacy and Safety of Moxifloxacin (MXF) vs Cephalexin (with or without Metronidazole) in the Treatment of Mild to Moderate Uncomplicated Skin and Skin Structures Infections (USSSI)

P. Leal Del Rosal, Hosp. Clin. Del Parque, Chihuahua, Mexico;* G. Fabian, R. Vick-Fragoso, Hosp. Gral. Manuel Gea Gonzalez; R. Martinez Y Zamora, Hgz 27 Imss; Jj Morales-Reyes, Nuevo Hosp. Civil Guadalajara; A. Rodriguez, Hosp. Gral. Occidente, Guadalajara; R. Lang, Meir Hosp, Israel; R. Malkani, Jaslok Hosp., Mumbai, India; H. Silm, Tartu Univ. Hosp. Tartu, Estonia; G. Lapinskaite, National Clin, Of Dermatology And Venereology, Vilnius, Lithuania; S. Zabielski, Central Clin. Hosp., Warsaw, Poland, Gm Hernandez-Oliva; R. Vivar; A. Torres, Bayer De Mexico And The Usssi Study Group.

A phase III trial conducted at the Jaslok Hospital & Research Centre in 1997.

Background: Empirical therapy for the treatment of USSSI is currently used due to difficulties in diagnosis and isolation of organisms, (3-lactams are used as standard treatment, but selection of rapid resistance to them is becoming a problem worldwide. Moxifloxacin, has been assayed because its Minimum Inhibitory Concentrations (MIC) are adequate to the most common causative organisms of the uSSSI including anaerobes.

Methods: This was a prospective, multicenter, multinational, controlled, randomized, double-blind trial in adult out- and in-patients with mild to moderate acute uncomplicated skin and skin structure infections. The endpoint was to compare the clinical and microbiological efficacy, and safety of 5-14 days oral regimens of 400 mg MXF once daily vs 500 mg cephalexin three times daily (tid) (with or without metronidazole 400 mg tid) (control) was. Clinical outcome was evaluated in 385 patients (191 MXF, 194 control) of 468 patients randomized.

Results: Clinical resolution was achieved in 92.7% (177/191) MXF-patients and 92.8% (180/194) of controls (95% CI: -5.2%, 5.0%);212 patients (55.0%) were valid for microbiological.The bacteriological success rate was 89.0% (89/100) for MXF and 93.8% (105/112) for the control (95% CI: -12.1%, 3.0%). MXF showed slightly higher eradication rates than the control vs the predominant pathogen Staphylococcus aureus (91.7% MXF vs 89.3% control) and Streptococcus sp (100% MXF vs 94.4% control). Tolerability of both treatments was good with comparable incidences of drug-related adverse events.

Conclusion: MXF proved to be effective clinically and bacteriologically and also exhibited a good tolerability compared to standard therapy in the treatment of USSSI, providing the clinician and the patient, another alternative of treatment leading to reduced possibility of resistance.

BACKGROUND:

Because the skin is the major interface between humans and their environment, it is not surprising that bacterial, fungal and viral infections of the skin and skin structures (SSSI) are the most common human infections(1). The skin presents a barrier to the external environment and has specific antibacterial mechanisms. Absorption through normal skin does not occur.

To be effective, host defenses require the integrated and efficient function of the component parts. The failure of any segment of the system due to trauma, maceration from excesive moisture, or other factors can result in an infectious process. The inflammatory response is the basic delivery system. The classic signs of inflammation rubor pain, tumor, and calor can be explained by examining the vascular, cellular and molecular components of the response(2). The natural history of each infection can be conceptualized on an anatomic basis, that is on the basis of the body's attempt to localize infection to the original site or, if that is not possible, to confine the process regionally. When regionalization fails, invasion of the bloodstream takes place, and bacteremia must be controlled using all homeostatic mechanisms.

Although the normal resident flora can sometimes cause the ensuing infectious complications, especially cutaneous abscesses, organisms acquired from elsewhere are usually responsible, particularly Staphylococcus aureus, and Streptococcus pyogenes(3).

Appropriate antibiotic therapy for established infection, in conjunction with early diagnosis reduces the incidence of failure when treating either an uncomplicated or complicated SSSI. The major current classes of these antibacterial agents include penicillins; extended spectrum penicillin derivatives and beta-lactamase inhibitors; cephalosporins; clindamycin; carbapenems and more recently quinolones(4). However, S. aureus and streptococci have shown increasing resistance trends to beta-lactams and other antimicrobials, so newer quinolones, especially Moxifloxacin, a new 8-methoxy quinolone, are offering a therapeutic option with low-resistance development in addition to adequate pharmacokinetic parameters that allows once-daily dosage, good tissue concentration, broad spectrum including gram positive organism as well as anaerobes, and Minimum Inhibitory Concentrations (MIC) above the ones required to kill causative SSSI pathogens. As a result, Moxifloxacin has challenged traditional concepts of treatment of SSSI.

MATERIAL AND METHODS

- This was a multicenter, multinational, prospective parallel group, randomized, controlled, double blind study of patients with treatment of mild to moderate uncomplicated superficial skin structure infections.

- The study was carried out from April 1997 to May 1998 in 5 centers in Mexico, 7 in Israel, 3 in India, 1 in Estonia, 2 in Lithuania, and 2 in Poland.

• The total number of patients enrolled were 468. All patients were randomized to receive either Moxifloxacin (MXF) 400 mg bid (234 patients) or the comparator Cephalexin (CPH) with or without metronidazole (234 patients).

• Treatment duration was 5-14 days based on response and investigator's judgement. Blinding was maintained by the use of placebo capsules and/or placebo tablets to match metronidazole active in the Moxifloxacin group for the afternoon and evening doses.

Inclusion Criteria:

• Male or female patients 18 years old and above were enrolled as in or outpatients.

• Diagnosis of mild to moderate skin and soft tissues infection was based on two or more of the following signs symptoms within 24 hours before enrolment:

• Fever >38°C or chills

• Edema of the Skin/soft tissues

• Erythema of the skin/soft tissues

• Purulent exudate

• Local pain or tenderness

• Local hypertermia

Plan:

(V1) Within 24 hours prior to treatment initiation; (V2) 3-6 days after start of treatment; (V3) 48 hours after visit 2 with clinical and laboratory evaluation.

(V4) 1-7 days after the end of treatment; (V5) 8-21 days after the end of treatment with clinical and bacteriological evaluation. Laboratory evaluation was done if necessary.

Evaluation:

• Clinical resolution was defined as the reduction or disappearance of all signs and symptoms related to the infection 1-7 days after the end of treatment.

• The microbiological efficacy, catalogued like eradication, persistence, superinfectionand indeterminate, was assessed on the basis of the cultures taken before treatmentand in comparison to those taken at visits 2,3 and 4 if microbiological material was available. If no adequate material to culture was available, the evauation was stated as "presumed eradication" if the patient was judged to be clinically well.

• Safety was evaluated on the basis of clinical and laboratory adverse events (frequency, intensity and relation).

Results:

The total number of patients enrolled in the study was 468, being 451 valid for ITT analysis (ITT population) and 385 for efficacy analysis (PP population). The distribution within groups is shown in Table 1 below:

Table 1. Distribution of patients enrolled.

Treatment	Valid for ITT analysis	Valid for PP analysis
Moxifloxacin	227	191
Ceph ± met*	224	194
Total	451	385

Ceph + met = Cephalexin with or without Metronidazole

Demographic and baseline characteristics of patients in the ITT and PP populations were comparable in respect of age, body weight, sex, medical history, concomitant medication, concomitant diseases and nature of skin and soft tissues infection. (Table 2)

Table 2.Demographic and baseline data. PP population.

Variable		Moxifloxacin N = 191	Ceph ± met N = 194
Sex	Male	112 (58.6%)	111 (57.2%)
	Female	79 (41.4%)	83 (42.8%)
Age (years)	Mean ± SD	45.9 ±19.5	41.8 ±18.5
	Range	18-93	18-94
Weight (kg)	Mean ± SD	73.2 ±16.2	69.9 ±17.1
	Range	41-135	40-150
Race	Caucasian	76 (39.8%)	69 (35.6%)
	Oriental	34 (17.8%)	38 (19.6%)
	Hispanic	1 (0.5%)	1 (0.5%)
	Other	80 (41.9%)	86 (44.3%)
Time since SSTI onset[a]	< 7 dayss	106 (55.5%)	117 (60.3%)
	8-14 day	55 (28.8%)	39 (20.1%)
	> 14 days	30 (15.7%)	38 (19.6%)
Hospitalised before therapy	No	160 (83.8%)	167 (86.1%)
	Yes	31 (16.2%)	27 (13.9%)

a) Refers topresent episodeonly

The great majority of patients suffering from a spontaneous infection experienced this in connection with cellulitis. (Table 3).

Table 3. Source of infection, PP population.

Source	Moxifloxacin N = 191	Ceph +_met N= 194
Hospital-acquired	20(10.5%)	14(7.2%)
Spontaneous	133(69.6%)	144(74.2%)
Wound	46(24.1%)	43(22.2%)
Ulcer	12(6.3%)	7(3.6%)

Clinical signs and symptoms of SSTI were analyzed and compared at the entry, end of therapy (EOT) and follow-up (FU). A marked reduction in severity of the signs and symptoms is shown for both groups at the EOT and FU in Table 4 below:

Table 4. Clinical signs and symptoms at end of therapy and at follow-up. PP population

Sign / symptom	Severity	Moxifloxacin N = 191			Ceph ± met N = 194		
		Entry	EOT	F-U	Entry	EOT	F-U
Erythema of skin/soft tissue	Moderate	113	5	1	108	2	1
	Severe	51	-	-	62	-	-
Oedema of skin/soft tissue	Moderate	97	5	1	92	4	4
	Severe	44	-	2	53	1	1
Local pain/tenderness	Moderate	91	4	3	96	1	2
	Severe	50	-	-	49	-	-
Local hyperthermia	Moderate	87	1	-	98	-	-
	Severe	25	-	-	28	-	-
	Moderate				"67		
Purulent exudate	Moderate	55	1	1	67	-	1
	Severe	20	-	-	21 13	-	-
ills	Moderate	13	1	-	13	-	1
	Severe	4	-	-	9	-	-
	Moderate	22	2	2	22	3	2
	Severe	9	-	-	14	-	_

y of the most common causative organisms is
le 5. In the Moxifloxacin group, 107 out of 191
patients gave identified causative organisms,
cephalexin/metronidazole group, 119/194
did so

Table 5.More common causative organisms

	Moxifloxacin N = 107		Ceph ± met N = 119	
	n	%	n	%
Number of causative organisms Identity of causative organism				
One organism identified	76	71.0	78	65.5
Two organisms identified	27	25.2	39	32.8
Three organisms identified	4	3.7	2	1.7
Total (any causative organism identified)	107	100.0	119	100.0
Any Gram-positive organism	98	91.6	112	94.1
Staphylococcus aureus	76	68.2	78	65.5
Staphylococcus epidermidis	6	5.6	5	4.2
Streptococcus sp.	14	13.1	21	17.6
Streptococcus pyogenes	6	5.6	13	10.9
Streptococcus agalactiae	5	4.7	4	3.4
Enterococcus faecalis	3	2.8	4	3.4
Staphylococcus haemolyticus	1	0.9	4	3.4
Any Gram-negative organism	19	17.8	19	16.0
Escherichia coli	3	2.8	7	5.9
Pseudomonas aeruginosa	3	2.8	5	4.2
Klebsiella pneumoniae	5	4.7	1	0.8

Numbers of patients with the respective number or identity of causative organisms are shown. The total number in each group is the number of patients with identified causative organisms at enrolment, and the percentages are calculated with respect to these.

The most numerous organisms isolated were Staphylococcus aureus and Streptococcus sp. and Streptococcus pyogenes. The MIC values obtained for these species from patients entering the studies are summarized in Table 6 below.

Table 6. Median MIC values and ranges for susceptibility testing with Moxifloxacin. PP population.

| | Moxifloxacin group | | | Ceph ± metgroup | |
	N	Median	Range	N	Me
Staphylococcus aureus	51	0.064	0.002-0.50	55	0.0(
Streptococcus sp.	11	0.250	0.032-0.50	15	0.5(
Streptococcus pyogenes	6	0.125	0.125-0.25	12	0.1:

Units: mg/L

The clinical response at the end of therapy was the primary endpoint of the study, and a secondary endpoint was the clinical response at FU. Results are given in Table 7. The measures of clinical response were: (1) 'resolution versus, failure' at the EOT visit; (2) for patients with resolution at EOT, continued resolution 'versus recurrence/ relapse' at the FU visit; and (3) for patients valid for the

combined EOT and FU analysis, 'continued resolution versus failure plus recurrence/relapse' at the FU visit
Table 7.

Time of assessment	Comparison (measure of clinical success)	Success rate		Estimated difference	95% Cl for difference
		Moxifloxacin	Ceph ± met		
a) EOT	'Resolution' versus 'failure'	92.7%	92.8%	-0.1%	(-5.2,5.0)*
b) Follow-up	'Continued resolution' versus 'recurrence/ relapse'	99.4%	98.2%	1.2%	(-1.1,3.5)*
c) EOT and follow-up combined	'Continued resolution' versus 'failure plus recurrence/ relapse'	91.8%	91.0%	0.8%	(-4.9,6.5)*

a. Population: all efficacy-evaluable (PP) patients; success-rate quotients are 177/191 and 180/194, respectively.

b. Population: all PP patients who showed resolution at end of therapy; respective quotients are 162/163 and 164/167.

c. Population: all PP patients valid for combined EOT and follow-up analysis; quotients are 167/182 and 171/188.

Table 8. Eradication rates for the most frequent organisms. PP population.

Causative organism	Treatment group	Eradication and presumed eradication vs. superinfection + persistence + non-reported + indeterminate (EOT)	Eradication and presumed eradication vs. superinfection + persistence (EOT)
Staphylococcus aureus	Moxifloxacin	55/76 (72.4%)	55/60 (91.7%)
	Ceph ± met	50/78 (64.1%)	50/56 (89.3%)
Streptococcus sp.	Moxifloxacin	14/14 (100.0%)	14/14 (100.0%)
	Ceph ± met	17/21 (81.0%)	17/18 (94.4%)
Streptococcus *pyogenes*	Moxifloxacin	0/6 (0.0%)	0/1 (0.0%)
	Ceph ± met	2/13 (15.4%)	2/2 (100.0%)

The eradication rates in the two treatment groups at EOT are shown in Table 8 above. Gram-positive organisms, as expected, were the most common infecting causative organisms of the superficial skin and skin structure infections. Among them, Staphylococcus aureus was the most common, with a total of 210 isolates. The percentage of eradication at EOT was slightly higher in the MXF group, except Streptococcus pyogenes. The number of *Streptococcus pyogenes* isolates was too small to draw valid conclusions.

Table 9. Incidence rates of AEs* by body system.

	Moxifloxacin N = 227 n(%)		Ceph ± met N = 224 n(%)	
Any body system	112	49.3	102	45.5
Body as a whole	53	23.3	40	17.9
Cardiovascular	20	8.8	18	8.0
Digestive	58	25.6	41	18.3
Haemic and lymphatic	12	5.3	9	4.0
Metabolic and nutrition	8	3.5	9	4.0
Musculoskeletal	7	3.1	6	2.7
Nervous	14	6.2	19	8.5
Respiratory	3	1.3	1	0.4
Skin and appendages	20	8.8	14	6.3
Special senses	1	0.4	2	0.9
Urogenital	9	4.0	9	4.0

Table 10.Incidence rates of AEs occurring in at least 2% of either treatment group.

	BAY 12-8039 N = 227 n%	Ceph ± met N = 224 n %
Any event ..	112 49.3	102 45.5
Nausea	29 12.8	10 4.5
Diarrhoea	15 6.6	8 3.6
Liver function tests abnormal	9 4.0	9 4.0
Infection	9 4.0	7 3.1
Rash	8 3.5	8 3.6
Headache	8 3.5	7 3.1
Asthenia	7 3.1	8 3.6
Dyspepsia Hypertension	9 4.0 6 2.6	5 2.2 7 3.1
Dizziness	5 2.2	7 3.1
Hypotension Pain	5 2.2 6 2.6	6 2.7 4 1.8
Somnolence	3 1.3	7 3.1
Urinary tract infection Diabetes mellitus	2 0.9 5 2.2	7 3.1 4 1.8
Edema	6 2.6	2 0.9
Vomiting	5 2.2	- 0.0

*AEs: Adverse Events

The incidence of AEs was rather greater in the MXF group (49.3%, compared with 45.5% in the ceph/met group). This was particularly clear for the systems 'body as a whole' and 'digestive' (Table 9). Other differences for body systems were small, and no other general trend was observed.

The types of AE with a conspicuously higher incidence in the BAY 12-8039 group were nausea, diarrhoea and dyspepsia (Table 10). The numbers of patients with abnormal results in liver function tests were the same in the two groups. The incidence of somnolence was slightly higher in the ceph/met group.

CONCLUSIONS

1. The demographic and baseline characteristics of patients in the treatment groups were comparable in respect of age, body weight, sex and concomitant diseases for both ITT and PP populations.

2. The clinical results showed that Moxifloxacin 400 mg od is at least as effective as Cephalex in with or without metronidazole 500 mg tid.

3. MIC for the three major pathogens isolated are better than the comparator and above the required to kill the organisms.

4. The bacteriological response demostrated that both treatment groups are equivalent in eradication and presumed eradication.

5. The overall incidence rates of adverse events was very similar between both treatment groups, apart from the digestive system, where Moxifloxacin had a rather higher rate. There were

more serious adverse events in the Moxifloxacin groups, (16 vs 6 in the comparator group) but the majority of these were not related to the study drug. Thus, both treatment groups were equivalent in safety and tolerability,

6.   Moxifloxacin, a novel 8-methoxi-fluoroquinolone becomes a new therapeutic option because of the once a day administration, MIC above those required to kill current pathogens causing superficial skin and soft tissues infections, possibility to develop lower levels of selection of resistance, and with a good safety profile.

REFERENCES:

1. Feingold DS, Hirschmann JV, Approach to the patient with skin ans soft tissue infection. In Gorbach SL, Bartlett JG, Blacklow NR editors: Infectious Diseases. W.B. Saunders. Philadelphia, 1998: 1262-3.

2. Meakins JL: Barriers to infection. In Howard RJ, Simmons RL editors: Surgical Infectious Diseases. Appleton and Lange, Connecticut, 1995: 237-40.

3. Hirschmann JV, Feingold DS: Staphylococcal and streptococcal skin or soft tissues infections. In Gorbach SL, Bartlett JG, Blacklow NR editors:

Infectious Diseases.W.B. Saunders. Philadelphia,
1998: 1265-6.

4. Solomkin JS, Howard RJ: Antimicrobial
agents. In Howard RJ, Simmons RL
editors:Surgical Infectious Diseases. Appleton
and Lange, Connecticut, 1995: 533-40.

Evaluation of clinical efficacy and tolerance of Tazarotene 0.05% gel in the treatment of Acne vulgaris & Psoriasis-March 2003 to June 2003.

Belinda Vaz, Ram Malkani

INTRODUCTION

Acne Vulgaris is usually a self limiting disorder of teenagers and young adults. The permissive factor for the expression of the disease is the increase in sebum release by sebaceous glands after puberty. Small cysts, called comedones are formed in hair follicles due to blockage of the follicular orifice by retention of sebum and keratinous material. The lipophillic yeast and bacteria within the comedones release free fatty acids from sebum, which causes inflammation within the cyst and results in rupture of cyst wall. An inflammatory reaction develops as a result of extrusion of oily and keratinous debris from the cyst.

Tazarotene is a retinoid prodrug which is converted to its active form tazarotenic acid by rapid deesterification in humans. Tazarotenic acid binds to and regulates gene expression through retinoid nuclear receptors.

Tazarotene has been shown to exert its multiprongal effect on gene expression, cell differentiation and inflammation, thereby alleviating the symptoms of acne vulgaris. Its efficacy and safety in the treatment of acne vuigaris has been reported in well controlled clinical trials conducted abroad.

The present study was planned to evaluate the clinical efficacy and tolerance of Tazarotene 0.05% gel in Indian patients of acne vulgaris.

METHODS

The study protocol was approved by the Drugs Controller General of India.

Fifteen patients of acne vulgaris, satisfying the inclusion and exclusion criteria set out in the protocol were enrolled. The informed written consent was obtained from each of them prior to the inclusion in the study. The general demography of the patients was recorded.

The history of acne vulgaris along with the treatment taken in past was noted. The family history of skin disorders, information on associated illnesses. if any and ongoing treatment for the same were also recorded.

The baseline efficacy parameters of acne vulgaris were evaluated.

All the 15 patients satisfied the inclusion/exclusion criteria and each of them was given 1 tube of 30 gms tazarotene 0.05% gel. The patients were advised to apply the gel over the affected areas, once a day and the method of application was demonstrated to them.

Patients were followed up on week 4, week 8 and week 12. During each follow up visit, efficacy and overall clinical severity parameters as well as global response to treatment and treatment success rate were evaluated. Cosmetic acceptability and global tolerance and acceptability were assessed at the end of week 12.

In the event when the follow up was missed, the patients were contacted telephonically and were pursued to visit the clinic for follow up.

Patients were interviewed for possible adverse events during each follow up visit. The detailedinformation of the adverse event along with details of follow up of the event, rescue medication given and outcome were recorded in case report form.

The data base was created in MS Excel programme and the data was statistically evaluated using appropriate test. Unpaired Student's 't' test was applied for objective parameters such as inflammatory, non inflammatory and total lesion count and Chi square test was applied for overall clinical severity grade.

The tolerance was evaluated on the basis of investigator's assessment of tolerance and patients rating of acceptability and also in terms of percent incidence of adverse events.

RESULTS

Out of total 15 patients enrolled, 2 patients were dropped out due to lost to follow up. Thirteen patients, 8 males and 5 females completed the study.

The baseline data of the patients is presented in table 1.

TABLE 1: BASELINE DATA

No. of patients   15
No. Of patients completing the study 13
Sex M: F ratio   8:5
Age range   6 - 38
Mean Age (Years)   22.30±1.65
Mean weight (Kg)   50.83±1.98
Mean Height (Cms)   161 .O4±2.27

The patients were between 16 and 38 years of age. The mean weight of the patients was 50.83±1.98 kgs and height was 161.04±2.27 cms.

Twelve patients were newly diagnosed patients of acne vulgaris. One patient (Patient No. 14) was known patient of acne and had used Erythromycin topically around 6 months before the Enrollment in the study.

Five patients were taking concomitant treatment for the: associated diseases at the time of enrollment. One patient (Patient No. 6) had mild psoriasis vulgaris, one patient (Patient N0. 8) had T. corporis infection, two patients (Patient Nos. 9 and 11) were suffering from acidity and one had dryness of skin and lips (Patient No. 12).

The associated medical conditions and concomitant medicines taken for these conditions, have been listed in table 2.

TABLE 2: ASSOCIATED MEDICAL CONDITIONS AND THERAPY

Associated Medical Condition	No. of Patients
Psoriasis Vulgaris	1
T corporis	L
Acidity	2
Dryness of skin and lips	1

No. of patients	Concomitant Therapy
1	Keratolytic treatment
1	Greisofulvin
	Hydroxyzine
	Clotrimazole
1	Ranitidine
	Digene
1	Omeprazole
1	Vaseline

All the medications were continued during the study.

The effect of Tazarotene 0.05% gel on inflammatory, non inflammatory and total lesion count is shown in table 3.

TABLE 3: EFFECT OF TAZAROTENE GEL ON LESION COUNT

Parameters	Day 0	Week4	Week8	Week12
No. of patients (n)	13	13	l3	13
		*	**	**
Inflammatory Lesion Count	17.26 ±2.98	7.30 ±2.25	7.18 ±2.41	5.15 ±1.26
		***	***	***
Non Inflammatory Lesion Count	80.26 ±12.69	44.69 ±12.07	37.72 ±10.58	17.92 ±5.38
		***	***	***
Total Lesion Count	97.53 ±13.11	52.00 ±13.53	44.90 ±10.62	23.07 ±5.97

* $p<0.05$, ** $p<0.01$, *** $p<0.001$

There was a significant decrease in lesion count, both inflammatory as well as non inflammatory, following treatment with Tazarotene 0.05% gel.

On week 0, the mean inflammatory lesion count was 17.26±2.98 whereas non inflammatory lesion count was 80.26±12.69.The mean inflammatory lesion count decreased significantly to 7.30±2.25, 7.18±2.4 and 5.15±1.26 on week 4, week 8 and week 12 respectively. Similar trend was seen also in non inflammatory lesion count .The mean total lesion count, which was 97.53±13.11 before initiation of the treatment, decreased to 23.07±5.97 ($p<0.001$) on week 12. The mean reduction in total lesion count on week 12 was whopping 76.34% on week 12 as compared to that at the initiation of the treatment.

The assessment of overall clinical severity grade of the lesions also showed Significant decrease from 1.46 ± 0.13 at the baseline to 1.07 ± 0.07, 1.09 ± 0.09 and 0.84 ± 0.10 on week 4, week 8 and week 12 respectively.

All the patients responded very well to Tazarotene therapy. At the end of 12 weeks of treatment, 7 patients showed excellent response with 75 to 99% improvement, 5 patients showed good response with 50 to 74% improvement, whereas one patient showed fair response with 25 to 49% improvement in the lesional severity.

Two patients reported adverse events, which were resolved without any treatment. One patient (Patient No. 3) reported burning sensation of skin of moderate intensity 7 weeks after initiation of the treatment . The event was related to the trial drug and was subsided within 2-3 days. One Patients (Patients no.11) experienced redness, burning and stinging sensation of the skin after 3weeks of the treatment. The symptoms lasted for 1 week and subsided spontaneously. The overall tolerance to Tazarotene was found to be excellent.

The cosmetic acceptability was observed to be favorable in as many as 10 patients, whereas 2 patients reported it to be neutral. Only one patient felt the cosmetic acceptability to be unfavorable.

The patients compliance to the treatment was also found to be good.

CONCLUSION

Tazarotene 0.05% gel was found to be effective in decreasing the intensity of lesions of acne vulgaris in all the 13 patients completing the study. The reduction in inflammatory as well as non inflammatory lesion count was highly significant.

The beneficial effect of Tazarotene was also reflected in clinical severity grade of the lesions as well as in overall response to treatment.

In our study, Tazarotene displayed excellent clinical tolerability and acceptability. Two patients reported adverse events viz. redness. burning and stinging, which were of moderate severity and were resolved spontaneously.

Tazarotene seems to be effective in the treatment of mild to moderate acne vulgaris and has good tolerability profile

Evaluation of azithromycin in the treatment of acute pyogenic skin infections

(Protocol AZM-II-92-002C)

Ram H. Malkani, MD, DVD, DDV

Consultant Dermatologist Jaslok Hospital and Research Center G. Deshmukh Marg Bombay 400026

Azithromycin (ZITHROMAXT) in Pyoderma R.H. Malkani

Summary

Azithromycin (ZITHROMAX,I* Pfizer) was used in a dose of 500 mg once daily, orally, for 3 days to treat 20 adult patients (14 M, 6 F) with acute pyogenic skin infections after obtaining their written informed consent. Diagnosis was made from symptoms, signs, and Gram's stain of the discharge when available. The patients were seen on days 1, 4, 7 and, if necessary, on day 14 to record their symptoms and signs, side effects if any, and compliance with the treatment by capsule count. WBC count and serum chemistry were done initially and at the end of trial. The patients' mean age was 33 years (range 15-55 years). The diagnoses included: folliculitis, 6; ecthyma, 2; infected eczema, 6; impetigo, 5; and infected scabies, 1. All 20 patients completed the trial. Of the 20 patients, 19 had Gram (+) organisms and one had Gram(-) organism in the smear; 8 of the Gram(+) organisms were identified as coagulase-positive Staphylococcus aureus. Clinically, all 20 patients (100%) were cured. None of the patients had any side effects. Serum chemistry did not show any abnormalities. Thus, Azithromycin was found to be highly effective, well tolerated, and convenient for treating acute pyogenic infections of skin and skin structures.

Introduction

Azithromycin, an azalide antibiotic resembling macrolides, is highly active against many Gram(+) and Gram(-) organisms, both aerobic and anaerobic (Peters et al, 1992). Its pharmacokinetic features of special interest are (i) a long half-life of about 50 hours, which makes once-daily dosage possible, and (ii) its propensity to be concentrated in tissues cells rather than serum and be released slowly, which permits a short, 3-day regimen with a longer in vivo availability for continued action (Lode, 1991). In a dose of 500 mg once daily for 3 days, it has been reported to he highly effective in pyogenic skin infections (Amaya-Tapia et al, 1993). This study was undertaken to verify the efficacy and tolerability of this regimen in our patients.

Patients and Methods

Selection Criteria: Adult patients, aged 18-60 years, with acute pyogenic skin infection were selected if they gave written consent to participate in the study after being explained its nature and purpose. Diagnosis of a skin infection needing antibiotic treatment was established from symptoms, signs, and appropriate investigations such as WBC count and Gram's stain smear of any exudate if available.

Exclusion Criteria: Patients were excluded if (i) they had known allergy to macrolides, hepatic or renal impairment, malabsorption, history of antibiotic treatment during previous 3 days, or participation in another study during the previous month; (ii) they needed concomitant treatment with ergotamine, carbamazepine or digoxin; (iii) they were pregnant females; or (iv) had donated blood during the previous 2 weeks.

Dosage Regimen: Azithromycin was used as 250 mg capsules (ZITHROMAX, - Pfizer). The dose was 2 capsules once daily for 3 days. Patients were instructed to take the capsules either 1 hour before a meal or 2. hours after a meal. The first dose was administered under observation if these conditions were satisfied. Compliance was checked by asking patients to bring the containers during follow-up visits and inspecting them. No other antibiotic was allowed concomitantly. Vitamin capsules (BECOSULES, - Pfizer) were given from day 4 onwards, one daily, as incentive for follow-up.

Observations: Each patient was seen at least 3 times, on days 1, 4 and 7, and if necessary a fourth time, on day 14, for proper assessment of response. Symptoms and signs were recorded on days 1, 4 and 7/14; investigations for diagnosis and response (Gram staining) and for safety (serum chemistry) were done on day 1 and 7/14. At each visit, inquiry was made about side effects or any concomitant illness using an open-ended question.

Assessment: First, none valuable patients, if any, were segregated into dropouts and exclusions, with cause for it as far as it could be determined. Each evaluable patient's response was classified as: cure, if the symptoms and signs were completely or almost completely relieved and investigations, if abnormal initially, had returned to normal; improvement, if the symptoms and signs were markedly relieved, investigations showed normalcy or near-normalcy, and no further treatment was needed; failure, if there was no change in or worsening of clinical condition, requiring change of treatment; relapse, if there was improvement on day 4/7 with worsening on day 7/14, requiring change of treatment.

Results

Patients: Of the 20 patients enrolled, 14 were males and 6 were females, with a mean age of 33 years (range 15-55 years, SEM 2.4 years). Their distribution by diagnoses, which included a variety of conditions, is shown in Table 1. Microscopic examination of pus or discharge was done in all 20 patients: 19 (95%) had Gram(+) organisms and 1 (5%) had Gram(-) organisms. Of the Gram(+) organisms, 8 were coagulase-positive Staphylococcus aureus.

Dropouts: There were no dropouts; all patients completed the trial.

Compliance: All 20 patients completed the 3-day treatment as prescribed, and thus compliance was 100%.

Table 1. Diagnoses of Patients

Folliculitis	6 (30%)
Ecthyma	2 (10%)
Infected eczema	6 (30%)
Impetigo	5 (25%)
Infected scabies	1 (5%)
Total	20 (100%)

Table 2. Clinical Efficacy

Cure 20 (100%)

Total 20 (100%)

Clinical Efficacy: As shown in Table 2, all 20 patients (100%) were clinically cured. The symptomatic relief at successive follow-up visits is shown in Table 3. As can be seen, most

of the symptoms were relieved in a majority of patients between day 4 and day 7, while in a few they were relieved by day 14.

Bacteriologic Efficacy: Gram's stain was negative in all 20 patients at the end of treatment, suggesting elimination of the initial organism, which was Staphylococcus aureus in 19 of the patients.

Table 3. Relief of Symptoms

Symptom	Day 1	Day 4	Day 7	Day 14
Itching	15	11	3	1
Fever	3	0	0	0
Purulent discharge	18	2	0	0
Pain	15	3	0	0
Crust formation	14	11	1	0
Papules 8	2	0	0	
Vesicles	5	1	0	0
Pustules	2010 0	0		
Scaling	1 1 0	0		
Pigmentation	4	4	3	2
Erythema	17	6	0	0
Edema	16	3	0	0
Regional lymph	3	1	0	0

(Figures are numbers of patients with symptoms on that day)

Table 4: Serum chemistry

Test	Initial	Final
Total WBC count/μl	7.1 + 0.3	7.0 + 0.3
Bilirubin, mg/dl	0.6 + 0.0	0.6 + 0.0
Alkaline Phosphatase, U/mi	67.8 + 3.7	66.5 + 3.4
SGOT, U/ml	24.0 + 1.1	24.0 + 1.0
BUN, mg/dl	12.2 + 0.8	12.0 + 0.8
Creatinine, mg/dl	0.8 + 0.0	0.8 ± 0.0

Side Effects: There were no side effects reported by any of the patients, so that tolerability was uniformly good. As shown in Table 4, there were also no adverse effects on serum chemistry variables pertaining to hepatic and renal function.

Discussion

For treating pyogenic skin infections in adults, azithromycin has been used in a total dose of 1.5 g given once daily over either 5 days (Peters et al, 1992) or 3 days (Amaya-Tapia et al, 1993) giving comparable success rates. We chose to study the shorter, 3-day regimen because of its convenience and found it to be clinically successful (Table 2) in 100% of patients with commensurate relief of symptoms (Table 3). It was also well tolerated, both in terms of subjective complaints and in terms of biochemical parameters of hepatic and renal function as reflected in serum chemistry (Table 4).

The efficacy of a short, 3-day regimen of azithromycin (500 mg daily for 3 days) in pyogenic skin infections seems to be due as much to its activity against the causal pathogens, especially Staphylococcus aureus, as due to its ability to get concentrated almost 300-fold inside phagocytic cells and fibroblasts (Panteix et al, 1993). Consequently, although drug administration is over in 3 days, the antibiotic resides in the tissues at the site of infection much longer to provide the necessary activity where it is needed. For these reasons, azithromycin seems to offer a definite advantage over other antibiotics that need to be given 2-4 times daily for 7-10 days. Treatment with it may not only ensure compliance by outpatients, but also enable early discharge of indoor patients as soon as their condition improves and treatment is completed.

Acknowledgements

Capsules containing 250 mg of azithromycin as dihydrate (ZITHROMAXTh) were supplied by Pfizer Ltd, Bombay, who also supported the study with a research grant.

References

1. Amaya-Tapia G, Aguirre-Avalos G, Andrade-Villanueva J, et al. Once daily azithromycin in the treatment of adult skin and skin-structure infections. J Antimicrob Chemother 1993; 31(Suppl E):129-135.
2. Lode H. The pharmacokinetics of azithromycin and their clinical significance. Eur J Clin Microhiol Infect Dis 1991; 10(10):807-812.
3. Panteix G, Guillaumond B, Harf R, et al. In-vitro concentration of azithromycin in human phagocytic cells. J Antimicrob Chemother 1993; 31(Suppl E): 1-4.
4. Peters DH, Friedel HA, McTavish D. Azithromycin: a review of its antimicrobial activity, pharmacokinetic properties and clinical efficacy. Drugs 1992; 44(5):750-799:

International Publications

Evaluation of Azithromycin / Zithromax for the treatment of skin infections

Ram H. Malkani, Vijay Aswani

At the International Congress for Infectious Diseases held at Prague, Czech Republic, 1994 July

Azithromycin, an azalide antibiotic resembling macrolides, is highly active against many Gram(+) and Gram(-) organisms, both aerobic and anaerobic (Peters et al, 1992). Its pharmacokinetic features of special interest are (i) a long half-life of about 50 hours, which makes once-daily dosage possible, and (ii) its propensity to be concentrated in tissues cells rather than serum and be released slowly, which permits a short, 3-day regimen with a longer in vivo availability for continued action (Lode, 1991). In a dose of 500 mg once daily for 3 days, it has been reported to be highly effective in pyogenic skin infections (Amaya-Tapia et al, 1993). This study was undertaken to verify the efficacy and tolerability of this regimen in our patients.

Patients and Methods

Selection Criteria: Adult patients, aged 18-60 years, with acute pyogenic skin infection were selected if they gave written consent to participate in the study after being explained its nature and purpose. Diagnosis of a skin infection needing antibiotic treatment was established from symptoms, signs, and appropriate investigations such as WBC count and Gram's stain, smear of any exudate if available.

Exclusion Criteria: Patients were excluded if (i) they had known allergy to macrolides, hepatic or renal impairment, malabsorption, history of antibiotic treatment during previous 3 days, or participation in another study during the previous month; (ii) they needed concomitant treatment with ergotamine, carbamazepine or digoxin; (iii) they were pregnant females; or (iv) had donated blood during the previous 2 weeks.

Dosage Regimen: Azithromycin was used as 250 mg capsules (ZITHROMAX,™ Pfizer). The dose was 2 capsules once daily for 3 days. Patients were instructed to take the capsules either 1 hour before a meal or 2 hours after a meal. The first dose was administered under observation if these conditions were satisfied. Compliance was checked by asking patients to bring the containers during follow-up visits and inspecting them. No other antibiotic was allowed concomitantly. Vitamin capsules (BECOSULES,™ Pfizer) were given from day 4 onwards, one daily, as incentive for follow-up.

Observations: Each patient was seen at least 3 times, on days 1, 4 and 7, and if necessary a fourth time, on day 14, for proper assessment of response. Symptoms and signs were recorded on days 1, 4 and 7/14; investigations for diagnosis and response (Gram staining) and for safety (serum chemistry) were done on day 1 and 7/14. At each visit, inquiry was made about side effects or any concomitant illness using an open-ended question.

Assessment: First, nonevaluable patients, if any, were segregated into dropou s and exclusions, with cause for it as far as it could be determined. Each evaluable patient's response was classified as: cure, if the symptoms and signs were completely or almost completely relieved and investigations, if abnormal initially, had returned to normal: improvement, if the symptoms and signs were markedly relieved, investigations showed normalcy or near-normalcy, and no further treatment was needed; failure, if there was no change in or worsening of clinical condition, requiring change of treatment; relapse, if there was improvement on day 4/7 with worsening on day 7/14, requiring change of treatment.

Results

Patients: Of the 20 patients enrolled, 14 were males and 6 were females, with a mean age of 33 years (range 15-55 years, SEM 2.4 years). Their distribution by diagnoses, which included a variety of conditions, is shown in Table 1. Microscopic examination of pus or discharge was done in all 20 patients: 19 (95%) had Gram(+) organisms and 1 (5%) had Gram(-) organisms. Of the Gram(+) organisms, 8 were coagulase-positive *Staphylococcus aureus*.

Table 1. Diagnoses of Patients

Folliculitis	6 (30%)
Ecthyma	2 (10%)
Infected eczema	6 (30%)
Impetigo	5 (25%)
Infected scabies	1 (5%)
Total	20 (100%)

Dropouts: There were no dropouts; all patients completed the trial.

Compliance: All 20 patients completed the 3-day treatment as prescribed, and thus compliance was 100%.

Clinical Efficacy: As shown in Table 2, all 20 patients (100%) were clinically cured. The symptomatic relief at successive follow-up visits is shown in Table 3. As can be seen, most of the symptoms were relieved in a majority of patients between day 4 and day 7, while in a few they were relieved by day 14.

Bacteriologic Efficacy: Gram's stain was negative in all 20 patients at the end of treatment, suggesting elimination of the initial organism, which was *Staphylococcus aureus* in 19 of the patients.

Side Effects: There were no side effects reported by any of the patients, so that tolerability was uniformly good. As shown in Table 4, there were also no adverse effects on serum chemistry variables pertaining to hepatic and renal function.

Discussion

For treating pyogenic skin infections in adults, azithromycin has been used in a total dose of 1.5 g given once daily over either 5 days (Peters et al, 1992) or 3 days (Amaya-Tapia et al, 1993) giving comparable success rates. We chose to study the shorter, 3-day regimen because of its convenience and found it to be clinically successful (Table 2) in 100% of patients with commensurate relief of symptoms (Table 3). It was also well tolerated, both in terms of subjective complaints and in terms of biochemical parameters of hepatic and renal function as reflected in serum chemistry (Table 4).

Table 2. Clinical Efficacy

Cure   20 (100%)
Total   20 (100%)

Table 3. Relief of Symptoms

Symptom	Day 1	Day 4	Day 7	Day 14
Itching	15	11	3	1
Fever	3	0	0	0
Purulent discharge	18	2	0	0
Pain	15	3	0	0
Crust formation	14	11	1	0
Papules	8	2	0	0
Vesicles	5	1	0	0
Pustules	20	10	0	0
Scaling	1	1	0	0
Pigmentation	4	4	3	2
Erythema	17	6	0	0
Edema	16	3	0	0
Regional lymph nodes	3	1	0	0

(Figures are numbers of patients with symptoms on that day.)

Table 4. Serum Chemistry

Test	Initial	Final
Total WBC count/^{1}	7.1 ± 0.3	7.0 ± 0.3
Bilirubin, mg/dl	0.6 ± 0.0	0.6 ± 0.0
Alkaline Phosphatase, U/ml	67.8 ± 3.7	66.5 ± 3.4
SCOT, U/ml	24.0 ± 1.1	24.0 ± 1.0
BUN, mg/dl	12.2 ± 0.8	12.0 ± 0.8
Creatinine, mg/dl	0.8 ± 0.0	0.8 ± 0.0

The efficacy of a short, 3-day regimen of azithromycin (500 mg daily for 3 days) in pyogenic skin infections seems to be due as much to its activity against the causal pathogens, especially Staphylococcus aureus, as due to its ability to get concentrated almost 300-fold inside phagocytic cells and fibroblasts (Panteix et al, 1993). Consequently, although drug administration is over in 3 days, the antibiotic resides in the tissues at the site of infection much longer to provide the necessary activity where it is needed. For these reasons, azithromycin seems to offer a definite advantage over other antibiotics that need to be given 2-4 times daily for 7-10 days. Treatment with it may not only ensure compliance by outpatients, but also enable early discharge of indoor patients as soon as their condition improves andtreatment is completed.

Conclusions

Azithromycin (ZITHROMAX,™ Pfizer) was used in a dose of 500 mg once daily, orally, for 3 days to treat 20 adult patients (14 M, 6 F) with acute pyogenic skin infections after obtaining their written informed consent. The diagnoses included: folliculitis, 6; ecthyma, 2; infected eczema, 6; impetigo, 5; and infected scabies, 1. Clinically, all 20 patients (100%) were cured. None of the patients had any side effects. Serum chemistry did not show any abnormalities. Thus, azithromycin was found to be highly effective, well tolerated, and convenient for treating acute pyogenic infections of skin and skin structures.

References

1. Amaya-Tapia G, Aguirre-Avalos G, Andrade-Villanueva J, et al. Once daily azithromycin in the treatment of adult skin and skin-structure infections. J Amimicrob Chemother 1993;31(Suppl E): 129-135.

2. Lode H. The pharmacokinetics of azithromycin and their clinical significance. Eur J Clin Microbiol Infect Dis 1991; 10(10):807-812.

3. Panteix G, Guillaumond B, Harf R, et al. In-vitro concentration ofazithromycin in human phagocytic cells. J Amimicrob Chemother 1993; 31(Suppl E):1-4.

4. Peters DH, Friedel HA, McTavish D. Azithromycin: a review of its antimicrobial activity, pharmacokinetic properties and clinical efficacy. Drugs 1992; 44(5):750-799.

Anonymous Counselling & Testing Centre, Bombay - an intervention strategy

Ram Malkani

At the World Congress on AIDS held at Vancouver, Canada in June 1996

ABSTRACT

In 1992, the Indian Association of Dermatologists Venereologists and Leprologists, Maharashtra Branch, established a Testing and counselling centre for HIV. The Dermatologists, Venereologists and Leprologists, were consulted by all those who had STD or had clandestine uprotected sex, as for STDs, they were the trained Consultants.

The Centre was conducting blood tests anddoing counselling to almost 300 patients per day. Qualified Dermatologists, who had undergone training in counseling were attending the clinic. Blood was collected for VDRL, HIV by Elisa testing. Viral load, CD4, Western Blot,was done in those, who were specially referred for the same and in those, who tested positive, oninnitial HIV Elisa testing.

Patients were counselled to avoid clandestine sex, have safe sex if at all, use condoms, avoid multiple partners, to settle down in a monogamous relationship.

Medico-politics and HIV related responses in India - impact, as a product of historicization with the epidemic

Vijay Thakur. Ram Malkani

At the 12th World AIDS Conference held at Geneva, Switzerland, June 28-July 3 1998.

POSTER

Epidemics galvanise a multitude of social forces and institutions. With the advent of modern medicine as an organised institution religious institutions which gazed upon epidemics and offered explanations and prescribed expiratory measures were displaced and with simultaneity the powers vested in the religious institutions were annexed by modern medicine.

The HIV/AIDS Epidemic did have feeble religious bigotry with its expositions but these were largely ignored. Globally though delayed the responses to HIV, except in the poorer countries where the World Health Organisation reigns supreme, were initiated by community groups, initially activist from the gay community and taken over by regional health institutions, like the Center for Disease Control (CDC)in the US,the Australian Federation of AIDS Organisation in Australia etc.

In India the initial call on "AIDS" was taken by an NGO, the Indian Health Organisation, now named Peoples Health Organisation, but was ridiculed by all and sundry with some specialists saying "Indian Culture would not permit the spread of AIDS"

The World Health Organisation with its miniscule bureaucrats in Delhi saw India as an opportunity to demonstrate its genius in preventing the spread of HIV. The Indian Council of Medical Research (ICMR) the Indian clone of CDC unleashed the first response to HIV by creating a quarantine facility for women in sex work who had tested positive for HIV, to be managed by a local NGO in Sangli a city in western Maharashtra. The women quarantined were given an allowance of Rs.1500/- (approx 30 $ US) per month as an incentive to "stay away from clients".

The WHO and Government of India negotiated a soft loan 100 million US $ from the World Bank for what was called the Phase 1. Controlled by the sagacity of WHO 80 million dollars were spent on IEC, Despite the knowledge accumulated globally the rapid community based targeted responses were the most effective and efficient strategy, Indian health authorities appointed advertising agencies and the in house health education machinery to print posters, wall papers, booklets and video clips over five years. Few NGOs, especially in Maharashtra and Tamil Nadu with funds from other agencies initiated targeted interventions. The prevalence of HIV increased alarmingly over these 5 years.

It is noteworthy that India which was and is one of biggest manufacturers of latex condoms and used to dump condoms at primary health centres for contraception, were not provided to NGOs' for free distribution. Instead under the expertise of WHO, Social Marketing of condoms was promoted with the wisdom the "people don't value anything that is free".Besides this the powder coated condoms failed lab tests of almost all parameters of "minimum quality" and it was only after fierce advocacy by few NGOs' that the government relented and provided free condoms and the much later improved the quality.

Thus the first phase response to the HIV epidemic in India was a mix of health politics and the control of financial aid.

The second Phase was again supported by loan from the World Bank and WHO in India was by now a shadow of itself, so local NGOs' shaped the plans which promoted targeted interventions and a supply of free condoms, but needle exchange and oral substitution for injecting drug users was still a dream though the HIV epidemic affected a large population.

The landscape seemed right for the Bill and Melinda Gates Foundation (BMGF) with its financial muscle to step in. They territorialised the control of responses and riveted on Karnataka, Rajasthan and in a small way Maharashtra. Karnataka and Maharashtra had by then developed targeted interventions to an advanced stage with the evolution of many sex workers and gay organisation, managed by community members.

BMGF had little to offer in terms of technical expertise, so they projected the need for instituting "modern managerial practices" within the existing intervention, which were operating on low cost effective models. In Karnataka after the BMGF take over the expenditure increased exponentially, almost to 10-15 times and this is besides the costs of the BMGF superstructure. The fact that they had invested in vaccine research is open to interpretation. It may be predicted that cost escalation in the name of modern management will neither be effective nor sustainable.

The aim of this presentation is that local and regional narratives which are the lighthouses to design and develop appropriate end effective responses are overridden by the power of institutions of health technology and the power of money. This is doubly true in situations like the HIV epidemic with its potential for public hysteria and in ecosystems like India which faces multiple challenges.

IADVL Maharashtra Branch's anonymous testing centre (ATC) at Bombay.

Vinay Gopalani, Ram Malkani

Presented poster at Kobe, Japan July 2005 Asia Pacific conference on AIDS.

The anonymous testing centre is a voluntary testing and counselling center at Dadar run under the auspices of IADVL with the aim to provide testing and coun-selling pertaining to HIV.

It is important for any project to know the basic facts about the community and the people they are working with. Many a times, the emphasis on information collec-tion and its use is fairly low because we firstly want to start intervention as soon as possible and also we are not even aware that this information can be of much value in the later stages of project development.

This study was therefore undertaken with the following aims and objectives:

Aims and objectives

1. To evaluate the basic facts about the patients presenting at our centre.
2. To test the questionnaire designed for the planned KABP survey.

Materials and Methods:

A serial lot of 100 questionnaires filled by our counsellor at the ATC were selected for the study. These were then analysed for

a. Socio-economic characteristics

b. Knowledge, attitudes, beliefs and practices towards sexuality and the effect of these on HIV spread in the community.

The questionnaire was designed to record basic demographic profile, relevant personal history, sexual history beliefs and practices, knowledge about HIV and AIDS, and general health profile. The answers were coded according to a key given in the questionnaire.

Results

On analysing the data we found that 87% of our patients were above 21 years of age, 9% in their teens, and 4% in the pediatric age group. Of the 87 adults 72 were males and 15 were females.

20% of the patients were illiterate, of whom 52% were HIV positive. 58% had completed schooling and 45% of these were positive. 22% had completed or were pursuing higher education, of which 30% were positive (Graph 1).

Percentage Positivity in different education groups

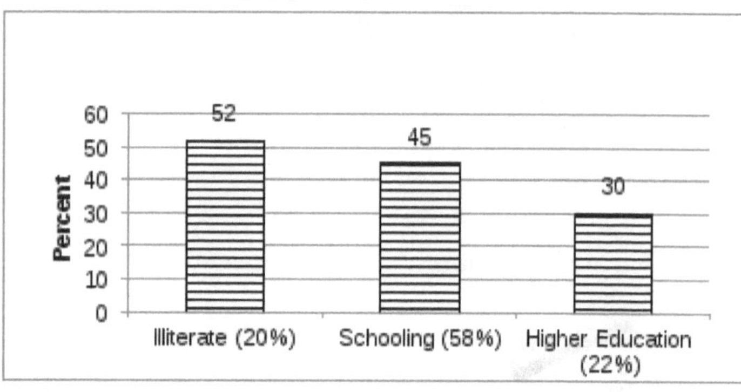

Graph 1

Considering the economic strata of our patients, 12% had a monthly income of less than 1500 rupees of which 50% were positive. 60% had an income of up to 4500 and of these 43% were positive and 28% had an income of more than 4500 and 45% of these were positive.

When the marital status of the patients presenting to us was considered, we found that 43.75% of our patients were married and 32% of them were positive compared to 47% amongst the unmarried group.

On comparing the positivity status with the history of addictions, we found that a significant 77% of patients were addicted to either alochol or tobacco or both. A majority of these were addicted to both alcohol and tobacco. (substance abuse)

On being questioned about the age of first sexual exposure, only 40% of the patients had responded. Of these 39.4% had their first sexual exposure between 15-20 years. (Graph 2)

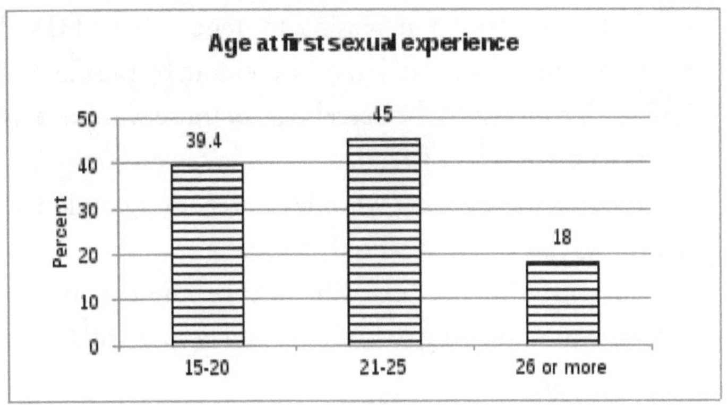

Graph 2

In our community, 95% of the patients had heard of HIV and 69% of them knew of intercourse as a mode of transmission, however only a marginal number of patients knew of Blood and blood products and vertical spread as a mode of transmission.

We found that only 7 patients with a history of exposure always used condoms. The positivity rate in this group was much lower than those who never or occasionally used condoms. (Graph 3)

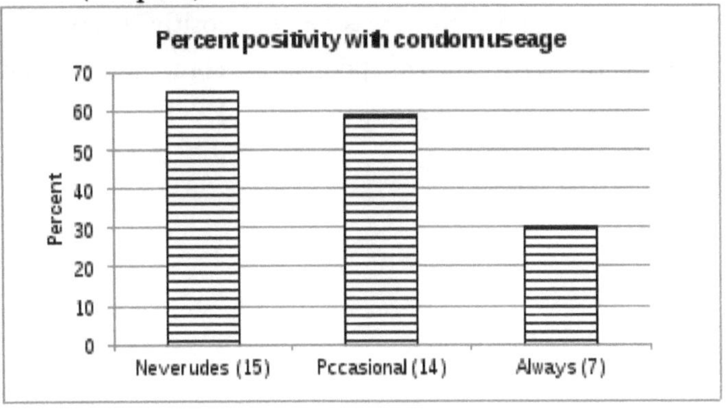

Graph 3

Reflecting on the increasing awareness about HIV, 33% of our patients were asked to use a condom by the CSW. This is in stark contrast to the percentage of those who were asked to use a condom by a friend.

65% of the patients who has never used condoms said that they were ignorant about its use.

On analysing the sexual habits, we found that 66% of the patients admitting to both pre and extramarital sex were positive. (Graph 4)

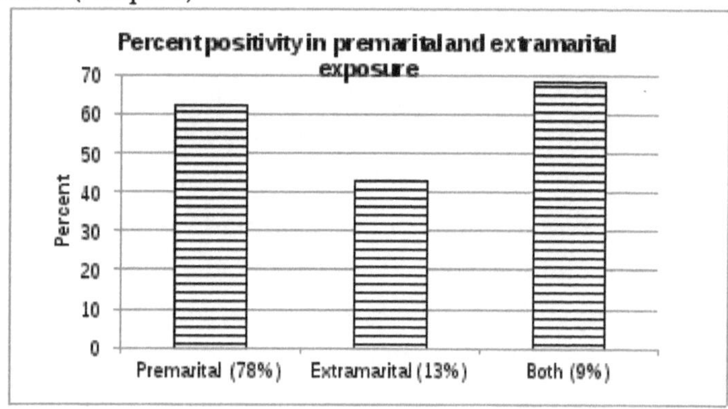

Graph 4

We found that there was a higher positivity rate amongst the habitually exposed people as compared to single/ occasionally exposed group. (Graph 5)

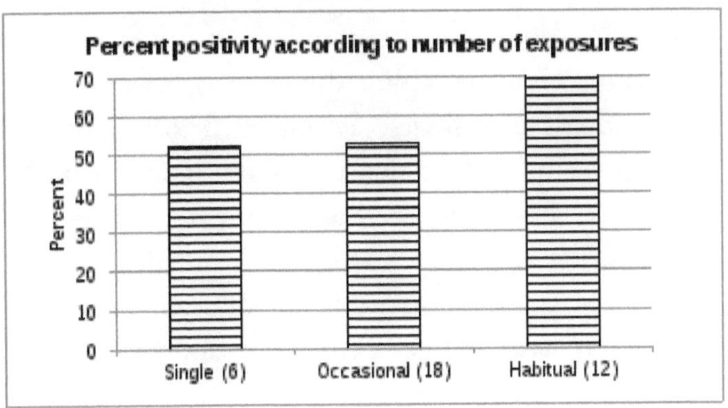

Graph 5

A high number of patients, on direct questioning, gave us a past history of STD. In the HIV positive group, 37% of the patients gave us a past history of STD.

Most of the patients that presented at our ATC were being tested for medical reasons. A sizeable number came for voluntary testing due to self-doubt.

The rest gave varied reasons such as getting married, going abroad etc.

The Elisa for HIV positivity rate in our community was high at 45%.

Discussion

The data analysis revealed a few thought provoking results.

We found that in our community as the education level increased the prevalence of HIV decreased. This was in concurrence with a study done in Ethiopian sailors by Demissie et al.

Oliviera L C in a study done in 1996 in brasil quoted that "we conclude that, at least for the moment, alcoholism per se, did not constitute an important risk factor for HIV infection. However, acquired immunodeficiency syndrome is a rather recent disease as compared to hepatitis B and C and, as the transmission routes are similar for HIV and hepatitis viruses, an increase in the incidence of HIV infection in alcoholics may be just a question of time." In our study we found that addiction of alcohol and smoking strongly related to the positivity status, thus proving his predictions true.

In our set up, we found the patients to be evasive on the questions pertaining to sexual practices. This was aptly demonstrated when only 40% of the patients responded when queried about the age of first sexual exposure. The percentage of patients that admitted to having the first sexual exposure in teen was quite high at nearly 40%. In a similar study done in Tanzania amongst school boys, 52% of them admitted to having a sexual intercourse.

To overcome this problem, a self filling questionnaire may probably be the best method.

A large number of our patients who admitted to having both pre and extramarital sex were positive. In a study done amongst schoolteachers in Jaipur, it was found that one third of unmarried and one fifth of married males had experienced premarital sex. The same for unmarried and married females was 11.8 per cent and 1.5 per cent, respectively. Since this study was done in the general population an coupling this with the high number of positivity (66%) we found in our patients having both pre and extramarital sex, we conclude that this situation is very conducive for the spread of HIV infection among general population.

Why this apathy?

Limited knowledge about psychoneurocutaneous diseases or the relation between stress and dermatology

No training to elicit neurological or psychological history

Not comfortable in prescribing psychotropic medications

Potentially, limited monetary benefits – particularly with a surge in cosmetic dermatology clinics in India

This often results in inadequate diagnosis and management of dermatological cases.

What should be done

It is important that the International Psychocutaenous Society should identify interested Dermatologists in India to start an India chapter

It should be accompanied with pilot funds for research grants, regular workshops, and conferences to improve the awareness and knowledge ofsychoneurodermatology

Theatre of the Soul

Issue 2   25 January 2012

Google hits on Suicidal ideation in Acne

ATOPIC profile / History of a patient

Psychometric testing

Psychotropic drugs

Passage About A Great Thinker

Hi, Colleagues,

You will be surprised there is not a single institute in India having a Department of 'Psychosomatic Medicine' where Doctors can impart their wisdom to the community about 'Good health being episodes between illnesses' and also by counselling, by giving information on the disease presented by the patient to the attending doctor, also dwelling on the 'Psychosocial history' of the patient, helping him to think rationally to lead a balanced, not 'reckless' but a life of manageable stress/ decisions.

In short, literally counselling the populace of the whole world, by the medical community.

Cheers!

regards

Ron.

The end of the disease era
Tinous ME, Fried T.

The time has come to elucidate disease as the focus of medical care. The changed spectrum of health, the complex interplay of biological and environmental factors, the aging population, and the interindividual variability in health priorities render medical care that is centered on the diagnosis and treatment of individual diseases at best out of date and at worst harmful.

A primary focus on disease may inadvertently lead to undertreatment, overtreatment, or mistreatment. The numerous strategies that have evolved to address the limitations of the disease model, although laudable, are offered only to a select subset of persons and often further fragment care. Clinical decision making for all patients should be predicated on the attainment of individual goals and the identification and treatment of all modifiable biological and psychological factors, rather than solely on the diagnosis, treatment, or prevention of individual diseases. Anticipated arguments against a more integrated and individualized approach range from concerns about medicalization of life problems to "this is nothing new" and "resources would be better spent determining the underlying biological mechanisms." The perception that the disease model is "truth" rather than a previously useful model will be a barrier as well.

Notwithstanding these barriers, medical care must evolve to meet the health care needs of patients in the 21st century.

Psychobiological Aspects of Atopic Dermatitis: An Overview

Center of Psychobiological and Psychosomatic Research, University of Trier, Germany.

While there is still little consensus on an AD-specific personality profile and its etiological significance, a growing number of reports support the role of psychosocial stress in the onset and the course of Atopic Dermatitis symptomatology.

Psychosomatic Medicine

In Germany Psychosomatic medicine is not a synonym for consultation-liaison Psychiatry but represents a comprehensive field (Fava GA et al. Curr Psychiatry Rep 2010;12:315-21) as well as a specialised medical field (Deter HC. Adv Psychosom Med2004;26:181-189.

The clinical care competency of German Psychosomatic medicine is centred on integrated care for the following disorders: somatoform / functional disorders, eating disorders, somatopsychic disorders including psycho-oncology, psycho-cardiology, neuro-psychosomatics, psychodiabetology and psychotraumatology. An overlap with psychiatry exists in the fields of depression, anxiety, and personality disorders. (Psychother Psychosom 2016;6:362-368).

Friedrich Wilhelm Nietzsche

15 October 1844 – 25 August 1900 was a German philosopher, cultural critic, poet, philologist, whose work has exerted a profound influence on Western philosophy and modern intellectual history.

Probably the greatest philosopher ever, or stirring up the thought process of the maximum no of human beings, agreement or disagreement with his ideas and opinions apart, was born in the family of clergy men and destined to become the staunchest critic of Christianity. Unfortunately, his concepts of 'will to power' and 'overman/superman' were badly distorted by many for their propaganda. Most remember him as only a nihilist. Still doubtful how many understood his most famous quote 'God is dead. You times I killed Him'.

His genius can be understood from the fact that he became a university professor of philosophy at the age of 24 ! He died as an insane man at the age of 56. Seeing the current world he might have died at much an younger age !

Google results on suicidal ideation in acne. About 1,82,000 results (0.15 seconds)

First Issue: Issue 1
Edited & published by the team us@atomhpsychosomaticdermatology.com

Regular newsletters to increase awareness about the
psychosomatic medicine

Despite the concentrated efforts to create awareness about the use of condoms, resistance to its use is still a major issue in our community. A silver lining to this problem is the increased promotion of condom usage by the CSW. The reason for not using condoms given by our patients was largely ignorance, which is correctable, followed by social stigma, which is more difficult to change. In a contrasting study by Roth J, lack of privacy and social stigma were the main issues.

We found that most of our patients were aware about the existence of HIV and also about its differentiation form AIDS, many of them also knew of the sexual mode of spread, but a very marginal number knew about the vertical and the blood and blood product mode of spread. This is a disturb-ing factor considering the vertical spread of HIV is the most important issue, with an average of about 1% of mothers presenting in an ANC being positive.

Most of the patient presented to us due to medical reasons and a marginal number due to self-doubt. In a similar study done in Bangkok, the reasons were high-risk behaviour (21%), feeling unwell (20%), checking a previous HIV test result (18%), a planned marriage or new relationship (10%), and planning a baby (5%). We believe that creating awareness amongst all sections of society about different modes of spread of HIV is the best method for ensuring selftesting by high-risk group.

References

1. HIV-l infection in relation to educational status, use of hypodermic injection and other risk behaviours in Ethiopian sailors. Demissie K, Amre D, Tsega E.East Afr Med J 1996 Dec; 73 (12): 819-22.

2. Prevalence of human immunodeficiency virus infection in alcoholics. Oliveira LC, Pereira.Mem Inst Oswaldo Cruz 2001 Jan; 96(1): 21-3.

3. KAP study results regarding HIV/AIDS, from primary school pupils in Tanga region, Tanza nia.Nesje, N. Millao, G. Mpaka.

4. Pre-and extra-marital heterosexual behaviour of an urban community in Rajasthan. Bhattacharjee J. J Commun Dis 2000 Mar; 32(1): 33-9.

5. Barriers to condom use: results from a study in Mumbai (Bombay), India. Roth J, Krishnan SP, Bunch E. New Mexico State University Las Cruces 88003-8001, USA.

6. Knowledge, attitudes and behaviour among HIV-Positive and HIV-negative clients of a confidential HIV counselling and testing centre in Thailand. Phanuphak P, Muller O, Sarangbin S, Sittitrai W. AIDS 1992 Aug; 6(8): 869-74.

Why is the Indian Dermatologist reluctant to acknowledge the magnitude of psychodermatology?

Ram H Malkani

Presented at the 17th Annual conference of the European Society of Dermatologists and Psychiatrists at Brest France, June 21 to 23, 2017

Background

Psychoneurocutaneous diagnoses are an important part of the dermatological practice.

Though the specialty has been recognized world-wide, it is yet to receive adequate recognition in India.

This apathy also often translates in clinical practice.

For example, Indian dermatologists talk about physical and clinical details are willing to treat patients with steroid, immunomodulators, and biologics.

However, they do not enquire about emotional state of the individual, relationship with family members, temperament, financial liabilities, sleep disturbances, or appetite and bowel movements.

Survey

An online cross-sectional survey

A preformed questionnaire sent to members of the Indian Association of Dermatologists, Venereologists, and Leprologists

Only 20 responded

Opinion on psychodermatology, training, history, use of psychotropic drugs in multiple dermatological conditions

Findings of the Survey - Opinion

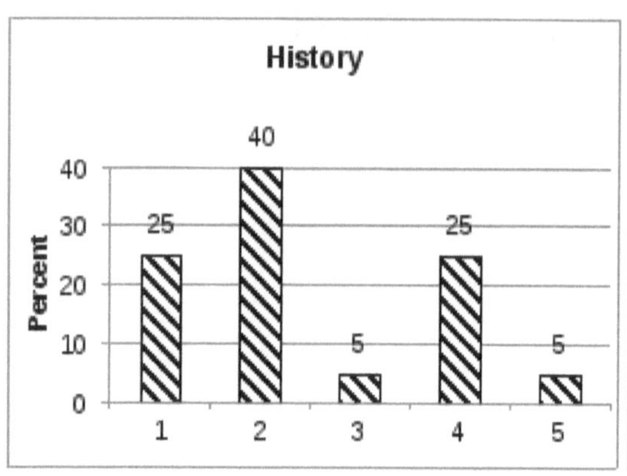

History
Percent
40
25
25
5
5
0 10 20 30 40
1 2 3 4 5

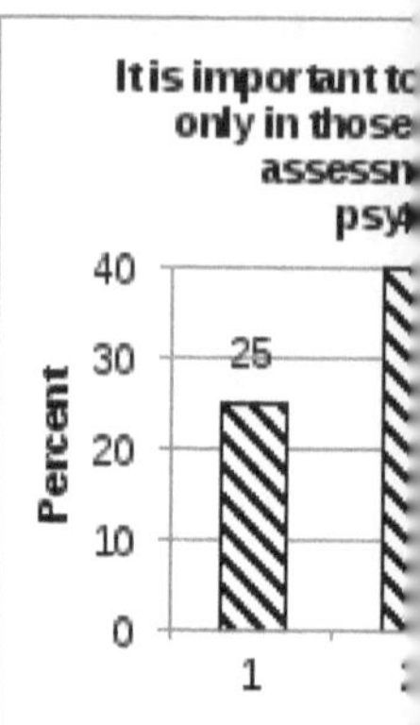

It is important to
only in those
assessn
psy
Percent
40
25
0 10 20 30 40
1

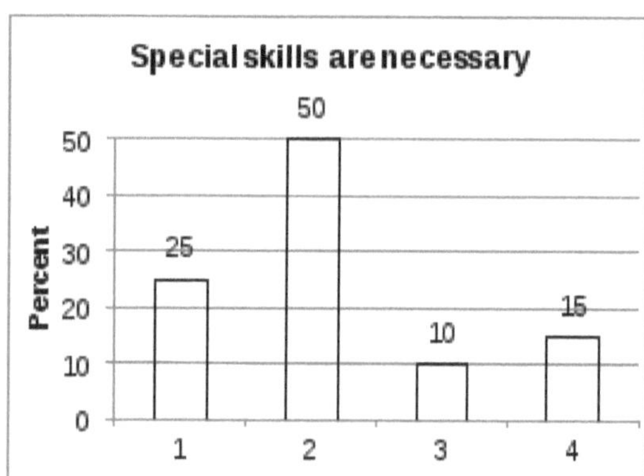

Special skills are necessary
Percent
50
25
10
15
0 10 20 30 40 50
1 2 3 4

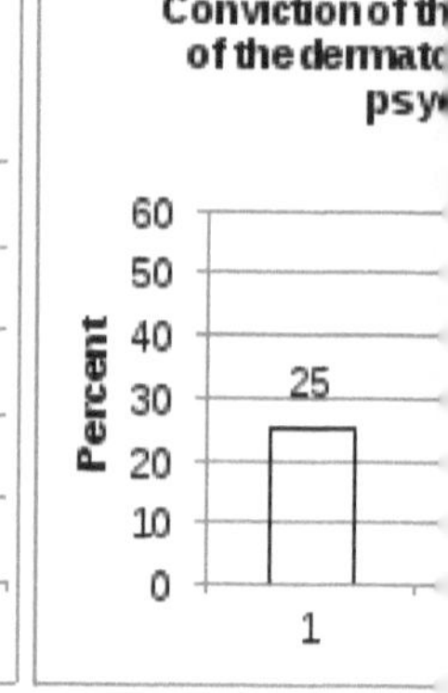

Conviction of th
of the dermato
psy
Percent
25
0 10 20 30 40 50 60
1

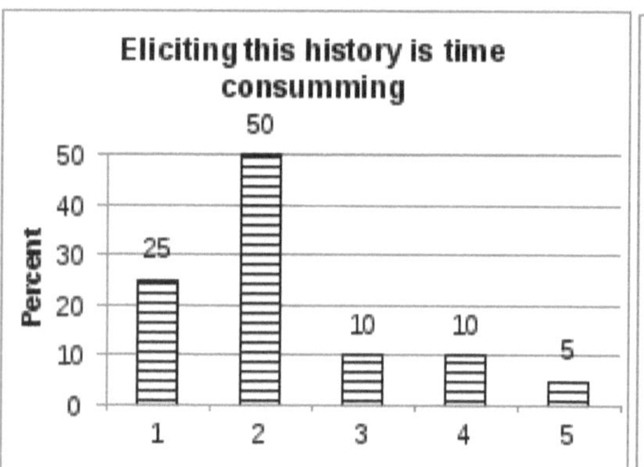

Eliciting this history is time
consumming
Percent
50
25
10
10
5
0 10 20 30 40 50
1 2 3 4 5

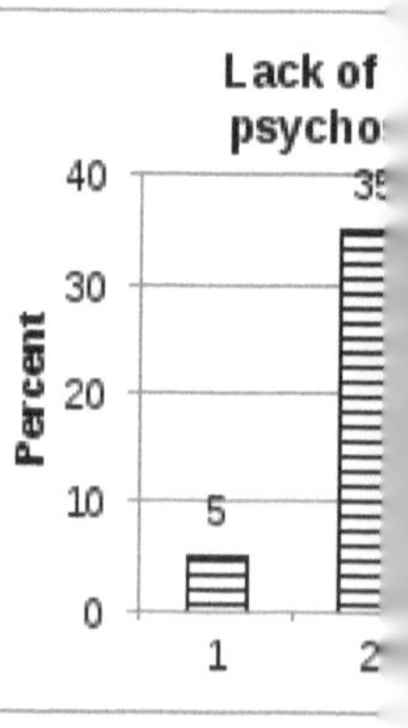

Lack of
psycho
Percent
35
5
0 10 20 30 40
1 2

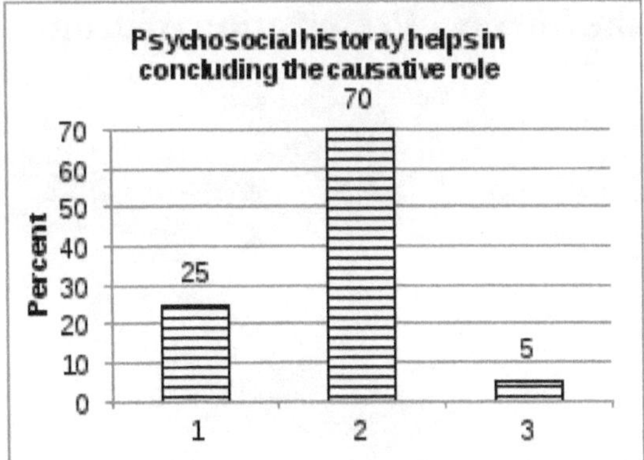

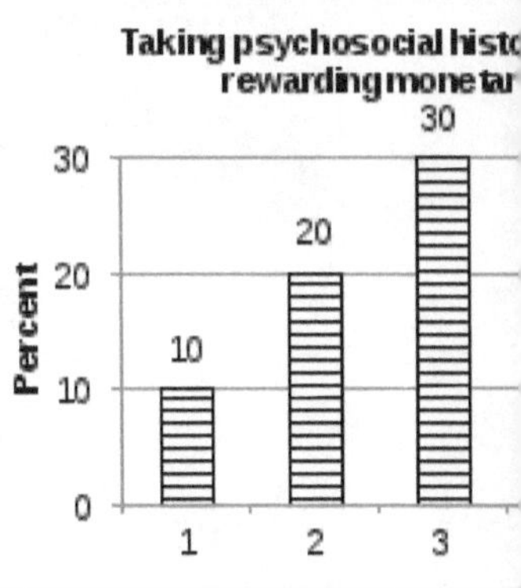

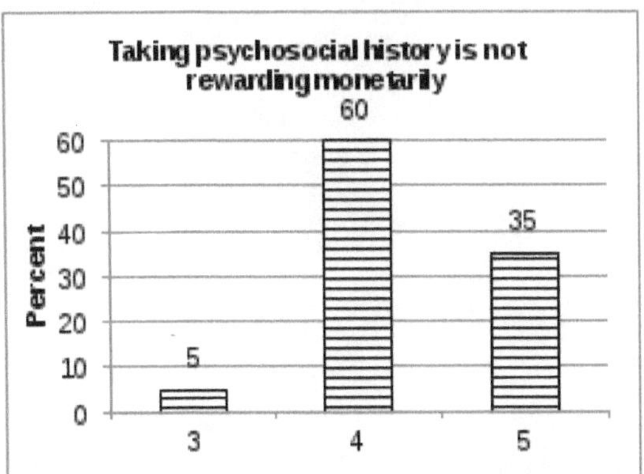

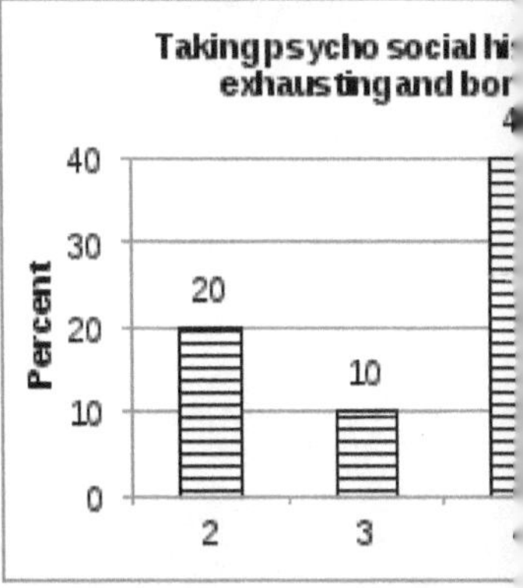

**1=Strongly Agree, 2=Agree, 3=Neutral, 4=Disagree,
5=Strongly disagree**

Findings of the Survey - Prescription of drugs

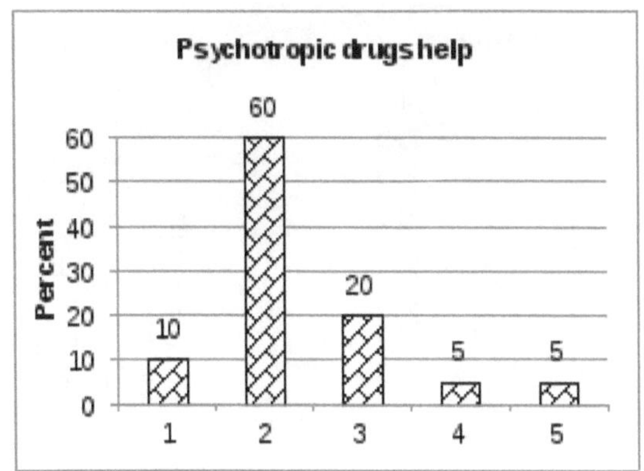
Psychotropic drugs help
Percent
60
50
40
30
20
10
0
10
60
20
5
5
1
2
3
4
5

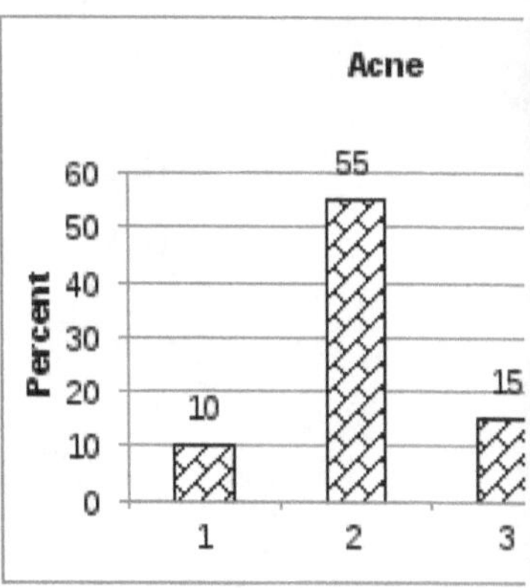
Acne
Percent
60
50
40
30
20
10
0
10
55
15
1
2
3

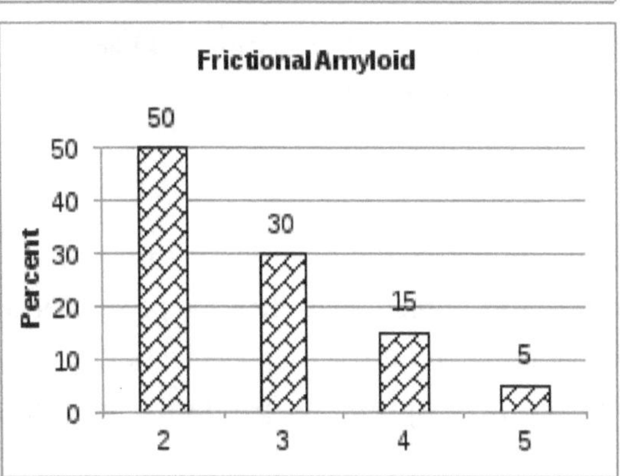
Frictional Amyloid
Percent
50
40
30
20
10
0
50
30
15
5
2
3
4
5

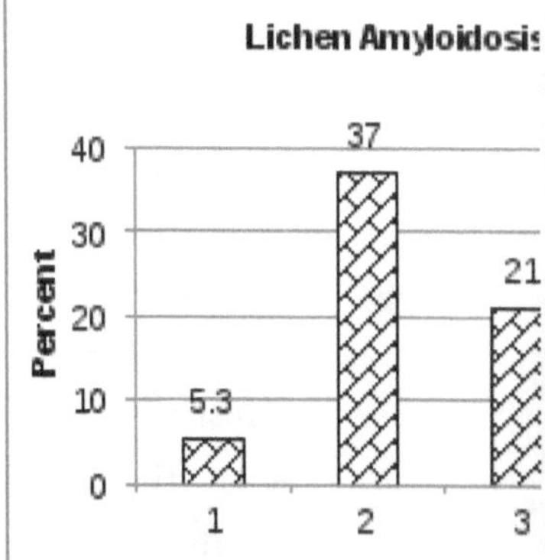
Lichen Amyloidosis
Percent
40
30
20
10
0
5.3
37
21
1
2
3

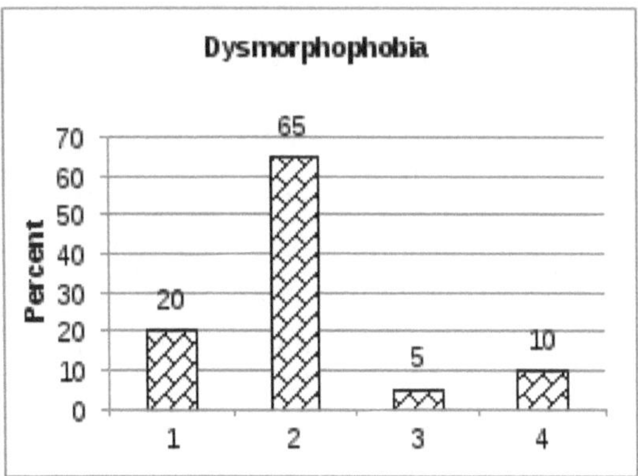
Dysmorphophobia
Percent
70
60
50
40
30
20
10
0
20
65
5
10
1
2
3
4

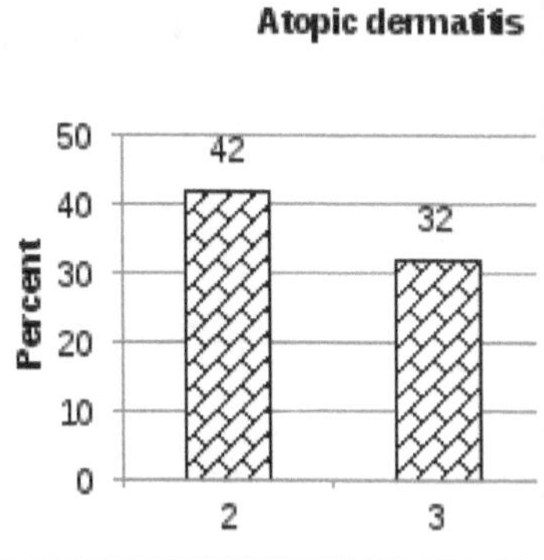
Atopic dermatitis
Percent
50
40
30
20
10
0
42
32
2
3

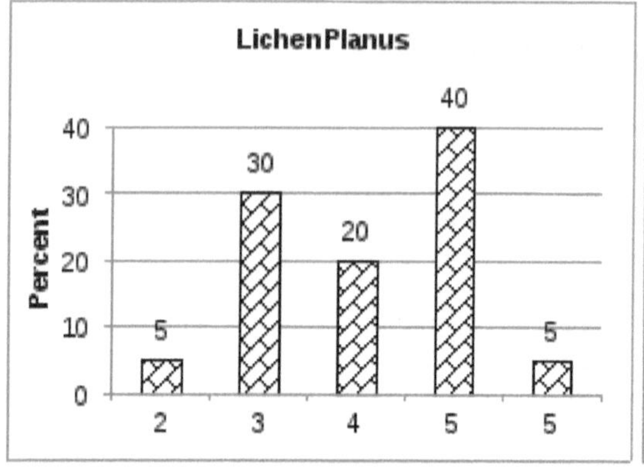

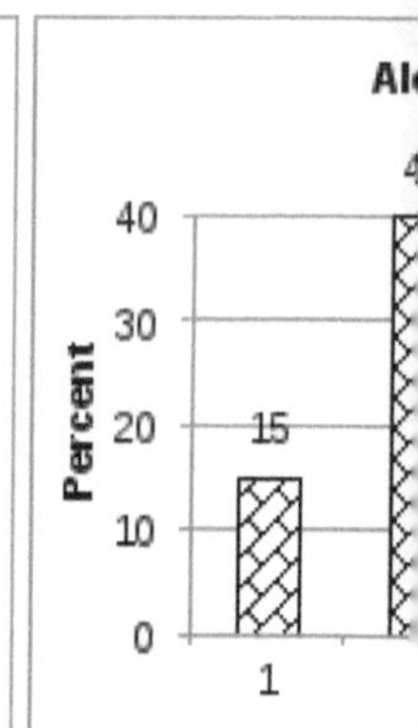

1=Strongly Agree, 2=Agree, 3=Neutral, 4=Disagree, 5=Strongly disagree

Findings

Most of them agreed that psychodermatology is important

However, many also agreed that eliciting psychosocial history is time consuming and it requires special skills

The opinion on prescription of psychotropic drugs differed by the condition

Other issues

In a recent National Dermatology Conference, though there was a complete session on medical management of urticaria, it did not include even a small talk on the psychoneurocutaneous aspects of urticaria.

This has also been observed in almost all dermatological conditions.

Acquired Zinc Deficiency in a Renal Transplant Recipient with Gastro-intestinal Tuberculosis Responding Promptly to Oral Correction

Priyanka Ghuge, Rusina Karia, Ram H. Malkani

Saudi J Kidney Dis Transpl 2018;29(5)

ABSTRACT. Zinc deficiency is an uncommon condition, known to occur in two forms: inherited type, known as Acrodermatitis enteropathica; and the acquired type. Cutaneous clinical manifestations observed include characteristic dermatitis on acral, periorificial, and anogenital areas through an unknown mechanism. The patient had a combination of causes which lead to a state of zinc deficiency. We are presenting it due to the rarity of acquired acrodermatitis in patients of gastrointestinal tuberculosis and renal transplant recipients. We emphasize the awareness about this condition, especially in resource-poor settings, where serum zinc levels may not be available, and a trial of oral zinc may be given.

Introduction

Acrodermatitis enteropathica (AE) is an uncommon autosomal recessive genetic dis-order of zinc malabsorption. Acquired zinc deficiency has multiple etiologies such as low nutritional intake, malabsorption, excessive loss of zinc, chronic diseases, or a combination of all these factors. Intestinal tuberculosis (TB) is the most common cause of malabsorption in India. Treatment with oral zinc gives prompt relief to the patient.

Case Report

A 46-year-old female patient presented with multiple, dark colored, itchy, scaly lesions involving both her upper and the lower limbs for one month. The lesions on the thigh were painful. She did not have a history of similar lesions in the past or in her family. She was a diagnosed with a case of ileocecal TB and was on anti-TB therapy for the past seven months. She was also a renal transplant recipient. The patient preferred a mixed diet (vegetarian and nonvegetarian), did not report any weight loss recently and did not show any features of malnutrition. There was no history of chronic diarrhea, decreased appetite, loss of hair, or alcohol abuse. On cutaneous examination, there was evidence of multiple, well-defined, hyperpigmented, scaly plaques, measuring of 3–7 cm (Figure 1a and b).

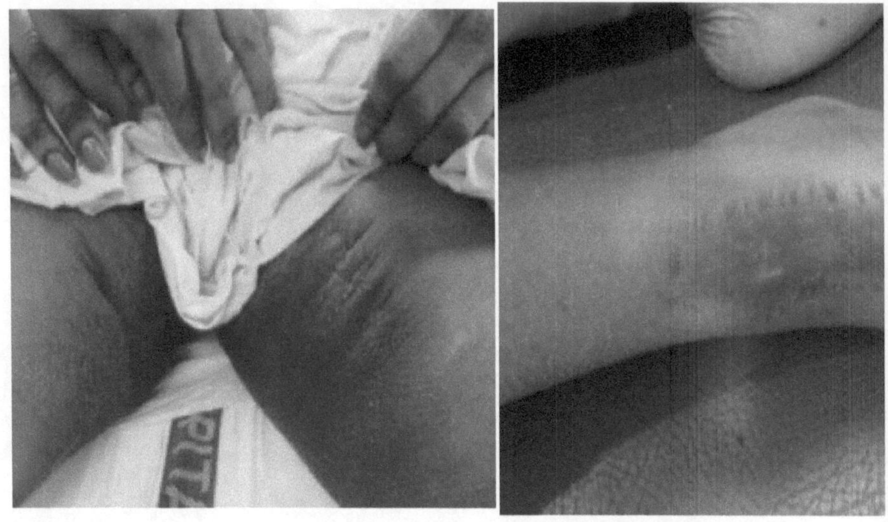

Figure 1a. Hyperpigmented scaly plaques on the thighs.

Figure 1b. Similar hyperpigment ankle.

A differential diag-nosis of atypical dermatophytic infection, psoriasis, seborrhoeic dermatitis and acquired Acrodermatitis enteropathica was considered. The laboratory investigations were as follows hemoglobin: 9.6 g%, packed cell volume: 28.3%, mean corpuscular hemoglobin concen-tration: 33.9%, red blood cell count: 2.95 millions/L, mean corpuscular volume: 95.9 fL, mean corpuscular hemoglobin: 32.5 pg, erythrocyte sedimentation rate: 103 mm/h, white blood cell count: 6150/mm3 (neutro-phils: 74.7%, lymphocytes: 18.3%, eosinophils: 1.0%, monocytes: 6.0%), and platelet count: 297,000/μL. The other investigations were as follows: blood urea nitrogen: 16.8 mg/dL, serum creatinine: 1.2 mg/dL, serum sodium: 133.2 mmol/L, serum potassium: 4.4 mmol/L, serum chloride: 98.3 mmol/L, serum bicar-bonate: 22.5

mmol/L, serum cholesterol: 1.43 mcg%, and dehydroepiandrosterone sulfate: 0.04 mcg/mL. She was negative for Hepatitis B virus and hepatitis C virus. Histopatho-logical evaluation of the skin lesions revealed hyperkeratosis, epidermal pallor, and psoria-siform hyperplasia suggestive of nutritional derma-tosis (Figure 2a and b).

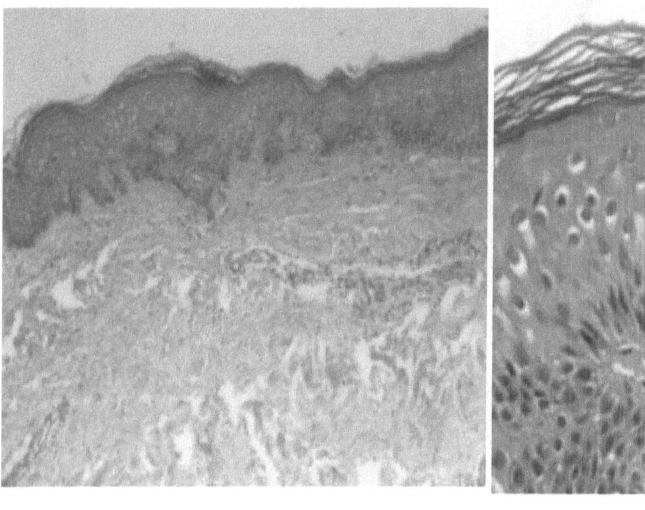

Figure 2a. High-resolution histopathology showing features suggestive of parakeratosis and psoriasiform hyperplasia.

Figure 2b. histopathology suggestive of para and cytoplasmic pal

The patient was treated with 3 mg/kg/day of elemental zinc (50 mg of elemental zinc per 220 mg zinc sulfate) along with topical emollients. The plaques showed reduced erythema and scaling by the end of one week, with decrease in their thick-ness by two weeks. There was complete clea-rance of the plaques by the end of three months (Figure 3a).

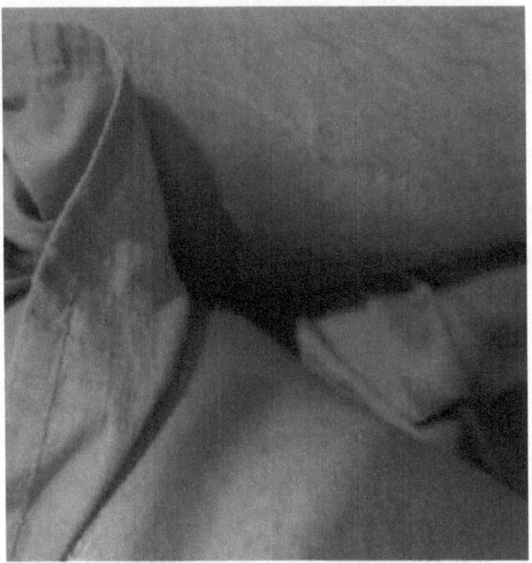

Figure 3a. Clearance of hyperpigmented and scaly lesions on the thighs after zinc treatment.

Discussion

Zinc deficiency is known to occur in two forms. The inherited type, known as Acro-dermatitis enteropathica or acquired by low nutritional intake (including parenteral alimentation, plant-based diets, alcoholism), malabsorption (including bariatric surgery, celiac sprue, and intestinal TB), excessive loss of zinc through the alimentary tract (such as diarrhea secondary to viral, protozoal, and bacterial pathogens), chronic diseases (liver or renal disease, diabetes, malignancies, sickle cell disease), or a combination of all these factors.[1]

Zinc absorption mainly occurs through the apical membrane of enterocytes with the help of diet-derived luminal factors. Malabsorption and possibly intestinal microbiota limit this zinc availability. The transporter ZIP4 present throughout the gastrointestinal tract is the main processor of dietary zinc for loading into enterocytes from the apical membrane.2 TB of the intestine is a common cause of malab-sorption in India, next only to tropical sprue.3

Intestinal TB is a common condition. Next, to tropical sprue, it is the most important cause of malabsorption in India.4 The other causes of malabsorption are: bacterial overgrowth proxi-mal to a stricture, bile salt deconjugation, diminished absorptive surface, involvement of lymphatics, and lymph nodes.5

The causes of Zn deficiency in kidney disease are not clear. Serum zinc levels are commonly found to be low in chronic kidney disease. After the renal transplant, the loss of zinc increases further, and the deficiency may become clinically apparent.6 The results of a study by Mahajan et al, suggested that zinc deficiency persist up to one-year post-transplant and may be related to increased urinary zinc losses.7

Zinc levels in plasma or serum are the most commonly used tests to evaluate for zinc deficiency. However, those levels do not necessarily reflect cellular zinc status because of tight homeostatic control mechanisms.8 Alkaline phosphatase is a zinc-dependent enzyme. Its levels can be used as an indicator of zinc deficiency.9

Treatment for zinc deficiency starts at 3 mg/kg/day of elemental zinc (50 mg of elemental zinc per 220 mg zinc sulfate) with rapid clinical improvement, even before changes in the serum zinc level are seem.10

Acknowledgment

We would like to thank Dr. B. V. Gandhi for his support for submitting the present case.

References

1. Bae-Harboe YS, Solky A, Masterpol KS. A case of acquired zinc deficiency. Dermatol Online J 2012;18:1.

2. Cousins RJ. Gastrointestinal factors influencing zinc absorption and homeostasis. Int J Vitam Nutr Res 2010;80:243-8.

3. Ranjan P, Ghoshal UC, Aggarwal R, et al. Etiological spectrum of sporadic malabsorp-tion syndrome in Northern Indian adults at a tertiary hospital. Indian J Gastroenterol 2004; 23:94-8.

4. Bhansali SK. Abdominal tuberculosis. Experiences with 300 cases. Am J Gastroenterol 1977;67:324-37.

5. Sharma MP, Bhatia V. Abdominal tuber-culosis. Indian J Med Res 2004;120:305-15.

6. Mahajan SK. Zinc in kidney disease. J Am Coll Nutr 1989;8:296-304.

7. Mahajan SK, Abraham J, Migdal SD, Abu-Hamdan DK, McDonald FD. Effect of renal transplantation on zinc metabolism and taste acuity in uremia. A prospective study. Transplantation 1984;38:599-602.

8. Maret W, Sandstead HH. Zinc requirements and the risks and benefits of zinc supplemen-tation. J Trace Elem Med Biol 2006;20:3-18.

9. Glover MT, Atherton DJ. Transient zinc deficiency in two full-term breast-fed siblings associated with low maternal breast milk zinc concentration. Pediatr Dermatol 1988;5:10-3.

10. Maverakis E, Fung MA, Lynch PJ, Draznin M, Michael DJ, Ruben B, et al. Acrodermatitis enteropathica and an overview of zinc metabolism. J Am Acad Dermatol 2007;56: 116-24.

Leprosy or sarcoidosis? A diagnostic dilemma!

Ram Malkani, Rusina Karia

Department of Dermatology, Jaslok Hospital and Research Centre, Mumbai, Maharashtra, India

J Family Med Prim Care 2018;

Abstract

There are two important differentials for non-caseating granulomatous inflammatory tissue—leprosy and sarcoidosis—which presents a diagnostic challenge due to their histological similarities and specific geographical distribution. This article describes a rare presentation of systemic sarcoidosis called Heerfordt's syndrome with the triad of parotitis, uveitis, fever, and optional paralysis of facial nerve. This case was initially diagnosed as leprosy.

Introduction

Non-caseating granulomatous inflammatory tissue has two important differentials—leprosy and sarcoidosis. Due to this shared similarity between the two, they often get misdiagnosed as one for the other.[1-4] The two diseases also have specific geographical prevalence and are often misdiagnosed in the countries where they are not prevalent. We present a rare case of systemic sarcoidosis in the form of Heerfordt's syndrome, which initially misdiagnosed as tuberculoid leprosy.

Case Report

In 2011, a 28-year-old male patient presented with asymptomatic pigmented lesions on dorsum of the left foot since 3–4 months. He gave a history of a solitary lesion that gradually progressing in number with no itching, burning, pain, or oozing from the lesions. There were no associated systemic complains. The cutaneous lesion on biopsy showed a non-caseating tuberculoid granuloma suggestive of tuberculoid leprosy and was, thus, diagnosed as tuberculoid leprosy on the basis of the clinical picture, burden of new leprosy cases in India,[5] and the biopsy report. He was started on paucibacillary leprosy treatment.

After anti-leprosy treatment, the patient seemed alright for 2 years but came back in February 2014 with symptoms of three cranial nerve involvement—difficulty in swallowing, suggestive of nerve IX and nerve X involvement, and drooping of right eyelid, suggestive of nerve V involvement. The patient also had hypotension - probably suggestive of X nerve involvement. He also had bilateral parotid swelling with fever and conjunctival redness. The fluorodeoxyglucose-positron emission tomography (FDG-PET) scan showed metabolically active bilateral, level IV cervical, mediastinal, hilar, and peribronchial lymph nodes with multiple lung nodules and left common iliac adenopathy [Figure 1a-c]. On the basis of this report, a differential diagnosis of sarcoidosis or lymphoma was given. The excision biopsy of the cervical lymph node showed as previously discrete and confluent typical tubercles with no caseous necrosis. Ziehl-Neelsen (ZN) stain was negative for acid fast bacilli (AFB). However, Fite-Faraco stain showed one stout bacillus. MRI BRAIN showed prominence of lateral ventricles with no other significant pathology identified. Due to the positive Fite-Faraco stain and previous diagnosis of leprosy, the patient was restarted on anti-leprosy treatment. The patient was continuously on anti leprosy treatment (as prescribed by the treating neurophysician) due to the reporting of AFB in histopathology. However, the patient did not get better and came back in October 2014 presenting with headache associated with nausea and vomiting since a month and a half, fever with chills for 8 days, and cough since 5 days. Patient was investigated and CT scan of chest showed right-sided basal pleural effusion and lower lobe subpleural consolidation with plate-like atelectasis with extensive mediastinal lymphadenopathy. The laboratory tests showed an elevated serum angiotensin-converting enzyme (SACE) level 62 U/L (normal range 8–53 U/L), raised serum calcium level 12.5 mg/dl (normal range 8.5–10.2 mg/dl), and urinary protein 976 mg/24 hours (normal range >80 mg/24 hours). The rest of the laboratory reports including peripheral smear for Malarial parasite, Dengue Serology, Widal, Mantoux, and Blood culture were negative. As the patient did not get better on anti-leprosy drugs and taking into consideration the triad of b/l parotid swelling, uveitis, fever along with neurological involvement, incriminating FDG-PET scan,[6] and elevated SACE levels,[7,8] the final diagnosis of systemic sarcoidosis in the rare form of

Heerfordt's syndrome[9] was made and patient was started on steroids.

Discussion

India has been saddled with leprosy for a long time and is one of the countries in which the highest number of new leprosy cases is detected every year. It is often the first diagnosis considered when the pathology of non-caseating granulomas is detected. Similarly, in our case, the patient was diagnosed with leprosy the first time as he presented no other symptoms or signs other than asymptomatic pigmented skin lesions, which on biopsy showed non-caseating granulomas. The patient came back after 3 years with symptoms of fever, b/l parotitis, uveitis, and neurological involvement. It is quite possible that this was a rare presentation of systemic sarcoidosis called Heerfordt's syndrome.[9] That this was systemic sarcoidosis, was also supported by the presence of b/l hilar lymphadenopathy [6,10] with nodes displaying non-caseating granulomas, on biopsy. When the tissue was subjected to Fite-Faraco stain, the pathologist felt he saw a single leprosy bacillus. In view of the fact that this patient was initially diagnosed as leprosy, and in view of the report of the pathologist authenticating a bacillus on Fite-Farraco stain, the neurophysician, the PETSCAN physician, felt convinced about the diagnosis of leprosy, the patient was restarted on leprosy treatment. The dermatologist, at that time, had categorically conveyed to the neurophysician, after consulting other colleagues expert in the knowledge of leprosy, that this case is unlikely to be leprosy, cranial nerves involvement and multiple glands in the chest seen on PETSCAN go against the diagnosis of leprosy. The patient came back the same year with headache associated with nausea and vomiting, weight loss, since a month and a half, fever with chills for 8 days, and cough since 5 days. This time the SACE levels were done and they were found to be very high. Thus, taking into consideration the previous history of cutaneous lesions showing tuberculoid granulomas, the cervical gland biopsy showing tuberculoid granuloma, the PETSCAN showing perihilar glands, the triad of b/l parotitis, uveitis, and fever along with neurological involvement and with the biochemical reports, a diagnosis of Heerfordt's syndrome which is a rare presentation of systemic sarcoidosis was established. He was started on steroids after which he showed continual improvement. Thus, this is a cautionary case history where the pathological evidence, if unsupported by clinical evidence, should not be taken as the sole basis of diagnosis. Pathology alone should not dictate the entire picture and a clinicopathological correlation should be made.

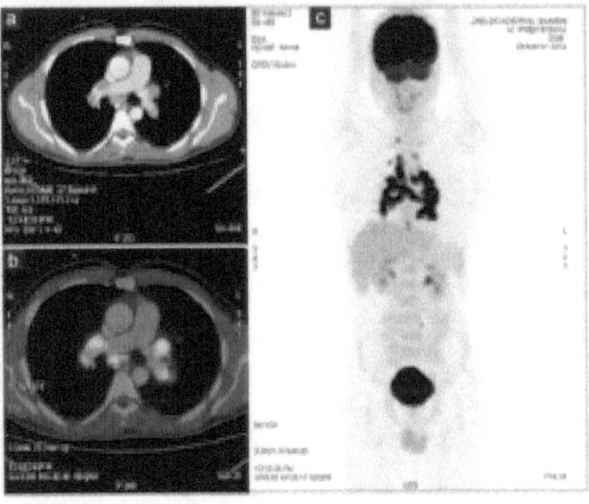

Figure 1: FDG-PET scan showing active lymph nodes with multiple lung nodules. a,b scan slice images, c - scan image

Declaration of patient consent

The authors certify that they have obtained all appropriate patient consent forms. In the form the patient(s) has/have given his/her/their consent for his/her/their images and other clinical information to be reported in the journal. The patients understand that their names and initials will not be published and due efforts will be made to conceal their identity, but anonymity cannot be guaranteed.

Financial support and sponsorship

Nil.

Conflicts of interest

There are no conflicts of interest.

References

1. Aftab H, Nielsen SD, Nielsen SL, Due E, Bygbjerg IC, Thybo S. A case of leprosy mistaken for cutaneous sarcoidosis. Acta Derm Venereol 2012;92:189-90.

2. Kaur S, Dhar S, Bambery P, Kanwar AJ, Khajuria A. Cutaneous sarcoidosis masquerading

as relapsed borderline tuberculoid leprosy? Int J Lepr Other Mycobact Dis 1993;61:455-8.

3. Ramanujam K. Tuberculoid leprosy or sarcoidosis? A diagnostic dilemma. Lepr India 1982;54:318-23.

4. Thaipisuttikul Y, Kateruttanakul P. Sarcoidosis mimics lepromatous leprosy: A case report. J Med Assoc Thai 2007;90:171-4.

5. World Health Organization. Leprosy: Regional elimination on the horizon. 2018;

6. Rubini G, Cappabianca S, Altini C, Notaristefano A, Fanelli M, Stabile Ianora AA, et al. Current clinical use of 18FDG-PET/ CT in patients with thoracic and systemic sarcoidosis. Radiol Med 2014;119:64-74.

7. Ainslie GM, Benatar SR. Serum angiotensin converting enzyme in sarcoidosis: Sensitivity and specificity in diagnosis: correlations with disease activity, duration, extrathoracic involvement, radiographic type and therapy. Q J Med 1985;55:253-70.

8. Romer FK. Clinical and biochemical aspects of sarcoidosis. With special reference to angiotensin-converting enzyme (ACE). Acta Med Scand Suppl 1984;690:3-96.

9. Walter C, Schwarting A, Hansen T, Weibrich G. [Heerfordt's syndrome — A rare initial manifestation of sarcoidosis]. Mund Kiefer Gesichtschir 2005;9:43-7. 10. Sehgal VN, Sehgal N, Jain S, Balal P. Hilar-lymphadenopathy predictive of cutaneous sarcoid. Indian J Dermatol Venereol Leprol 2002;68:161-3.

Psychodermatology

Institute of Psychosomatic Dermatology

Ram Malkani

About us

It is an organisation to promote a holistic approach in both clinical management and research in Dermatology. The Institute was formed in 1982 by DR. Ram Malkani one of the seniormost Dermatologist in India and Dr. Vijay Thakur a psychotherapist practitioner and researcher in 1982.

The seeds of the idea of such an Institute were sown by the clinical experience of Dr. Ram Malkani since increasingly he observed moderate to severe dermatosis were either triggered or accompanied by unresolved psychological distress. This was possible since Dr. Malkani had been sensitized through his experience of fifteen years in Psychoanalyses.

A clinical Psychologist joined the Institute in 1983 and selected patients were tested with internationally standardized Instruments for both simple and complex psychological distress and dysfunctions. The Institute was further inspired by the findings of the "Study on Psychological Profile of Common Dermatosis"a thesis conclude at the Jaslok Hospital and Research Center in 2008

With the emergent field of psychoendocrinology laboratory tests were included in the research protocols. The first landmark study was done with the levels of prolactin in acne and the results were encouraging

AIMS:

- Research; involve Psychiatrist, Psychologists, Neurologists, Endocrinologists, Immunologists

- Create awareness amongst the Medical fraternity and community

- Offer help to Dermatology Psychosomatic patients through counselling, guidance

- Network world over to improve our services.

- Liasion with the European Society of Dermatologists and Psychiatrist(ESDaP), Academic Medical Centre)AMC) Amsterdam, Association of Psychocutaneous Medicine of America, Psychodermatology Association of India(PDAI)

- Any other activity that will promote the aims of the organisation publications, original research, establishing the connect of body symptoms and psyche media education

- Solicit more consults Divide amongst consults experts

VISION:

To provide the highest quality of holistic treatment for patients with dermatosis through both research and practice.

MISSION:

To use the resources both financial and human to promote research and practice of a psychosomatic an integrative approach in the management of dermatosis.

GOAL:

To sensitise dermatologists and other branches of medicine in the psychosomatic approach, to conduct at least 4 research in psychosomatic dermatology and to provide holistic treatment to as many patients with dermatosis

At present the Institute has to centers one at Sion and another at Peddar Road Mumbai

The Institute grants free membership to all practitioners of holistic medicine free of cost and would welcome their contributions to the present team.

ACTIVITY

A thesis on Psychological profile of Lichen Planus, Lichen Amyloidosis,Acne Excoriee completed. Published in Acta Dermatologica,two publications related to the thesis. An survey carried out by an online questionnaire to the Indian Dermatologists on their Reluctance to be involved in the practice of psychodermatology.

Another survey is ongoing, where Chemists, Pharmacists are investigated about their Knowledge,

Attitude and Behaviour(KAP)in relation to the prescriptions of psychotropic drugs by the Dermatologists. A series of talks on 'Practical Psychodermatology' delivered to Family Physicians,at different venues and locations which includes an oration on the same was organised by a medical institution of a suburb of the city.

In one of the private consultation clinics, a Psychologist, interviews willing selected Dermatology Patients, about,by a specially designed questionnaire, on Body Image, Self Image, Anger, Social phobia, Sleep patterns, Post traumatic stress .A publication planned of both the surveys.

WEBSITE

www.instituteofpsychosomaticdermatology.com

Case histories and some interesting articles shared. A monthly online letter 'Theatre of the soul' circulated amongst family Physicians,Dermatologists and Medical Consultants for the last 18 months,to sensitise the medical fraternity on some interesting features of the mind, body.

Conceptualising Institute For Psychosomatic Dermatology

Dr. Ram Malkani Dr. Vijay Thakur

The inspiration to develop an Institute of Psychosomatic Dermatology draws from our personal experience of being in psychoanalyses, the observation of psychic distress in patients with long standing dermatological conditions like Atopic Dermatitis, Psoriasis, Lichen Planus. Alopecia Areata, the puzzle of recurrence and remission patterns in many of our patients presenting with these conditions, and our hope to discover psychic determinants of such dermatological conditions.

An institute for research with the setting of private practice which is essentially service driven presented us with some problems:

1. Why should the patient have to pay for extra-dermatological services like counselling and psychometrics?

2. How does the referral to a counsellor create a burden of stigma(both for the patient and the dermatologist due to its reflex socialized association with " mental illness")

3. Uncertainty that is universal to all research situations. We rationalized that some of the issues

could be resolved by developing all services under
a single roof and including facilities for laboratory
investigations.

The test for us would be to observe a relief from the psychic and social distress, the Somatopsychic aspects of these dermatological conditions, that almost always accompany long term dermatological condition through a emotionally supportive approach of the team members.

Occasionally more focused psychotherapy could also be accessed or at least offered an opportunity to access this service to address issues like social embarrassment, self esteem issues, anger and relationships issues. Sub therapeutic dosage with psychopharmacological agents were also prescribed when appropriate and under long term observation.

We translated our concept in to reality by integrating dermatological consultation with services of psychotherapy, psychometrics which included a battery of inventories, rating scales and projective tests. The Institute is also associated with hi-tech laboratories for assaying biochemical markers which usually consisted of Endocrinology and Immunology Profiles and HLA's typing in addition to the conventional baseline biochemistry. Though these were expensive, our associates offered a sliding scale for payments so patients with limited financial resources were not left out. Occasionally we were found strange anomalies but rejected these findings due to both their stochastic appearance and the unacceptable sample size.

However we found consistent high ratings on Depression Ratings and on Scales and Tests for Internalised Aggression, we are yet to make sense from these findings.

1980's was time when the momentum of the search for genetic causation of long term conditions like Psoriasis, Atopic Dermatitis and Lichen Planus and Alopecia Areata, gained momentum and its discoveries aroused more of a curiosity in us, than an assurance of any certainty, at least not a sufficient certainty for us to abandon seeking solutions within psychic dimensions.

This was the ecology that at the Institute of Psychosomatic Dermatology. After more than three and half decades we revisit our Dermatological Weltanschauung.

1. The Development Of Empirically Tested And Structured Psychotherapy: in the last two decades creates an opportunity to focus on offering relief to the psychic distress accompanying long term dermatological conditions through brief techniques of psychotherapy.

2. To Look At These Dermatological Condition/S as a Multifactorial Trait (1) with our attention directed at both, the intrapsychic phenomena and environmental conditions. After acknowledging the possibility that the underlying cause of these dermatological conditions stem from immune system, yet by holding this evidence in a self-conscious suspension, we can pose a research question: What are the trigger

factors? What factors aggravate these conditions and how the effect of these could be minimised ?

3. What Models are available or can be constructed to accommodate the two conditions, above? The Diathesis Stress Model, (2) which looks for factors that include Genetic, biological, physiological, cognitive and personality-related factors, may prove to be useful for the purposes of understanding the susceptibility to these conditions throughout the lifespan.[3] and offer a pragmatic paradigm for both treatments and research in Psychosomatic Dermatology in our future work This would allow us to locate "Protective factors", such as positive social networks or high self-esteem, that can counteract the effects of stressors and prevent or mimimise the effects of the condition(4)

4. The more recent and perhaps exotic models developing at the frontiers of contemporary psychotherapy drawing from the works of Stanislav Groff - "Holotropic Mind" (5) also offer exciting possibilities for those adventurous in our team and our clients, who seek to understand not only the problems in dermatology but also the age old problem of the Mind and the Body. Within this, our evolution, we should be able to offer the best possible service to our patients and with a simultaneity contribute to our knowledge and

understanding of some of the long term dermatological conditions.

"You may say I'm a dreamer, but I'm not the only one. I hope someday you'll join us. And the world will live as one."
John Lenon

1.   Diathesis–stress   model.
https://en.wikipedia.org/wiki/
Diathesis%E2%80%93stress_model

2. Multifactorial Traits. Genetic Disorders, Chapter 13

3. Sigelman, C. K. & Rider, E. A. (2009). Developmental psychopathology. Life- span human

development (6th ed.) (pp. 468-495). Belmont, CA: Wadsworth Cengage Learning

4) Administration for Children and Families (2012). Preventing child maltreatment and promoting wellbeing: A network for action. Department of Health and Human Services. Retrieved from

http://www.childwelfare.gov/pubs/guide2012/
guide.pdf#page=9

5. The Holotropic Mind. The Three Levels of Human Consciousness and How They Shape Our

Lives. Stanislav Grof, M.D. with Hal Zina Bennett, Ph.D. Harper Collins EBooks.1991

A study of stress in patients with acne excoriée, lichen and macular amyloidosis, and lichen planus

Dr. Ram Malakani, Dr. SakinaRangwala, Dr. Amit Desai, Dr. Maninder Singh Setia

Poster presented at the 16th annualconferenceof the European Society of Dermatologists and Psychiatrists, St.Petersberg, Russia, 2015

Objectives:

The present study was conducted to compare stress scores and types of reported stress in three dermatological conditions (acne excoriée, lichen and macular amyloidosis, and lichen planus) and those without any dermatological condition.

Methods:

We assessed stress by Gurmeet Singh's Presumptive Stressful Life Events Scale (by a psychiatrist) in 20 cases of each condition each of acne excoriée, lichen and macular amyloidosis, and lichen planus, and 20 controls. We collected demographic data and stressors in all participants, and clinical data in 60 cases. We used multivariate linear regression models to study the factors associated with stress scores.

Results:

The mean age (standard deviation [SD]) in acne excoriée, lichen and macular amyloidosis, lichen planus, and controls were 25.2 [5.5], 39.4 [12.7], 35.7 [14.1], and 38.5 [11.6] years respectively (p<0.001).

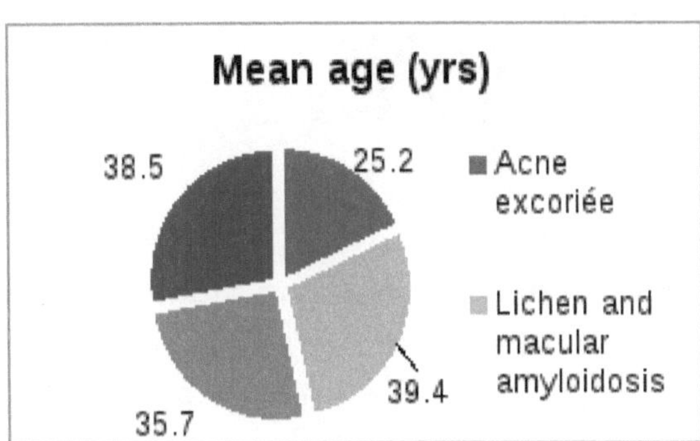

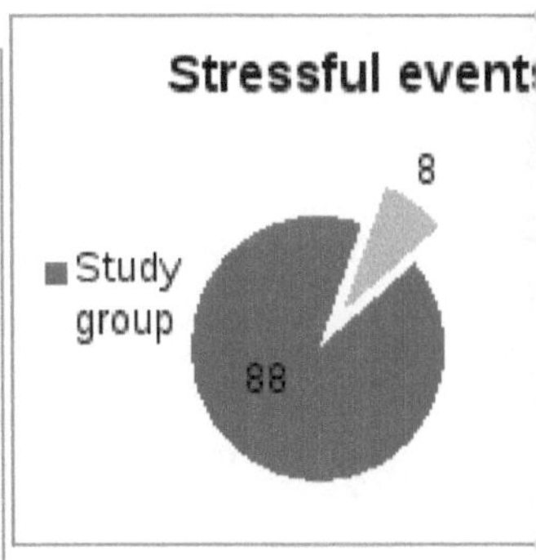

Stressful life events were significantly more commonly reported by cases compared with controls (88% vs 8%, p<0.001).

The common stressful financial problems (51%), f (40%), marital conflicts (3 (32%).

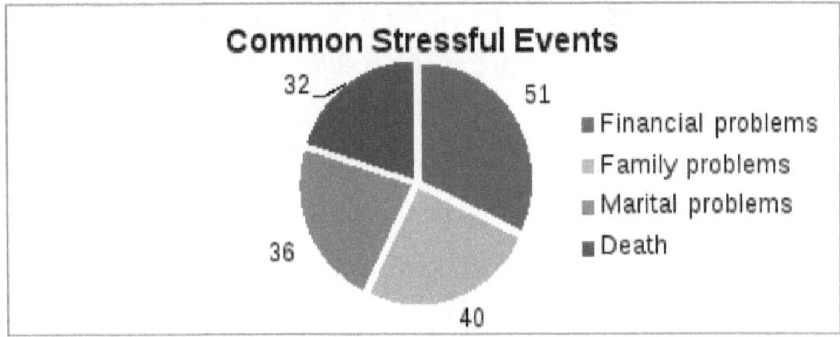

The Median (Interquartile range [IQR]) stress scores were highest in patients with lichen and macular amyloidosis (230 [210, 284.5]), followed by acne excoriée (189 [130, 234.5]), lichen planus (154 [105, 200.5]), and controls (0

[0, 65]); the differences were statistically significant
(p<0.0001).

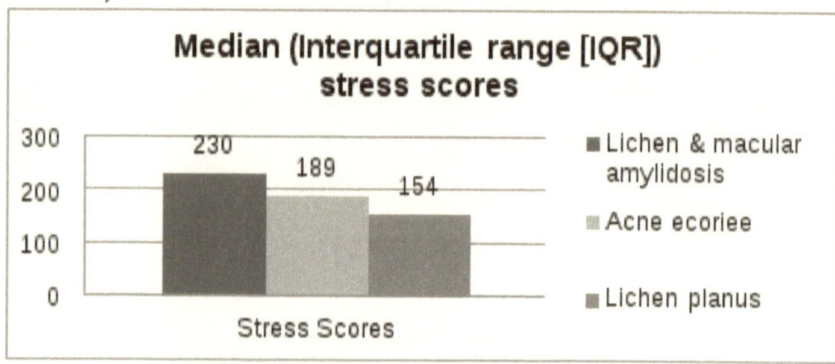

In the adjusted models, the mean stress scores were
significantly higher in patients presenting with lichen and
macular amyloidosis (201.4, 95% confidence intervals [CI]:
157.1, 245.6; p=0.001), acne excoriée (156.4, 95% CI:
107.4, 205.5; p<0.001), and lichen planus (128.5, 95% CI:
84.2, 172.7) compared with controls.

Financial stress was reported by 70% of acne excoriée,
65% of lichen and macular amyloidosis, 50% of lichen
planus cases, and by 20% controls (p=0.007). Marital
conflicts were reported by 60% of lichen and macular
amyloidosis, 45% of acne excoriée, 30% of lichen planus
cases, and by 10% controls (p=0.007). Similarly, family
conflicts were reported by 70% of lichen and macular
amyloidosis, 50% lichen planus, 40% of acne excoriée cases,
and none of the controls (p<0.001).

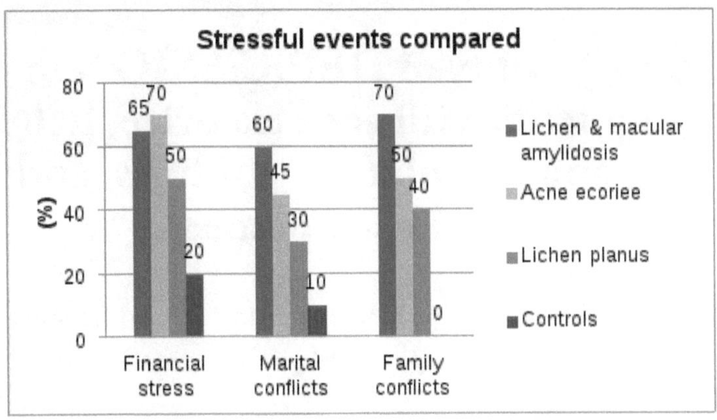

Conclusions:

Stressful life events were more commonly reported by cases compared with controls. Stress scores were highest in lichen and macular amyloidosis, and acne excoriée patients.

These dermatological diagnoses were associated with different types of stressful events in life.

A study of DEPRESSION in patients with acne excoriée, lichen and macular amyloidosis, and lichen planus

Ram Malkani, Sakina Rangwala, Amit Desai, Maninder Singh Setia

Presented as a poster at the IADVL National Conference, DERMACON 2016 held at Coimbatore

Reflections

While treating patients with dermatological diseases, it was realised that, in a lot of dermatosis, Psychological issues were responsible in the genesis of the presenting 'Symptom'. While taking history, most of the patients would deny any stress or accept the possibility of the mind set being responsible for the symptom. Hence a need was felt to assess objective evidence in selected, dermatosis, where it was a foregone conclusion about the role of the mind.

It was felt to read the mind of the patients, in view of the strong denials, by the patients, of the existence of psychological issues, the best objective way to go about was, to subject them to psychometric testing. Since controls were also subjected to psychological tests, it was possible to conclude that the coping mechanism of patients with symptoms was inadequate as compared to those in controls.

Going beyond the research protocol, reflecting on the report about the 'coping mechanism', it was realised, that coping mechanism depend a lot on the logical thinking, philosophical way of living life, accepting limiations in capabilities, having a provision for failures, being realistic and willing to feel sad about the fact of inevitable frustrations. One should by pass the denials, explain the existence of psychosomatic symptoms to the patient and go ahead with eliciting a good psychosocial history.

Psychological Pofiles in Selected Three Dermatosis

The skin is the mirror which reflects the state of the mind. Skin is one of thetarget organ of the stress reaction.(1) The skin and the nervous system have a common embryological origin; this supports a positive connection between skin changes and psychological phenomenon. Stress and other psychological factors trigger the onset and exacerbation of many dermatological diseases. Every person has a shock organ that is sensitive to stress, which is defined by environmental and genetic factors and this shock organ is the skin, in people who display dermatological symptoms under stress.(3)

Most dermatologic disorders influenced by psychosocial factors are associated with both psychosocial stress, which exacerbates the condition, and body image problems Psychodermatology focuses on the boundary between psychiatry and dermatology. Understanding the psychosocial and occupational context of skin disease is critical to the optimal management of psychodermatologic disorders.

Aims and objectives

To study the psychological profile of patients of acne excoriee, lichen planus and macular amyloidosis and lichen amyloidosis.

- To study various psychological disorders such as anxiety and depression and stress as the etiological factors for causing acne excoriee, lichen planus and macular amyloidosis and lichen amyloidosis.

- To compare the stress levels of the cases and controls.

- To analyze the psychological problems in patients and controls by various psychiatric scales.

Materials and methods

The study included80 cases i.e. 20 cases of acne excoriee, 20 cases of macular amyloidosis and lichen amyloidosis, 20 cases of lichen planus and 20 controls. Patients with previously diagnosed psychiatric disease and those on any psychiatric medications were excluded from this study. Controls were normal people who were not suffering from any skin disease.

All subjects included in the study were subjected to a detailed history including history and examination. Detailed psychological evaluation was done using the following scales with the help of a psychiatrist-

1) Hamilton rating scale for depression.(134)

2) Hamilton anxiety rating scale.(135)

3) Gurmeet Singh's Presumptive Stressful Life Events Scale.(136)

Skin biopsy was performed for confirmation of diagnosis for patients of lichen planus, macular amyloidosis and lichen amyloidosis.

The data was analyzed statistically using various tests like Pearson's(chi)2, Fischer's, t-test and p-value of < 0.05 was considered significant.

Results

- The mean age (standard deviation [SD]) in acne excoriée, lichen and macular amyloidosis, lichen planus, and controls were 25.2 [5.5], 39.4 [12.7], 35.7 [14.1], and 38.5 [11.6] years respectively (p<0.001).

- Sex distribution of cases

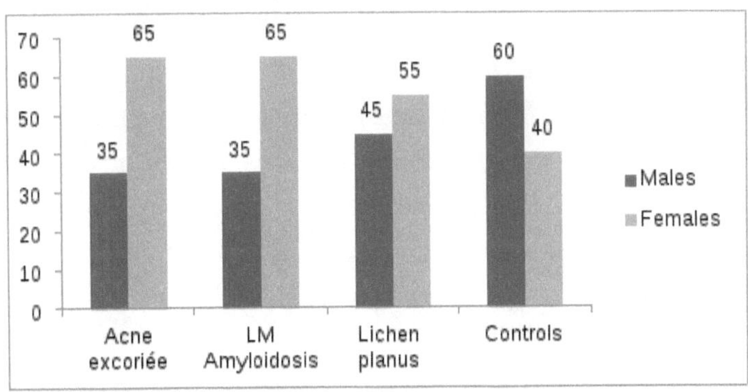

Out of total 80 subjects, 41.2 % are males while 58.8 % are females.

Since the p-value is 0.528 which is greater than the significance level (0.05), we conclude that there is no relationship between sex and cutaneous diagnosis groups.

- The differences in the mean depression scores were statistically significant($p < 0.001$) across these four groups.

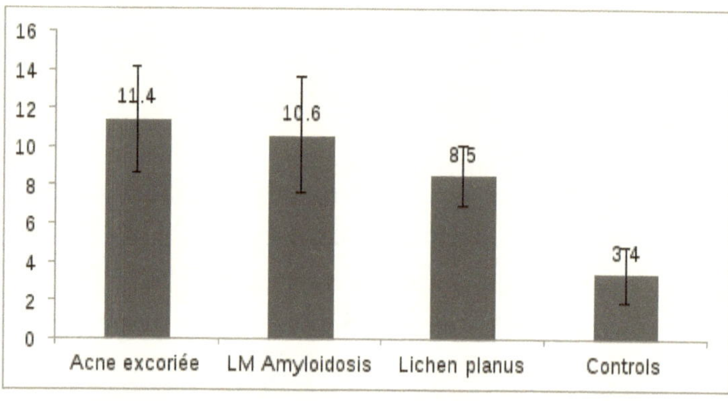

Financial stress was reported by 70% of acne excoriée, 65% of lichen and macular amyloidosis, 50% of lichen planus cases, and by 20% controls (p=0.007). Marital conflicts were reported by 60% of lichen and macular amyloidosis, 45% of acne excoriée, 30% of lichen planus cases, and by 10% controls (p=0.007). Similarly, family conflicts were reported by 70% of lichen and macular amyloidosis, 50% lichen planus, 40% of acne excoriée cases, and none of the controls (p<0.001).

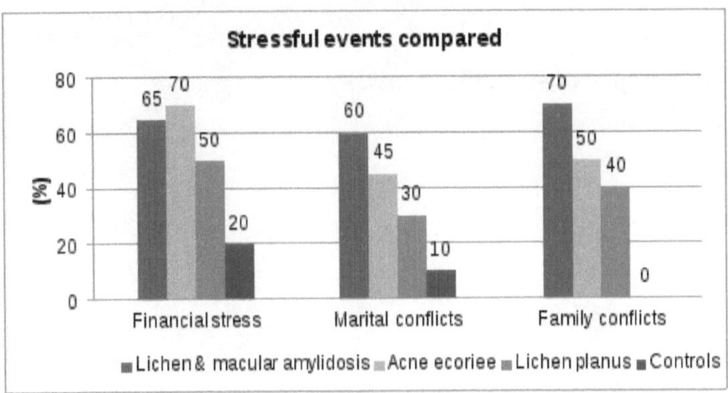

In the adjusted models, the mean depression scores were significantly higher in patients presenting with lichen and macular amyloidosis (6.03, 95% confidence intervals [CI]: 0.73, 11.34, p=0.03), and lichen planus (5.87, 95% CI: 1.60, 10.15, p=0.008) compared with controls.

There were no significant differences in mean depression scores in patients with acne excoriée compared with controls (3.25, 95% CI: -1.70, 8.19, p=0.19).

None of the stressful events (death, marital problem, family concerns, financial concerns, others) were significantly associated with high depression scores. Among clinical cases, the mean depression scores were significantly higher in those who had lesions on the scalp (11.83, 95% CI: 3.60, 20.07, p=0.006) and oral cavity (7.01, 95% CI: 1.58, 12.44, p=0.01).

Conclusions:

Lichen and macular amyloidosis, and lichen planus were independently associated with high depression scores.Interestingly, such an association was not found in acne excoriée patients. Thus, regular screening and management of depression, irrespective of the presence or absence of stressful events, may be warranted.

KAP of pharmacists to the prescription of Psychotropic drugs prescribed by the Dermatologists in Mumbai

Ram Malkani, Komal Parekh, Manindersingh Setia

Accepted as a Poster at the Annual conference of the European Society of Dermatologists and Psychiatrists (ESDaP) at Giesson, Germany, on June 20,2019

Background:

The present study was conducted to assess the attitudes and behaviours of pharmacists towards dispensing psychotropic medications to patients who have been prescribed these medications by dermatologists in Mumbai, India.Methods: We conducted structured interviews in 81 pharmacists across various geographical regions in Mumbai. The responses to statements were collected on a 5-point Likert Scale (strongly disagree to strongly agree). The means were compared using t-test or Analysis of Variance, and the proportions using chi square test.Results: The mean (SD) age was 32.4 (10.9) years; 72 (89%) were male and nine (11%) were female. The median (IQR) years of experience was 5 (2, 14.5) years. About 45% of pharmacists received prescription of psychotropic drugs from dermatologists; however, 32% of these were not comfortable that they are prescribing them. About 68% were agreed that psychological factors can lead to skin conditions including eczema and itching. About 46% agreed that they have a right to refuse the prescribed medication; of these, 41% refused to give medication to patient. Pharmacists who disagreed with statement that psychological stress can lead to skin conditions were more likely to discourage psychotropic prescription from dermatologists (33% vs 11%, p<0.001).Conclusion: Awareness and education among pharmacists will be an important intervention for appropriate dispensing of psychotropic medications in patients with dermatological conditions in India. This can be done by including them in psycho-dermatological conferences and teaching programmes.

Psychological profile of patients presenting with dermatological complaints:
A cross-sectional study

Ram Malkani, Komal Parekh, Suman Karmarkar, Maninder Singh Setia

Accepted as oral presentation at the Annual Conference of the European Society of Dermatology and Psychiatry (ESDaP), Giesson, Germany, June 20-22, 2019

Objectives:

The present study was conducted to evaluate the psychological profile in patients presenting to a dermatological clinic in Mumbai, IndiaMethods: We evaluated anxiety, depression, stress, anger, body image, and relationships in63 patients presenting with dermatological complaints. We used linear regression models formultivariate analyses for co-efficient and 95% confidence intervals [CI].Results: The mean age (standard deviation [SD]) was 37.4 (14.9) years; 30 (51%) were females and 31 (49%) were males. The common diagnoses were papulosquamous conditions (24%), acne (18%), hair fall (15%), pigmentary conditions (11%), pruritus (10%), and infection (8%). Mean (SD) anxiety scores were highest in pigmentary conditions (11.6 [13.9]), depression (15.0 [5.0]) and post-traumatic stress scores (16.3 [25.6]) in pigmentary conditions, social phobia scores in allergy (21.8 [17.0]), and anger scores in acne (25.4 [6.3]). Mean (SD) family scores were lowest in pruritus (8.0 4.2]), body image in infection (3.6 [0.9]), self-image in pigmentation (6.0 [2.3]). Mean social phobia scores were significantly higher in allergy compared with acne (12.2, 95% CI: 1.6, 22.8, p=0.02). Body images scores were lower in pruritus (-7.7, 95% CI: -14.5, -0.9, p=0.03).Conclusion: The psychological parameters differ in various dermatological conditions; hence a complete profile analyses will be useful for designing interventions in these patients.

Genodermatosis

Congenital Lip Pits

Vandana Punjabi, Ram Malkani

Presented at the clinical meeting of Jaslok Hospital & Research Centre on Nov' 21 -2003

Definition - Congenital Lip Pits

- Congenital Lip Pits are hereditary, developmental defects which are found clinically as unilateral or bilateral depressions, most commonly located on the lower lip vermilion border

- Small accessory or heterotopic salivary glands empty into sinuses or fistulas in the lip

Family History

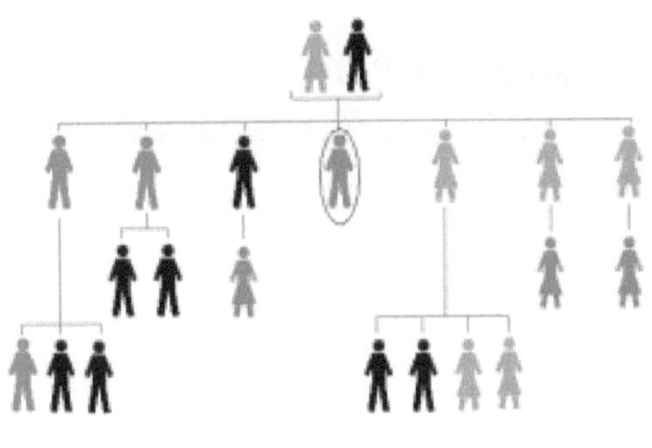

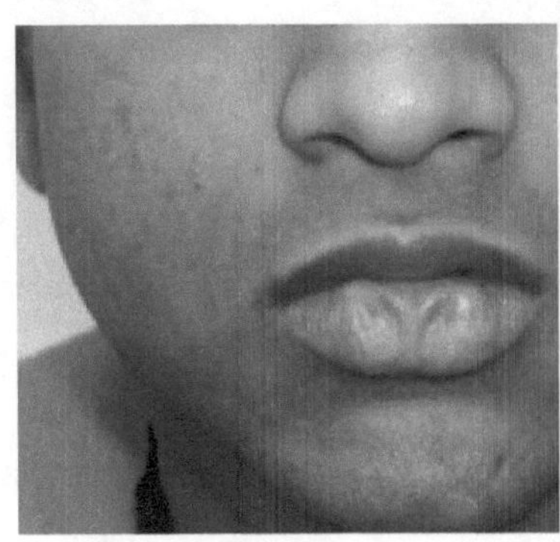

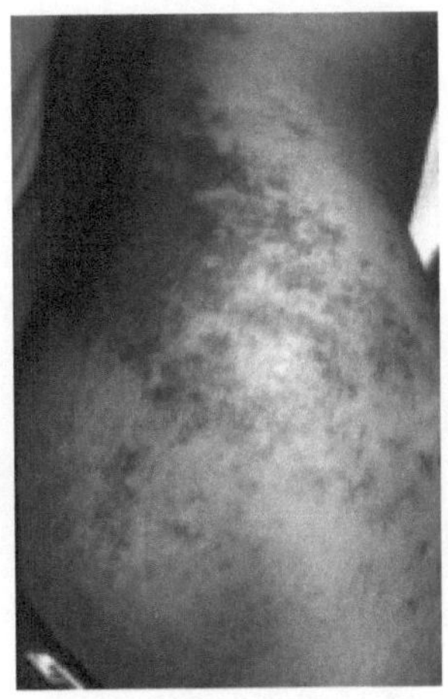

Etiology & Treatment
Etiology

- Hereditary
- Autosomal Dominant Trait

Treatment

• Surgical Correction for Cosmetic Purposes

Occurance of Congenital Lip Pits

May be seen as an isolated defect or with other associated congenital anomalies as

Hypodontia

Absence of second premolars

Natal teeth

Ankyloglossia

Syndactyly

Equinovarus foot deformity

Congenital heart disease

Kindler Weary Syndrome

Priyanka Ghuge, Rahul Bade, R. H. Malkani

Presented at IADVL Mahahrashtra Annual Conference; CUTICON2012

We present you a case of a 17/M who presented to the dermatology OPD with chief c/o multiple fluid lesions over extremities since childhood. H/o exacerbation of the lesions especially during summers. H/o mottled pigmentation all over body since several years. H/s/o photosensitivity since childhood. The lesions started over the dorsum of the hands and the feet, 16 yrs back, gradually involving the forearms and the legs. The lesions would heal gradually with scarring.

The frequency of occurrence of the blisters is gradually decreasing since 3-4 yrs.No h/o similar complaints in the family. No h/o facial erythema, recurrent infections, weight loss. No h/s/o any neurologic abnormalities. No h/s/o any eye or ear involvement. O/e reticulate hyper pigmented and hypo pigmented areas all over the body, marked especially in the sun exposed regions, also associated with telengectasias. Nasal/oral mucosa: normal.

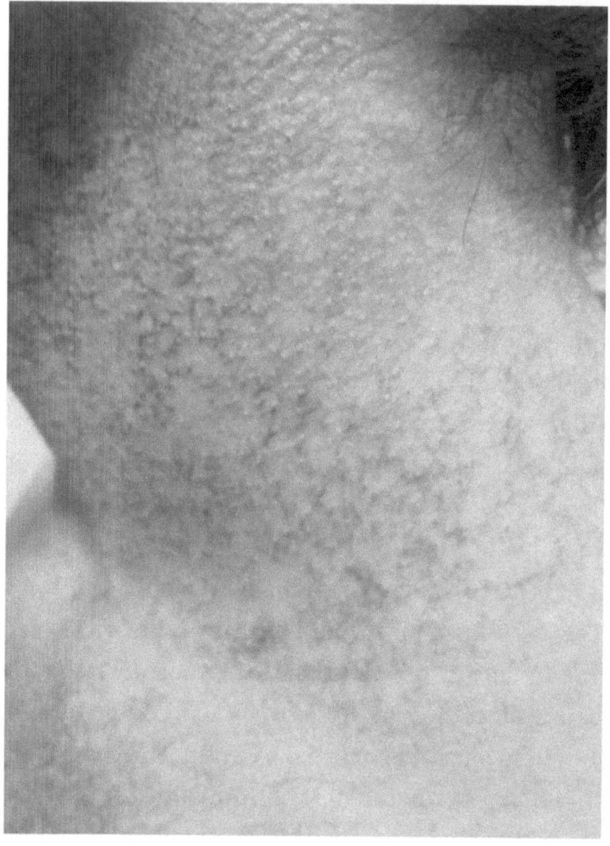

The major criteria for diagnosis of Weary Kindler Syndrome are acral blistering in infancy and childhood, progressive poikiloderma, skin atrophy, photosensitivity, and gingival fragility, and/or swelling. According to the proposed criteria, the presence of four major criteria makes the diagnosis certain. Thus the diagnosis of Weary Kindler Syndrome was considered based on the clinical criteria. Sample for genetic mapping was sent to confirm diagnosis.

We present this case for its rarity.

Skin and Systemic Disease

Case of Pyoderma Gangrenosum

Ram H Malkani

Clinical meeting of the Jaslok Hospital & Research Centre, Mumbai on April 25 1983

ABSTRACT:

We present a case of pyoderma gangrenosumfollowing folliculitis of legs

CASE REPORT:

A Patient presented to the dermatology OPD with an ulcer over the medial aspect of left leg since 45 days which started as a small pus filled lesion with the hair in the centre which he handled andpressed it manually and removed the pus following which over a period of 1 week another similar lesion developed adjacent to it which also was handled.

The boil broke open and became an ulcer which stared to increase in size. He had taken oral medications and applied topical medications for the same. However the ulcer increased in size inspite of treatment and gradually progressed to the present stage.

No H/O DM/ HTN/TB/ATOPY

On eaxamination Ulcer was seen over the medial aspect of the left leg around 5 inches above the medial malleolus. Ulcer is well defined punched out with raised margins with slough in the centre. Tender to touch. Patient is a chronic smoker (1-2 cig per day) and occasionally consumes alcohol. No h/o DM OR Hypertension Investigations:

HB – 18.3 gm%

PCV – 55

WBC – 7450

NEUTROPHILS   –   57%
LYMPHOCYTES – 33%

PLATELET COUNT – 1,44,000

MONOCYTES   –   5%EOSINOPHILS – 5%

RBC – 6.04 MILLION

ESR – 03 MM/HR

TOTAL BILIRUBIN2.2mg/dl (0.2 – 1.4)

SGOT- 61.3SGPT – 59.8(5-40)

GAMMA GT 87.2 (5 - 75)

G6PD – 5199 (4600 – 13500)

RETICULOCYTES 1.0 (0.2 – 2.0%)

GLCOSYLATED HB – 14.5% (4 – 7%)

HBsAG- NON REACTIVE

HIV 1& 2 – NON REACTIVE

HCV –NONREACTIVE

URINE   ALBUMIN   – PRESENT(+)

URINR SUGAR – 0.5g/dl

PUS CELL – 5-6/ hpf

Rbc – 1-2 /hpf

GRANULAR CASTS OCC SEEN IN URINE

CHEST X-RAY AND ECG - WNL

CONCLUSION:

The focus of this case report is to create awareness towards presentation of diabetes mellitus as a pyoderma gangrenosum as an initial finding without any medical complaints.

Reiter's Syndrome

Ram Malkani, Ajay Kumar

Bulletin of the Jaslok Hospital & Research Centre Vol XIII Vol 1 July 1988.

DEFINITION

Reiter's Syndrome is classically defined as the triad of nongonococcal Urethritis, Conjunctivitis and Arthritis(1,2) These symptoms are present concomitantly or sequentially in 90% of the patients. Mucocutaneous lesions are present in 80% of the patients and thus constitute the rationale for considering it a clinical tetrad. Incomplete Reiter's syndrome oc-curs when all features are not expressed.(3) The recent definition of American Rheumatism Association is an episode of peripheral arthritis of more than one month's duration occuring in association with urethritis and/or cervicitis.(4) A more mechanistic concept is that of a reactive arthritis following enteric and possibly sexually transmitted infection in the genetically predisposed host. More recent findings have however made broader definitions necessary.

HISTORICAL ASPECTS

In 1784 association between urethritis and arthritis was first reported by Swediaur.(5) Brodie in 1818 described the association with conjunctivitis.(5) Keratoderma blenorrhagica was introduced as a term in 1896. In 1916 Fiesinger and Leroy observed a conjunctivo-urethro-synovial syndrome in four French soldiers following dysentry. One week later Ham Reiter described the same syndrome along with dermititis in a young German Officer.(1) Paronen in 1944 established the link with Shigellaflexneri. A genetic predisposition was established in 1973 with demonstration in asssociation with HLA B27.

EPIDEMIOLOGY

The disease affects predominantly males between the ages of 15 and 35 years. Females account for 5-10 percent of cases. Caucasions are more commonly affected. It is rare in orientals and blacks. Due to its sporadic occurence, self limited course and incomplete forms true incidence is difficult to estimate.'9'

Two types of the disease occur the epidemic form of the disease linked to post dysentry usually occurs in Europe and North Africa. Endemic disease often attributed to venereal exposure is the major form reported from the United States and United Kingdom.(9) 1-2% of patients with non-specific urethritis develop Reiter's Syndrome. The risk is similar after dysentery.

ETIOLOGY AND PATHOGENESIS

The etiopathogenesis of Reiter's syndrome includes a genetic risk factor and an infectious triggering agent but, the mechanism underlying the inflammatory process is not yet elucidated. The skin and joint lesions are typically sterile.

It is currently presumed that the mechanism is one of immunologically mediated tissue injury.

GENETIC PREDISPOSITIONS

There is close clinical and genetic interrelationship between Reiter's syndrome, ankylosing spondylitis, psoriasis and psoriatic arthritis.(10) HLA-B27 occurs in 63 to 75 percent of Caucasians with Reiter's syndrome and in 8 percent of normal whites.(8) B27 negative patients have significantly less sacroilitis uveitis and carditis and generally the disease pursues a milder course. B27 individuals exposed to causative enteric pathogens have a 20 percent risk for Reiter's disease. There is a 10 percent prevalence of Reiter's disease among relatives of proband with the same disorder.

INFECTIOUS AGENTS

The list of enteric pathogens that trigger a reactive arthritis include *Shigella flexneri* (but not S. sonnet) *Salmonella enteriiidis, Salmonella typhimurium* and *Salmonella Heidelberg, Yersinia enterocolitica* and *Yersinia pseudotuberculosis* and Campylobacter fetus.(1-n<n) No antigenic factor common to all of them has been identified. A formalin killed strain of Yersinia which adheres to the lympocyte at the HLA antigen site has been shown in vitro to stimulate T lymphocytes.(13)

The hypothesis of veneral transmissions has not yet been proved and pivots on the presence of urethritis and the assumption that it is sexually acquired.(4) Urethral inflammation, is however an inherent mucocutaneous manifestation occuring even in post dysenteric cases with no evident sexual exposure. *Chlamydia trachomatis* is found in 37 percent of the cases. *Ureoplasma urealyticum* is also implicated.

CLINICAL FEATURES

The disease is characterised by active episodes that last an average of 3 months but may remit as early as 2 weeks and may last as long as one year. Recurrances occur in 40% cases and are often multiple.

Only one third of the cases have the complete triad and 40% will have arthritis as the only feature.

MUSCULOSKELETAL

The arthritis is typically oligoarticular and is the most constant clinical feature. It is asymmetric and involves 1-6 joints, more often in the lower limb heel with pain as a common feature.

GENITOURINARY

Mild to moderate dysuria with a transient mucopurulent discharge is usual. Pyuria and haematuria often occur. Cystitis, pro-statitis and seminal vesiculitis occasionally occur. Cervicitis and vaginitis may be noted.

OCCULAR

A mild, evanescent, usually bilateral non bacterial conjunctivitis is noted. Acute anterior uveitis is seen in 20% and Keratitis may also occur.

MUCOCUTANEOUS

Keratodermia blennorrhagica - It is seen in about 30% of the cases and occurs most frequently on the soles, toes and glans penis. It most often begins as an erythematous pinpoint macule that vesiculates, becomes purulent and develops a thick keratotic cover. Enlargement and papule formation is accompanied by a pustular centre, thickening hyperkeratosis and crusting. Heaped up lesions may resemble musk shells. Scaling plaques may develop on the scalp and over elbows, knees, buttocks and any other area. Erosive, exudative patches often are found on the penile shaft. Involvement may be widespread and may be indistinguishable from pustular psoriasis. Keratoderma may last from weeks to months

BALANITIS

It occurs independent of urethritis and is the most common mucocutaneous lesion occuring in 23-50% of patients. A small vesicle appears and later ruptures to form a painless superficial erosion of the coronal margin of the prepuce and nearby glans. Coalescence results in circinate pattern. In circumcised patients a hard crust may form whereas lesions remain moist in non circumcised patients. The duration varies from days to years.

Oral mucosa shows typically painless erythema, vesicle, erosion on the palate, tongue, buccal mucosa, lips or gums. Pharnynx or nasal mucosa may be similarly involved. These lesions lasting only a few days are seen in 40% of the patients.

NAIL CHANGES

They appear in the form of small yellow pustules below the nails, which enlarge dessicate and show brownish discolouration and become ridged and brittle and may later shed. Surrounding erythemia and scaling are seen (Pseudo paronychia).

OTHER FEATURES

The patient often presents with fever. Cardiovascular involvement includes conduction defects and aortic insufficiency.(15) Neurological disease(15) consisting of acute meningoencephalitis, acute pyschotic reactions and polyneuritis may occur. Amyloidosis rarely occurs.(16)

LABORATORY FEATURES

There is no specific laboratory test for Reiter's syndrome. The haematological abnormalities in order of frequency are, elevated E.S.R., Anaemia, Leucocytosis and thrombocytosis. 73%of cases are positive for HLA-B27 the Rheumatoid factor is absent. Synovial fluid is turbid and yellow with increased protein, elevated complement and leucocytosis. Rarely Reiter's cells Macrophages containing ingested polymorphs may be found in it. Serum proteins may show no abnormality or there may be non specific decrease in albumin and increase in alpha 2 globulin. Radiography may reveal periostitis and sacroilitis. The urine culture is usually sterile. A circulating antibody to prostatic fluid has been demonstrated.(8)

PATHOLOGY

Keratoderma exhibits the presence of elongation and hypertrophy of rete ridges. There is neutrophilic epidermal and dermal infilteration. There is hyperkeratosis and parakeratosis with microabscesses and spongiform pustules. Differentiation from pustulae psoriasis is difficult.

DIFFERENTIAL DIAGNOSIS

Gonococcal urethritis has to be excluded by smear and cultures. Rheumatoid, gonococcal and psoriatic arthritis require consideration. Behcet's disease has deeper and more painful orogenital ulcers and a vasculitic skin rash. Acute rheumatic fever and serum sickness mimic the clinical picture.

COURSE AND PROGNOSIS

Arthritis is the most serious and disabling feature. Most of the cases are self limiting in three months to one year. A third of patients have recurrent attacks. Deformities rarely develop. Death may rarely occur from cardiac involvement or amyloidosis. Repeated uveitis may impair vision.

TREATMENT

The aim of therapy should be to suppress articular inflamation and prevent deformities. During the acute phase, bed rest and joint splinting may be necessary. Non steroidal and inflammatory drugs are more useful than salicylates. Response to phenylbutazone is often dramatic. Metho-trexate usage may be necessary to control skin and joint disease. Physiotherapy prevents deformity and maintains function, A trial of Tetracycline or Erythro-mycin may be warrented though it is unclear whether it alters the course of the disease.

CASE I

A male patient aged 50 years, working in a Veterinary Hospital for the last 20 years was admitted to the hospital with complaints of multiple skin lesions all over the body for over the last two months, swelling of knee and ankle joints for the last 1½ months and fever for the last 15 days.

Swelling first appeared in the knee joint and then in the ankle joint. The swelling had been gradually increasing and the patient found it extremely difficult to walk because of the pain and swelling.

The skin lesions were asymptomatic. There were many isolated skin lesions on the scalp and upper extremity, few on the upper trunk and upper extremity and a large geographic plaque covering the whole of lower abdomen and perineum. In the past, personal and family history presented nothing significant. There was no history of exposure. The patient was poorly built and poorly nourished and looked cachexic. The patient had high fever which was intermittent in nature and there were no accompanying symptoms. The systemic examination showed no abnormality. Both the knees and ankles showed tender swelling with moderate effusion. The movements at both the knees and ankles were restricted and extremely painful. The skin lesions were hyperpigmented, with hyperkeratotic plaques with circular collarrete scaling at the periphery. There were many such isolated lesions on the scalp and lower extremity, few on the upper extremity and upper trunk. The lower abdomen and the perineum were covered with hyperpigmented and hyper keratotic scales with extremely well demarcated borders, Patient had moderate phimosis with purulent discharge seen at the tip. There was evidence of Tinea pedis between two toes in the right foot.

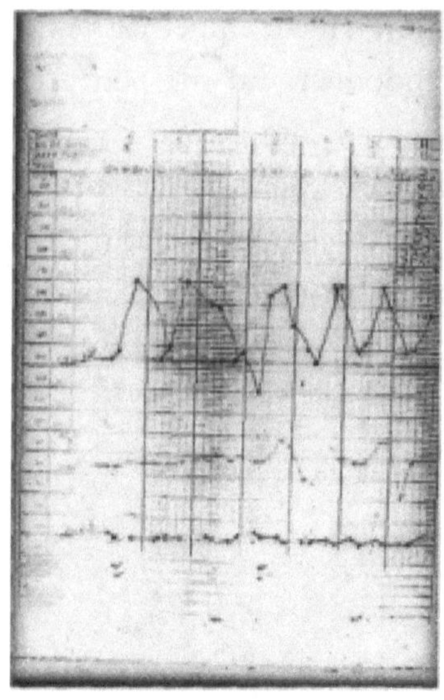

Fig 1 temperature pattern of the patient

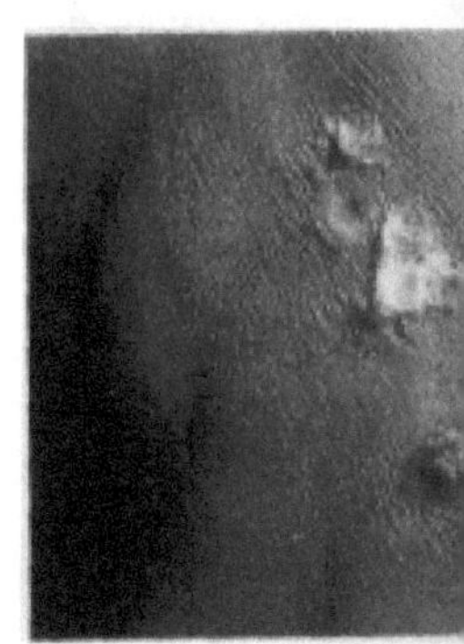

Fig. 2. Papule with Kerato

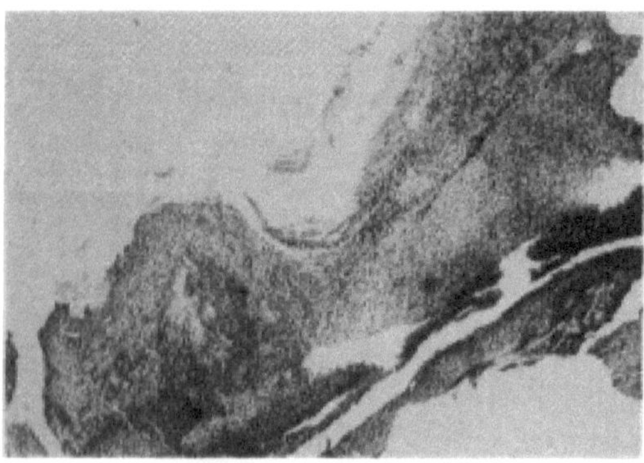

Fig. 3 Histopathology under lower power

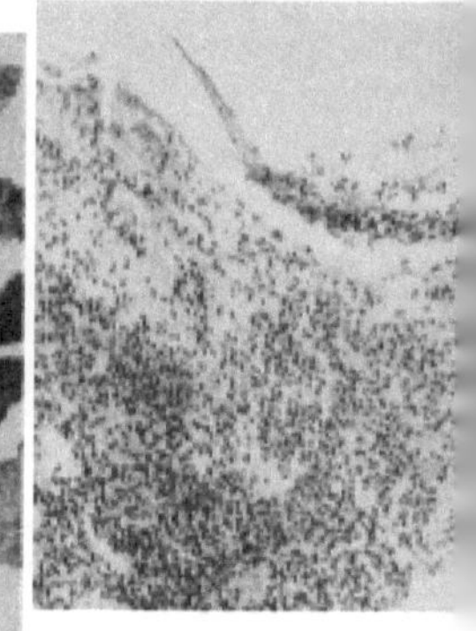

Fig. 4 High power view
polymorphonuclear absces.

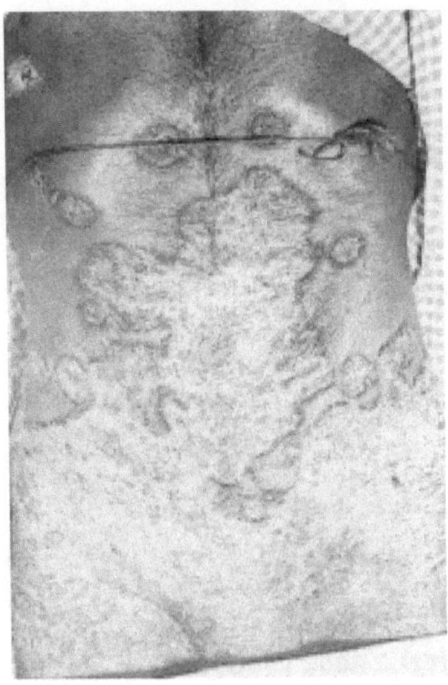

Fig. 5 Lesions resolving with therapy

The patient was investigated his Haemoglobin was 10.8 gms% and E.S.R. was 56 mm, in 1st hour. Total and Differential W.B.C. counts were normal. Urine analysis revealed 2-3 W.B.G. per HPF and Urine culture revealed growth of *Eschericha coli* and *Proteus mirabilis*. L.E. Cell test and Rheumatoid factor were found to be Negative. Serum Protein Electrophoresis revealed Total Proteins to be; 7.2 gms%, Albumin 2.0 gms, Alpha globulin 0.6 gm%, Alpha2 globulin 2.8 gms%. Radiologically the knee ankle and sacroiliac joints and chest were normal. There was no growth in his blood culture. His ECG was normal. HLA typing studies revealed HLA B2?. His VDRL was 1:8 positive. Skin biopsy revealed hyperkeratosis with evidence of corneal abscesses consisting of polymorphs, with evidence of spongiform pustule of Kogoj at one place and hence diagnosis of Reiter's syndrome was arrived at. He was given aspirin and oxypenbutazone initially, upon which his articular inflammation came down. Indomethacin was later added but the patient had recurranees of his joint complaints. Subsequently the patient was put on oral corticosteroids with prednisolone being given in the dose of 60 mg daily in 2 divided doses for three weeks on which the patient showed complete remission of articular complaints. His cutaneous complaints also improved markedly. Injectable long acting penicillin once a week for three weeks and oral Tetracycline 250 mg thrice a day for one week were also administered. Supportive therapy with Vit. C and B Complex was also instituted. Penicillin was given in view of the positive V.D.R.L. report. In the absence of lack of facility for specific test for syphilis, he was treated for syphilis. Tetracyclines were given for treating Chlamydia infection in the urethra emperically, as the specialised tests for confirming the presence of Chlamydia were not available.

CASE 2

A 27 year old resident of Saudi Arabia presented with the complaint of generalised rash on the body of eight months duration. The Psoriasiform scaling plaques initially manifested on the genitals and later spread to the elbows, trunk and the scalp. He gave a positive history of exposure three years prior to this, following which he had a complaint of purulent discharge from urethra which was not subjected to any investigation but responded to therapy with antibiotics. Few weeks after this episode the eruptions occurred on the genitals. His systemic examination did not reveal any positive finding. He gave no history of joint or eye complaints. He had no evidence of balanitis or nail changes.

The patient was investigated. His Blood counts, Urine analysis and E.S.R. were normal, V.D.R.L. and Rheumatoid factor were Negative and his Serum biochemistry profile (SMA 6/60) was within normal limits. Serum Protein Electrophoresis revealed Total Proteins 7.2 gms%, Albumin 2.5 gms% and Gamma Globulin 2.1 gms%. His urine culture was sterile. Biopsy of the skin lesions showed the rete ridges to be elongated with epidermal neutrophilic infilteration forming microabscesses. Stratum corneum showed hyperkeratosis and parakeratosis.

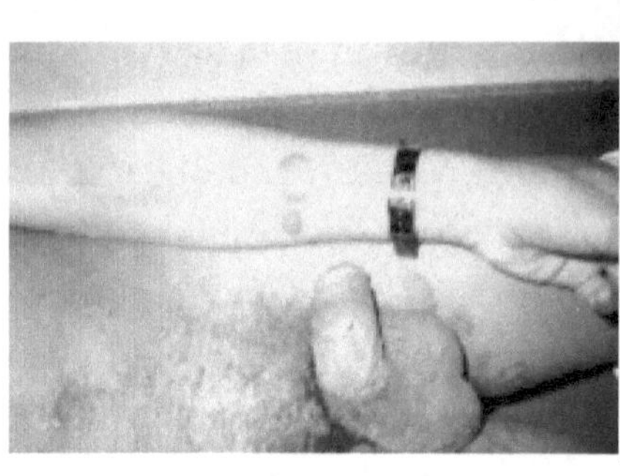

Fig. 1 Keratotic papule on the arm

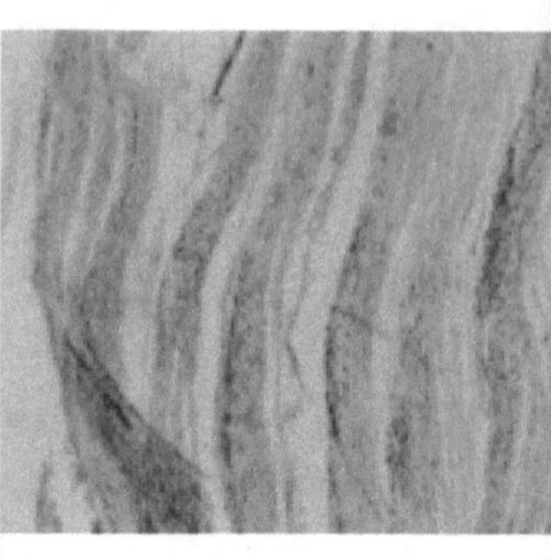

Fig. 2 Low power view of his. showing nuclear dust in pe epidermis

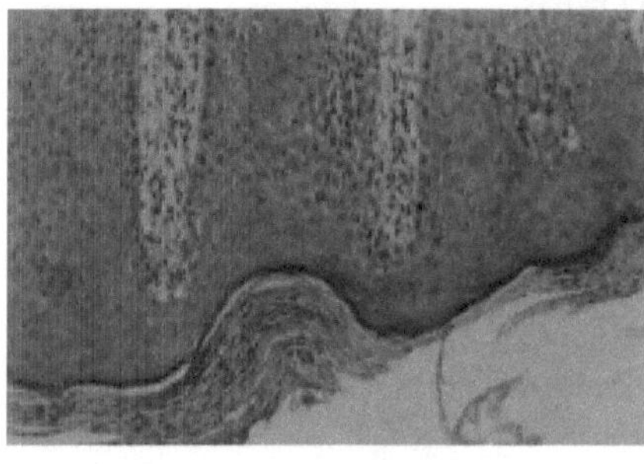

Fig. 3 Histopathology showing elongated rete ridges and epidermal neutrophil infilteration

The patient was given PUV/ with 2 Tab. Melanocyl folk hours later with sun exp 10-15 minutes. The patien respond satisfactorily to thi He was then put on Met orally in the dose of 2.5 mg 3 doses 12 hours apart repea week for 12 weeks. The lesions disappeared on this schedule.

REFERENCE

1. Reiter H: Dentsch Med Wochenschr 42: 1536, 1916.*

9. Masi A T, Medsga A Jr: Clin Orthop 143 1979.

10. Moll JMH et Medicine (Baltimore) 343, 1974.

2. Baner W., Engleman EP: Trans Assoc Am Physicians 57:307, 1942.*

3. Arnett F C et al: Ann Interm Med 84:8, 1976.

4. Willkens R F et al: Reiters syndrome Ar thritis Rheum 24:844, 1981.

5. Brodie B C: London, Longman, Hurst, Rees Orme and Brown 1818 P 54.

6. Benedek T G., Rodman G P: Bull Rheu dis 32:59, 1982.

7. Paronen I: Acta Med Scand (Suppl) 212:1, 1948*

8. Brewerton D A et al: Lancet 2:996, 1973.

11. Neer H R: JAMA 198: 693, 1966.

12. Aho K et al: Arthritis Rheum 17:521, 974.

13. Bremer M B et al: Arthritis Rheum 25: 563, 1982.

14. Ford D.K., Rasmussen G: Arthritis Rheum 7: 220, 1964.

15. Good A.E.: Arthritis Rheumatol 3:253, 1974.

16. Miller L D et al: J Rheumatol 6: 225, 1979.

17. Csonha et al: BMJ 1:243, 1958.

18. Bartholomew L E: Arthritis Rheum 8:376, 1973.

Pyoderma Gangrenosum

Ram Malkani, Ajay Kumar

Bulletin of the Jaslok Hospital & Research Centre Vol XIV No. 4 April 1990 p.41.

Definition:

Pyoderma Gangrenosum (PG) is a rare destructive, inflammatory necrotising, idiopathic ulceration of the skin which presents as a nodule or pustule which breaks down to form a progressively enlarging ulcer with a raised tender undermined border. Lesions may be solitary or multiple and may be associated with systemic disease such as ulcerative collitis, Crohn's disease, polyarthritis or gammopathy.

History:

Brunsting, Goeckerman and O'leary discribed Pyoderma Gangrenosum PG in 1930(1) Four of the five cases described had chronic ulcerative collitis. Staphylococci and haemolytic Streptocicci were cultured from the ulcers and the disease was therefore thought to be an infection.

Etiology and Pathogenesis:

Although bacteria can be easily cultured from the ulcers, the fact that initial pustules are consistently sterile proves that the infection is secondary. The phenomenon of pathergy which describes the development of new lesions following trivial trauma suggests altered, exaggerated and uncontrolled inflammatory response to non specific stimuli. A circulatory dermonecrotic factor described in serum of PG patients, is capable of inducing necrosis in guinea pig skin, but its pathogenic significance in humans is not clear. PG has been considered an example of Schwartzman's reaction but the idea has been abandoned. The most impelling evidence of a defective immune mechanism lies in the considerable number of cases that have now been reported with associated gammopathies, paraproteins and other disorders of the reticulo endothelial system such as T-cell imbalances or failure of phagocytosis by monocytes. No consistant pattern of immunological disturbance has emerged so far. Thus although evidence suggests that disturbances of immunoregulation and immunologic effector functions occur in some patients with PG, they are not detectable disorders, and it is not at all clear whether they represent an epiphenomenon only.

Clinical Manifestations:

The disease can occur at any age and involves females by almost two to one ratio. Although the lesions may occur anywhere they favour lower extremities and are usually multiple and painful. The early lesion is a red papule or plaque that evolves with a papulovesicle or pustule with central necrosis within hours. Ulceration follows within 1-2 days. This rapid evolultion is a distinctive but inconsistent feature.

The Salient feature of PG is an irregular, ulcer with a raised inflammatory border and a boggy necrotic base . The borders of the ulcer are well defined because of their striking blue colour, and are boggy and undermined. A halo of bright erythema surrounds the margin of an advancing ulceration which may extend rapidly in one direction and more slowly in another so that a serpigenous configuration of the ulcer results. The base is partially covered with necrotic material, is irregular and granulating and studded with small abscesses. The ulcers may extend into the fat and fascia.

Healing usually occurs spontaneously, resulting in a thin atrophic, usually cribriforms scar. Almost invariably the lessons are painful. Considerable toxicity and a sustained fever may occur in the course of the active disease.

The term pathergy describes the phenomenon of trivial trauma provoking new lesions or aggravating existing ones. It occurs in about 20 percent of the patients and pricks, needles, biopsies or operations may induce new lesions. Potassium iodide may also induce an exacerbation.

Associated Diseases:

Pyoderma gangrenosum may occur as a disease confined to the skin in 40 to 50 percent of the cases (idiopathic PG)(5). It may also be associated with a variety of conditions, the heterogenecity of which makes pinpointing of a common denominator responsible for such associations difficult. Chronic ulcerative collitis is noted most frequently. Other associated gastrointestinal diseases include Crohn's disease, diverticulitis, diverticulosis, and chronic active hepatitis. Arthritis, Paraproteinemia, myeloma, leukemia and Behcet's Syndrome have also been reported to be associated.

Histopathology:

The histopathologic findings are non diagnostic and serve only to exclude other diagnostic possibilities. Ulcerative lesions are characterised by loss of epidermis centrally and acanthesis laterally. There is extensive necrosis centrally and edema haemorrhages and mixed inflammatory infilterate peripherally. Immunoreactants (Ig M C3 and fibrin) in the papillary and dermal vessels of 46 per cent of 37 patients have been demonstrated. The findings confirm a pathogenic role of immune complex vasculitis in the evolution of PG lesions.

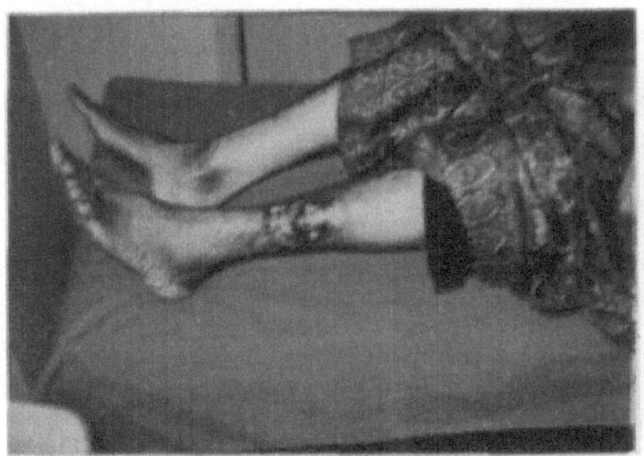

Fig. 1. Large irregular ulcer with necrotic base.

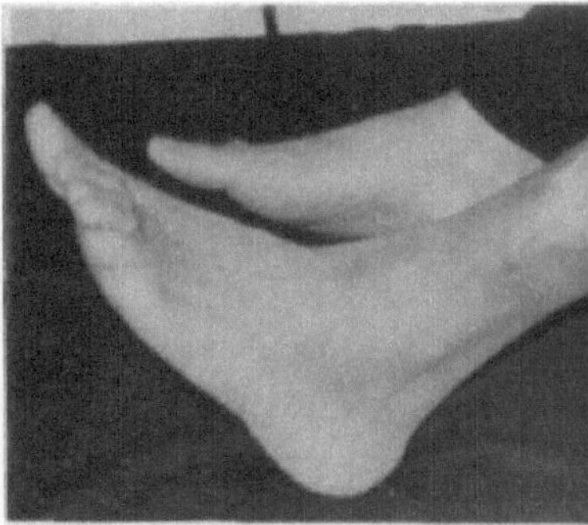

Fig. 3. Resolving Lesion

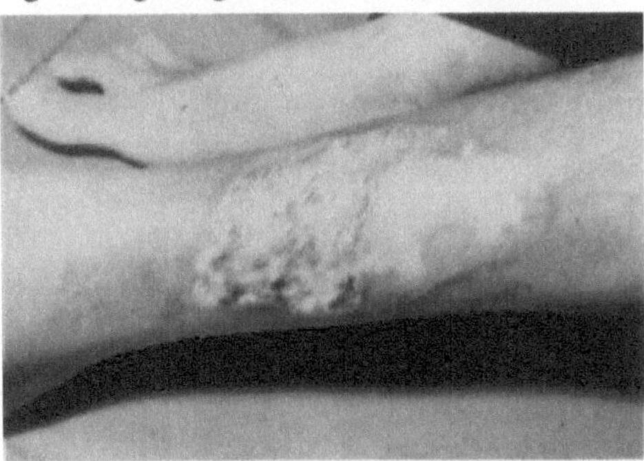

Fig. 2. Lesion showing signs of improvement on therapy

Treatment:

In patients with underlying disease, therapy should be directed not only to PG but also to control the systemic disorders. Since the pathogenesis is unknown specific therapy is not available. Bed rest and adequate nutrition are essential. Soaks with potassium permangnate or acetic acid help maintain cleanliness. Injection of triamcinolone, 10 mg/ml into the rim of the ulcer is often helpful. Grafting and vigorous debridement should be avoided as trauma may aggravate the disease. If local measures are inadequate, systemic corticosteroids are indicated. They may be used alone or with cyclophosphamide and azothiaprim. Pulse therapy with suprapharmacological doses has been successfully tried. Clofizamine has given good results recently. Hyperbaric oxygen has been occassionally found helpful.

Prognosis:

Although eventual prognosis is good, the disease persists for years with remissions and exacerbations.

Case 1:

A 49 year old female patient presented with a non healing, painful tender ulcer on the lower third of her left leg. The ulcer was large, irregular is shape with whitish necrotic base, reddish blue margins and a rough undermined edge. She also had complaints of pain in multiple joints. Investigations revealed her haemoglobin level to be 9.2 gm%. E.S.R. was 62 mm/hr. Her Rheumatoid factor was positive 320 dilutions (more than 40 is significant). Radiograph of the chest, abdomen and barium studies of intestines were normal. Serum protein electrophoresis revealed low albumin and raised globulins. Serum Iron was 88mg percent. Biopsy of the lesion revealed neutrophilic abscess with dilated, blood vessels in the dermis. She was prescribed prednisolone 20mg per day, potassium permangnate soaks and cortisone cream. Supportive therapy with oral iron was instituted. The ulcer healed in 8 months but recured 9 months later. As oral and topical steroids did not help her she was advised dapsone 200mg/day and later cyclophosphamide 100mg/day upon which the ulcer showed signs of healing.

Case 2:

An Eighteen year old girl presented with multiple ulcers on different sites of the body of two years duration. Initialy, she had developed a single module on her right leg which ulcerated and later similar multiple lesions developed elsewhere. She was diagnosed as a case of vasculitis earlier and given oral steroids, dapsone, cyclophosphamide, besides carrying out multiple skin grafts. The borders of the ulcer were well defined, blue red, edematous with undermined edges. The margins were studded with pustules. The base was moist, purulent and covered with granulation tissue. Her systemic examination was normal. Investivations revealed haemoglobin level of 8.4 gm. Reticulocyte count 20% E.S.R. of 41 mm/hr, and Leucocytosis. Biopsy revealed large neutrophilic micro abscesses surrounded by granulation tissue with no evidence of vasculitis. She was treated with oral prednisolone 15mg/day, dapsone 100 mg/day and supportive therapy with iron and vitamins. The ulcer showed signs of healing in 4 months time.

References:

1. Brunsting LA et al: Pyoderma gangrenosum: Clinical and experimental observations in five cases occuring in adult. Arch Dermato], 22:635, 1930.

2. Delesclure J et al: Pyoderma gangrenosum with altered cellular immunity and dermonescrotic factor. Br. J. Dermatol, 87:529, 1972.

3. RostenbergAJr:ThedSchwartzman phenomenon: A review with consideration of some possible dermatological manifestations. Br. J. Dermatol, 65 : 389, 1953.

4. Perry O, Brusting LA: Pyoderma gangrenosum: A clinical study of nineteen cases. Arch Der matol, 75 : 380, 1957.

5. HickmanJG,LazarusGS:Pyoderma gangrenosum: a reappraisal of associated sys temic diseases. Br. J. Dermatol, 102: 235, 1980.

6. Schroeter AL, SV PD: The vasculitis of pyoderma gangrenosum: Dermatolpathologic and im-munopathologic study (abst). Arch Dermatol, 116: 1388, 1980

Behcet's disease

Ram Malkani, Ajay Kumar

Bulletin of the Jaslok Hospital & Research Centre Vol XIV No. 4 April 1990 p. 34.

Behcet's disease is a chronic, multisystem disease consisting of at least three of the following (1) Recurrent aphthous stomatitis, which is the most important criterion (2) Recurrent genital ulcers (3) Uveitis, both anterior and posterior (4) Vasculitis of either cutaneous or large vessels (5) Meningoencephalitis (6) Cutaneous hyperreactivity to minor trauma. These diagnostic criteria are not universally accepted but are favoured by most authors.

Hulusi Behcet (1889-1948), a Turkish professor of dermatology described the classic triple symptom complex of iritis and ulcers of oral and genital mucosa in 1937. At the International Congress on Behcet's disease in Istanbul in 1977, the majority present used the diagnostic criteria listed in the definition and favoured the term Behcet's disease over Behcet's syndrome.

The disease is idiopathic. There is a suggestive but as yet inconclusive evidence that Behcet's disease may be caused by a virus. A hereditary predisposition in some ethnic group associated with histocompatibility antigen A5 is reported.

The diagnosis is essentially clinical in the absence of pathognomic laboratory tests. Behcet's disease is a multisystem syndrome of variable duration characterized by exacerbations and remissions. It primarily affects young adult males in 20-40 years age group in Japan and Middle East but may occur almost anywhere. It is twice as frequent in men.

The four major manifestations of the disease are oral and genital ulcers and eye and skin lesions. Mucocutanous ulceraton is the keystone to the diagnosis because of its universal presence at some stage and is usually the first manifestation. Recurrent aphthous ulcers are indistinguishable from the common aphthous stomatitis. Lesions start as red papules and quickly evolve into painful round or oval ulcers covered with white or yellow pseudomembranes, bordered by erythema. They may be found on the lips, gums, tongue, palate and posterior pharynx. Most heal in about 10 days without scarring but some may increase in size for weeks and heal after several months, and may resolve with scarring. The tendency is towards recurrence in crops. Ulcerative haemorrhagic lesions may also occur in stomach, intestine and anus.

Genital ulcers occurring in 90 percent of patients are similar to those in the month but are smaller and deeper and more likely to scar. They occur mainly in the scrotum, around the root of the penis or on the labia majora. They are the source of extreme discomfort and anxiety to the patient.

Ocular manifestations develop in most patients and is bilateral in 80% patients. It includes recurrent conjunctivitis and uveitis. The earliest changes are photophobia and irritation and in some cases only conjunctivitis develops in successive attacks. The onset is commonly an acute pan uveitis. There is development of hypopion, which is transient and recurrent being a hallmark of anterior uveitis. There is marked reduction in binocular vision because of inflammation of macular retinal and choroidal vessels resulting in vitreous haze with dilatation of the retinal venules. Fluorescein angiograpy reveals leakage in both small and large veins initially in peripheral but extending to central vessels. The appearance reflects widespread damage to the endothelium of the retinal veins and capillaries of the retina and optic disc. Areas of retinal infiltrates and non perfusion are seen in later stages of the disease. This periphlebitis may lead to branch retinal vein occlusion. Complications may include cataract, glaucoma, hyphema, retinal detachment and vitreous haemorrhage. Ultimately blindness may occur.

Among the skin lesions which are present in 80% patients at some stage, erythema nodosum is a frequent clinical feature. It appears on the legs and ankles but also on the neck, face and buttocks. Erythema nodosum predominates in women and when present in men, Behcet's disease should be thought of as a possible cause. Other skin lesions include acneform papulopustular erruption seen on face, neck and trunk, maculopapular rashes, blister and widespread recurrent pyoderma. Very characteristically when the disease is active, sterile pustules develop at the site of skin punctures as for example for therapeutic injections. Dermopathia is frequently elicited by a needle prick and read, not as an immediate type hypersensitivity reaction but as a delayed type reaction at 24-48 hours. Polymorphonuclear chemotaxis may be responsible for this delayed tuberculin like response.

Minor, less frequent manifestation includes arthritis, neurological, cardiovascular lesions and psychogenic symptoms.

Arthritis is non migrating, recurrent and seronegative and present in about 60 percent of patients. It is seen in the knees, ankles and wrists. It is non destructive.

Neurological involvement, seen in 25% of cases carries a grave prognosis. Clinical picture of stroke, Meningoencephalitis, brainstem dysfunction and confusional state leading to dementia are seen.

Cardiac involvement also carries a poor prognosis. The principal vascular lesions are venous and arterial occlusions and aneurysms. Superficial thrombophlebitis is common, and recurrent. Deep veins occlusion leads to renal and bone involvement.

Fever and constitutional symptoms are variable histopathologically. A perivascular mononuclear infiltrate is seen in all organs. A vasculitis with endothelial swelling, fibrinoid necrosis, occlusion and perivascular inflammatory infiltrate is seen in many organs. The oral and genital ulcers show non specific inflammatory changes.

The diagnosis is mainly clinical based on multiple physical signs. An arbitrary point scoring system in which at least 14 points are necessary for confident diagnosis, is used to differentiate this condition from sarcoidosis, seronegative arthritis multiple sclerosis, inflammatory bowel disease, Stevens - Johnson syndrome and syphilis.

Needle reaction (hyperirritability) is seen in 60-70% of cases and is highly characteristic but not specific.

An acute phase is characterised by high ESR, acute phase proteins, circulating immune complexes and compliment levels.

There is no specific treatment. Steroids are the mainstay of treatment in low dose both orally and locally such as eye drops, Cyclophosphamide, azothioprim and chlorambucil may be combined. Colchicine prevents recurrence. Livamisole also reduces the frequency and severity of oral and genital ulceration. Prostacycline and cyclosporine may be helpful.

CASE REPORT

A 22 year old male student was admitted with complaints of recurrent ulcers on the tongue and on the scrotum and pain in various joints on and off. The complaints were of five years duration. The first complaint was the painful ulceration of oral cavity, on and off on the tongue about once a month on an average. Other areas of oral cavity were spared. They healed in 10-15 days time. They were associated with presence of fever and malaise.

The scrotal ulcers were always multiple and appearance showed no relation to appearance of tongue ulcers. Joint pains involved the same joints recurrently and there were no other signs of inflammation. He gave history of watering and redness of eyes on two occasions in the past 18 months, which recovered in about two weeks. He had recurrent attacks of erythema nodosum over the limbs. There was no history of other skin lesions of neuro psychiatric manifestations.

On admission he had 3 ulcers on the tongue margins, 2 small punched out ulcers on the left side of scrotum, pain in the wrist and knee joints bilaterally and fever of 101° F with malaise. Ophthalmological examination was normal. Investigations revealed HB-12.8 gms% WBC count - 18,100, ESR -128 mm in first hour, VDRL was negative. Immunoglobulin levels showed raised IgM and IgA, and serum protein electrophoresis pattern showed high alpha 1, and gamma globulins. EGG showed tachycardia. Serum biochemistry profile was normal, L.E. cell and rheumatoid factor were negative.

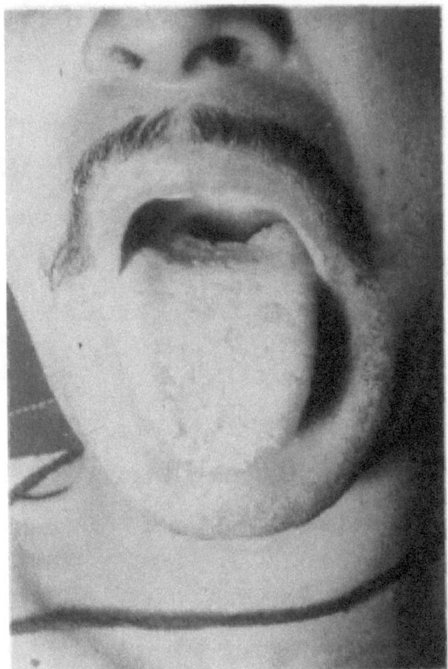

Fig. 1. Oral Lesions

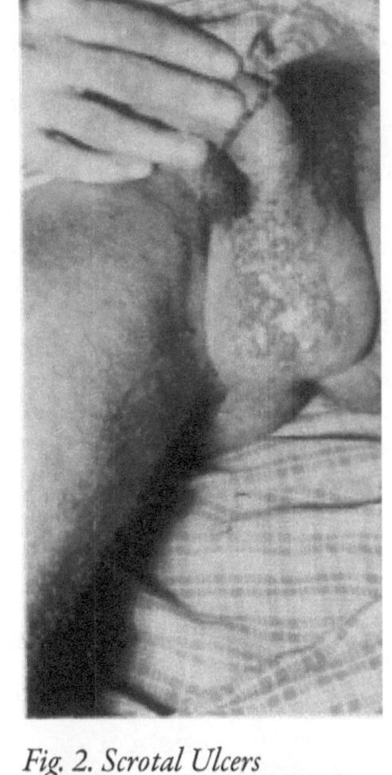

Fig. 2. Scrotal Ulcers

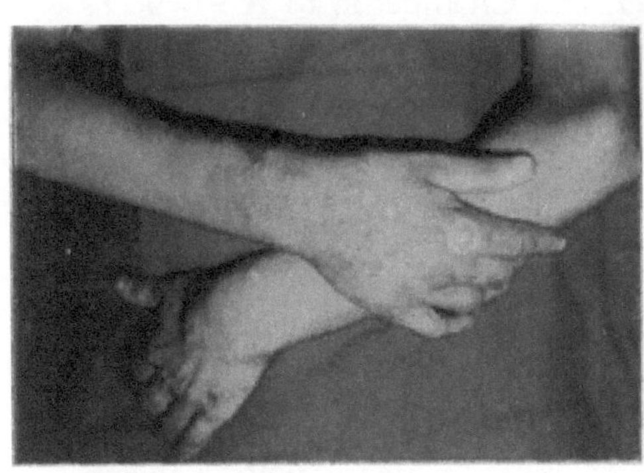

Fig. 3. Erythema nodosum on the upper limbs

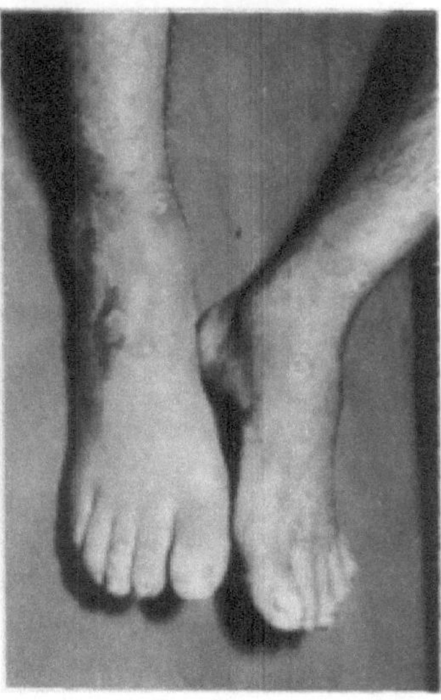

Fig. 4. Erythema nodosum on lower

limbs.

Considering these features a diagnosis of Behcet's disease was made. He was given prednisolone 30 mg per day orally. The complaints showed improvement in about 2 weeks time, upon which the dose was reduced to maintain at 10 mg/ day. He had a symptom free period of 6 months after which he was lost to follow up.

REFERENCES

1. Waong R C, Ellis L N, Diaz L A : Behcet's Disease, Internat J Dermatol 23:25 - 32, 1981.

2. Moftonghi A V : Symposium on haemotological and immunological aspects of Behcet's Disease: Opening remarks. Haematologica, 65:374, 1980.

3. Wright V A and Chamberlin M A : Behcet's syndrome, Bull Rheuma Dis, 29:972, 1978-79.

4. Watson P G : Behcet's Syndrome In: Recent advances in ophthalmology, No. 5 (Edited by P D Trevor Roper) Churchill Livingstone, London. P 249, 1975.

5. O' Duffy J D, Goldstein N P : Neurologic involvement in seven patients with Behcet's disease. AmerJMed 61:170, 1976.

6. Callan J P:Behcet's syndrome in : Cutaneous aspects of internal medicine, Editor, Callan J P : Year Book Medical Publishers, Chicago, p 93, 1981.

7. Teizlin Y, Attac M Yazici H : Non specific skin hyperreactivity in Behcet's disease, Haematologica, 65 : 395 - 399, 1980.

8. Miyachi Y, Taniguchi S, Ozaki et al: Colchicine in the treatment of Behcet's disease, Brit J Dermatol, 104:67, 1981.

Impetigo Herpetiformis - A Case Report

Ajay Kumar, Ram H. Malkani

Bulletin of the Jaslok Hospital & Research Centre Vol XIV No.4 April 1990 p.47.

SUMMARY:

A 23 year old female patient presented in her thirty sixth week of gestation with classical features of impetigo herpetiformis. This is considered a rare disorder. It was well controlled by giving systemic cortico steroids. She delivered a normal child at term.

INTRODUCTION:

Impetigo herpetiformis is a form of pustular psoriasis usually occurring during pregnancy but not restricted to pregnancy alone. It may be life threatening. It was first described by Hebra in 1872. The frequency of its relationship with psoriasis had led us to believe that it is a form of pustular psoriasis. A personal or family history of psoriasis may or may not be present. The disease mostly occurs in the third trimester of pregnancy. Recurrence during the subsequent pregnancies may be expected.

The lesions progress from erythematous macules studded with pustules, to crusting, more often in the flexoral areas. Mucosal areas may be involved. Constitutional symptoms are common. Tetany due to hypocalcaemia is sometimes reported. Low titres of urinary sex steroids have suggested associated placental insufficiency. The histopathology is similar to generalised pustular psoriasis. The characteristic lesion is the macro pustule formed as the neutrophils move up into the horny layer and become pyknotic. The treatment of choice is systemic corticosteroids, prednisolone upto 60 mg per day being necessary with judicious tapering of dose after effective control. Death may occur from hypothermia, renal and cardiac failure in days to weeks.

CASE REPORT:

A 23 year old female primiparous patient, in her thirty fourth week of gestation developed an erythematous patch in her left axilla. This was studded at its periphery with multiple small pustules. She had complaints of intense itching, burning and irritation at the site of her lesion. The pustules showed crusting and later she developed similar lesions on the trunk, limbs and flexures. Some of the patches showed oozing and crusting. She had low grade fever and malaise.

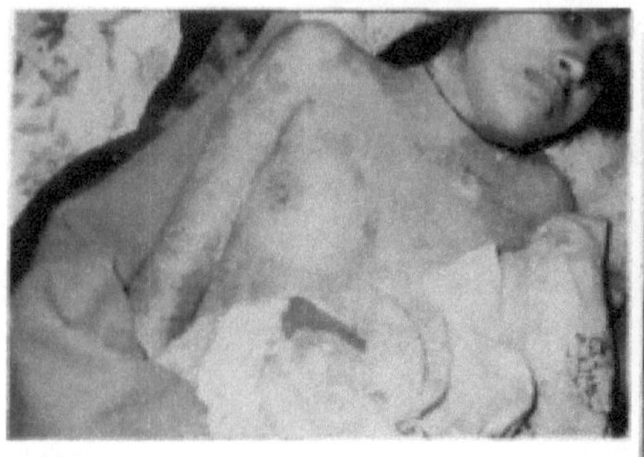

Fig. 1. Lesion showing patches of crusting on the chest and upper limbs

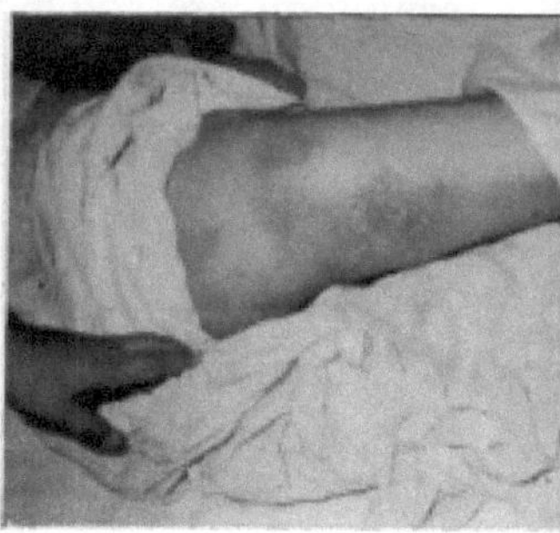

Fig. 2. Close up of lesion on lower li

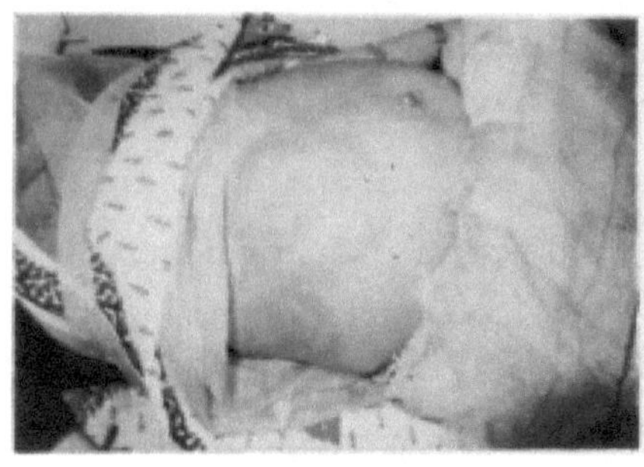

Fig. 3. Resolving lesions on the abdomen

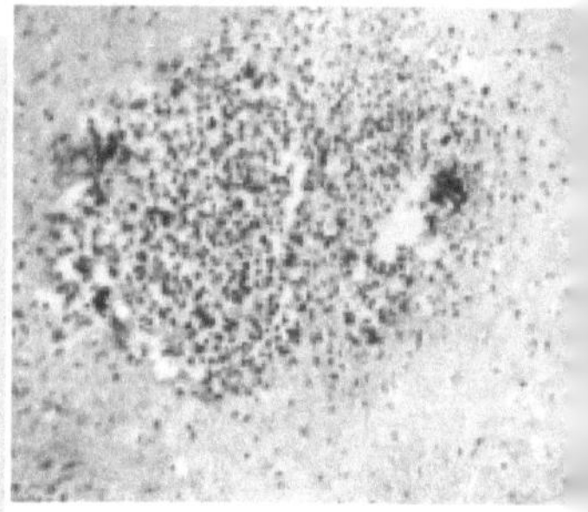

Fig. 4. Intraepidermal r microabscess. (H and E x 100)

Oral cloxacillin and topical application of antibiotic and antifungal medication did not give her any relief. Clinically a diagnosis of Impetigo herpetiformis was made. She gave no personal or family history of psoriasis. Her blood counts, urine analysis and serum electrolytes were within the normal range. Serum calcium was 8.5 mg %. She was taking calcium tablets routinely for the past three months. Pus from the lesions was sterile on culture. Biopsy of the lesion showed intraepidermal neutrophilic macroabscess. She was administrated prednisolone orally in the dose of 10 mg twice a day along with topical application of betamethasone cream. Within seven days, the lesions showed signs of resolution and cleared by the fifteenth day. She delivered a healthy male child per vaginum at term. Prednisolone was tapered over a period of two weeks thereafter.

DISCUSSION:

Since its first description in 1872, impetigo herpetiformis is considered a rarity. It is now considered a form of pustular psoriasis occurring mainly in the third trimester of pregnancy. Prompt remission after delivery is seen. Recurrence in subsequent pregnancies is noted. Recognition of the disorder and prompt and adequate therapy by corticosteroids can bring down maternal mortality but foetal prognosis is still poor.

REFERENCES

1. Bavermen IM: Pregnancy and the menstrual cycle, In Skin signs of systematic disease, Philadelphia, WB Saunders, p 761, 1981.

2. Schelly WB, Kirshbaum JO: Generalised pustular psoriasis. Arch Dcrmatol, 84: 73-78, 1962.

3. Mullet S A Kilzillcr KW: Generalised pustular psoriasis. Act Dcrmatol (Stockh), 42: 504-12,1962.

4. Baveridge GW et al: Impetigo hcrpctiformia in two successive pregnancies. Br. J. Dcrmatol, 78:106-08, 1966.

5. Oumeish OY et al. Some aspects of impetigo herpetiformis.   Arch   Dermatol,118:103-105 1982.

Refsums Disease A Case Report

Ram Malkani, Ajay Kumar

Bulletin of the Jaslok Hospital & Research Centre Vol XIV No.4 April 1990 p.31.

SUMMARY:

A 37 year old female patient presented with icthyosis which had appeared about three months after her birth. During the course of her illness, she had episodes of facial palsy, developed ataxia, visual impairment and sensory loss below the knees. EMG revealed sensory motor polyneuropathy. On dietary management she stabilised clinically.

INTRODUCTION:

Heredopathic atactia polyneuritiformis (Refsum's disease) is a rare autosomal recessive multisystemic disorder of lipid metabolism. It was first described by Refsum, a Norwegian Neurologist. The underlying abnormality is the deficiency in the alpha hydroxylation of certain branch chain fatty acids, notably phytanic acid (3,7,11,15 tetra methyl haxade canoic acid) which is exclusively of exogenous origin, being a normal constituent of green vegetables. As a consequence of this, phythanic acid accumulates and appears to displace some of the unsaturated fatty acids such as linoleic acid from the lipids. There is involvement of the nervous system, eyes, skin and the bones. Serum levels of phytanic acid are high and these correlate well with the raised levels of diphenylated triglycerides. Serum linoleic and arachidonic acid levels are low. Prenatal diagnosis is possible by demonstrating decreased phytanic acid oxidation in cultured amniotic fluid fibroblasts. No animal model for the disorder has yet been identified.

There is degeneration of myelin sheath of axons and the retinal cells. Skin biopsy of the icthyotic skin reveals non membranes bound epidermal lipid containing vacuoles, preferentially at the level of the basal cell layer4. Further, the epidermis is slightly thickened and appears hyperprolifertive. There is increased epidermal turnover as shown by radioactive labelling studies under scanning microscope. Disruption of stratum corneum and keratinocytic microvilli is observed. Phytanic acid has been biochemically demonstrated in the epidermal cells.

Clinically, neurological manifestations are most marked and these include progressive flaccid paralysis resulting from hypertrophic chronic polyneuritis, cerebellar degenerative disorder and sensory deafness. Spinal fluid shows a normal cell count with increased protein. Cutaneous findings are those of acquired icthyosis of the trunk and extremities, clinically resembling autosomal dominant icthyosis. Finding in the eye include retinitis pigmentosa, lenticular opacities and cataracts. Cardiomyopathy is common. Skeletal changes include deformities of the tubular bones of the hand and feet. Urinary findings include lipiduria, cylinderuria, proteinuria and mild azotemia. Fat emboli may develop. The course of the disease is variable but progressive and fatal if not treated. Diagnosis can be made by lipid analysis of the blood or the skin.

The major aspects of the treatment is the use of low phytanic acid diet. High caloric diet must be maintained to prevent mobilisation of endogenous phytanic acid from fat stores. Major foods to be avoided are beef, lamb, grilled liver and margarine. Serum phytanic acid and diphenylated triglyceride levels are shown to decrease after such diets and the serum levels are helpful in monitoring the dietary management. Clinical improvement is seen following diet therapy. Plasmapheresis has been shown to be beneficial. Dialysis is ineffective as the phytanic acid is bound by lipoprotein.

CASE REPORT:

A 37 year old female school teacher presented with ichthyosis which had developed about three months after her birth and she was delivered normally at term. At the age of fourteen, she developed alopecia universalis which did not respond to treatment with systemic corticosteriods. A year later she developed a right sided lower motor neuron facial nerve palsy preceeded by headaches, redness and watering of the eyes. The facial palsy cleared in about two weeks. At the same time she developed blurring of vision in the right eye. It has been progressive since then. Two years later she developed a left sided lower motor neuron facial palsy which cleared in ten to twelve days.

In course of time she developed complaints of cramps in the right lower leg followed by burning, tingling and numbness and difficulty in walking. She had ataxia which was worse in the dark. The condition remained static for a few years. She developed a swelling on the left foot, the radiograph of which revealed multiple fractures of small bones. It was painful and tender and about one litre of pus was drained out from the swelling which was diagnosed as osteomylitis.

Two years prior to presentation, she complained of burning, tingling and numbness in the left lower limb and inability to walk. Fifteen days prior to admission she expressed heaviness in the right upper limb and used to drop objects like cups and glasses occasionally. Her bladder and bowel functions were normal. There was no history of fits, headache, vomiting, fever or head injury. She was not born out of consanguinious parentage.

On examination her skin was icthyotic over her trunk and extremities with presence of alopecia areata on the scalp. Examination of her neurological system revealed normal intellectual functions. She had impaired visual acuity bilaterally. Pupillary reaction was sluggish bilaterally due to iridocyclitis. Her hearing was normal. She had pseudo athetoid movements of the left upper limb, gross sensory ataxia and Rhombergs sign was positive. There was no muscular wasting. There was presence of sensory impairment below the knees.

Investigations revealed her hematological parameters to be normal. Her ESR was 15mm per hour. Serum biochemical values were in the normal range, urine examinations was normal. Her lipid profile was normal. EMG revealed sensory motor polyneuropathy of upper and lower limbs, sensory involvement being more than motor involvement.

Keeping in view of these findings a diagnosis of Refsum's disease was made.

She was advised dietary management for her problem, with exclusion of foods containing phytanic acid. As a consequence of this she showed no further deterioration.

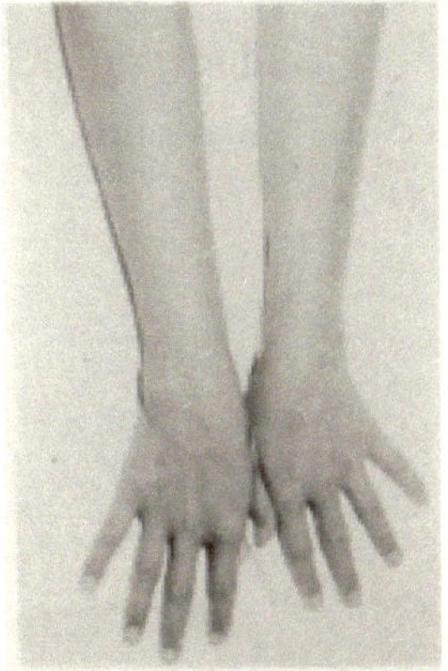 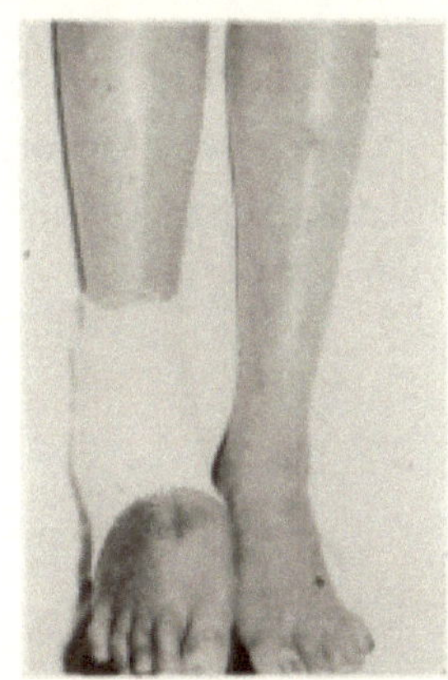

Fig. 1. Icthyosis involving the upper extremities

Fig. 2: Icthyotic skin of the lower limbs

REFERENCES

1. Davies MG, Marks R, Dykes PJ et al: Epidermalabnormalities in Refsums disease. BJ Dermatol97:401, 1977.

2. Stenby et al: Refsums disease - a recently characterised lipidosis involving the nervous systems, Ann Int. Med, 66:365, 1967.

3. Maize CE et al: Phytanic acid storage in Refsums disease is dueto defective alphahydronylation. Clin Res. 16:346:1968.

4. Blanchet, Bardon CL et al: In the ithyoses, E.Marks and R Dykes P.J. Lancaste MTP Press,1978 p 65.

5. Gibberd F B et al: Heredopathic actactiapolyneuritiformis treated by diet and plasmaexchange. Lancet, 1:575 1979.

Hypereosinophilic Syndrome - A report of two cases

Ram H. Malkani, Balnath Bhandary

Bulletin of the Jaslok Hospital & Research Centre, Vol XVI No. 2 October 1991.

Eosinophils:-

Ever since its description 100 years ago by Paul Ehrlich, eosinophils have been associated with a wide variety of diseases. They normally constitute a small proportion of the circulating leucocytes with normal values ranging from 0-350 m.

Human Eosinophils measure 10-15um in diameter. A unique morphological feature of the eosinophil, is its content of distinctive cytoplasmic granules. These membrane bound granules have a unique structure, a crystalloid core, which is composed of Major Basic Protein (MBP). The other basic proteins are Eosinophilic cataionic protein (ECP), Eosinophilic peroxidase and Eosinophil derived neurotoxins. An enzyme histaminase is associated with granules in the eosinophil. A number of lysozomal hydrolases are present in the eosinophilic granules. Another enzymatic constituent of human eosinophil is lysophospholipase. This protein which is associated with membranes but not granules of human eosinophils is shown to be sole protein constituent of charcot leyden crystals. Two neutrophil granule proteins, lysozyme and phagocytin are not detected in the eosinophils. The external plasma membrane of the eosinophils express receptors for several immunoglobulins and complement moeties.

The Fc receptors for IgG and a receptor for IgE are the important ones. A receptor for C3b complement component is also present.

Production

Augmented marrow production of eosinophils is under T lymphocytes control. There are certain substances incompletely characterised which stimulate eosinophil production.

1. Eosinophil colony stimulating factor
2. Eosinophil growth stimulating factor

After about a week in the marrow where they develop and form a mature pool of cells, eosinophils circulate in the blood only briefly with a half life in the order of 6-12 hours. Eosinophils then enter the tissues and persist for atleast several days. For each eosinophil present in the blood, there are about 300 in the marrow and about 100-200 in the tissue.

Functions

Eosinophil is a motile, phagocytic cell. Eosinophils engage in exocytosis, a process whereby the contents of cytoplasmic granules are released extracelluraly. Stimulated eosinophils are capable of an oxidative burst and can release a number of oxidative products including hydrogen peroxide, superoxide ions and hydroxyl radicals. An activated eosinophil undergoes morphological alterations like cytoplasmic vacuolization and partial degranulation. Increased expression of membrane receptor for IgG, IgE and Cab have been found on eosinophils from patients with eosinophilias of diverse aetiologies.

Helminthotoxic effector cell

The cytotoxic interaction between eosinophils and the large non phagocytosable parasite requires direct contact. Eosinophils binding to the parasite may be mediated by parasite bound Cab or predominantly by specific antiparasiteIsG Following this initial attachment,subsequent binding of the eosinophil to theparasite becomes firmer; in association with deposition of granule contents on the surface of the parasite. Products of the eosinophil that are helminth toxic include the granule derived catatonic proteins, MBP, EOF, oxidative derivatives such ashydrogen peroxide and those fromeosinophil peroxidase H_2O_2 halide enzymesystem.

Modulators of Immediate hypersensitivity reactions

The accumulation of eosinophils at sites of immediate hypersensitivity reactions and their potential recruitment by recognized eosinophils chemoattractants (ECF-A) released by mast cells and basophils have led to the studies of the cellular functions Ibf; the eosinophils in these reactions. A number of findings have suggested a role of eosinophil in modulating or down regulating an ongoing IgE mediated mast cell dependent reaction.

Eosinophils as mediators of disease

The cytotoxic effect of eosinophil granular basic protein of parasites has led to the recognition of their potential cytotoxicity on mammalian cells.

The eosinophils maybe directly or indirectly responsible for liberating mediators of immediate hypersensitivity reactions. Eosinophil peroxidase can cause mast cell degranulation. Eosinophil itself can generate leukotrine which possesses potent vaso constricting activity.

Clinical Features of Hypereosinophilic syndrome

There are three main criteria for diagnosing HES

1. Persistent esonophilia of more than $1500mm^3$
for 6 months
2. No known specific cause for eosinophilia
3. Signs and syptoms of organ involvement

Presenting symptoms of HES frequently include anorexia, weight loss, fever, night sweats, dyspnea, cough, chest pain, pruritic rash, neurologic abnormalities, diarrhoea and arthralgias. These are accompanied by hepato splenomegaly, lymphadenopathy and signs of cardiac disease. Multiple organ involvement may include neurologic, pulmonary, gastro intestinal, cardio vascular or skin.

Cardio vascular system

Cough, dyspnea, chest pain with signs of mitral regurgitation with congestive cardiac failure. EKG changes include T wave inversion and left atrial enlargement. Echocardiography showed left ventricular wall thickness and increased mass.

Dermatological changes

50% of the patients suffer from skin manifestations. These are not specific and have differing morphologic appearance. They are most often located on the extremities followed by the trunk and the face. It may vary from pruritic erythematous papular eruption or an urticarial eruption with angioedema. Dermographia may be present in 75% of people.

Central Nervous system

May be of two types 1. Associated with peripheral neuritis such as parasthesias and dysesthesias. 2. Those associated with diffuse CNS dysfunction, such as coma, confusion, ataxia, slurred speech, hemiparesis.

Pulmonary system

Pleural effusions, interstial non lobar infiltrates associated with a persistant non productive cough.

Other systems:

Diarrhoea with or without hepatic dysfunction or malabsorbtion may occur. Renal involvement is infrequent but may manifest as persistant hematuria. In most cases cardiac disease was the cause of morbidity and mortality. Autopsy findings included increase in heart size, endocardial thrombi and fibrosis, valvular damage, myocardial fibrosis and early eosinophilic infiltration of the myocardium. Infections, renal hepatic failure have been identified as causes of death. Vasculitis is rarely seen.

Investigations

Majority of the laboratory tests include a complete blood count, differential count, E.S.R., serum electrolytes, blood sugar, calcium, alkaline phosphatase, iron, total protein, protein electrophoresis, immunologic parameters, EGG, chest Xrays and stool examination. These are usually within normal limits. Essential for diagnosis are, increased eosinophil count, bone marrow infiltration by eosinophils. Also found are anaemia thrombocytopenia, abnormal liver functions and EGG changes especially T wave inversion. Uric acid levels are high. Negative tests include serologies for collagen vascular disease, negative direct immuno fluorescence of skin. Factors associated with a poor prognosis include a peripheral leucocytosis myeloblasts in peripheral blood, signs of CHF. Skin biopsy of a skin lesion demonstrates eosinophilic and is an easy, convenient tool for infiltrates confirming the diagnosis.

Treatment

Indications for treatment include documentation of organ involvement and prognosis of the disease. The treatment of choice is corticosetroids. The dosage is Prednisone 60 mg/day daily intially and then switched to every other day therapy. An elevated IgE, frequent angioedema or a prolonged eosinopenia following a single dose of Prednisone are indicators of good response. Patients not responsive to steroids respond well to hydroxyurea 1-2g daily. It has been shown that early and aggressive treatment of HES may minimise cardio vascular complications. Other modalities of treatment include Vincristine 1-2 mg IV followed by hydroxyurea or steroids with the intention of reducing the leukocyte count.

Case Report No. 1

Mr. G.K. 38 years, male, office clerk, normotensive occasional smoker, non alcoholic, diabetic came with a history of low grade fever, chills and rigors and night sweats. He had associated vomiting, productive cough, loss of appetite, loss of weight and joint pains. He had rashes all over the body, with associated itching. His past history was not significant.

He was poorly nourished, moderately built with maculopapular rashes all over the body. Scratch marks were present. Lymph nodes were palpable in the axillary, submandibular and inguinal region. His respiratory and cardiovascular system was normal.

Investigations done: Total count: 30, 150

Differential count: Neutrophils: 73 cells/cumm, Eosinophils: 24 cells/cumm

Mantoux test: Negative

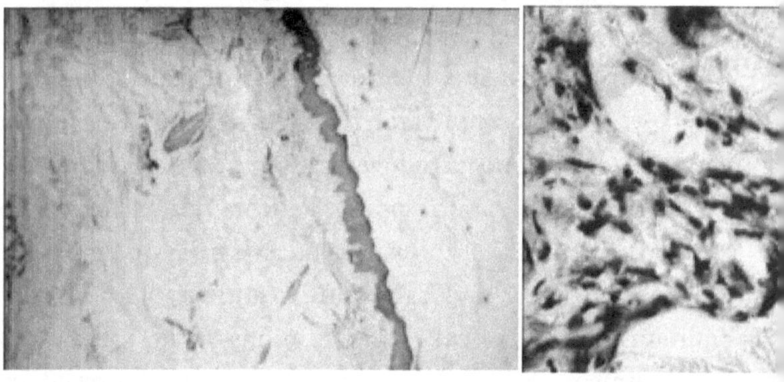

Fig 1 Scanner of skin biopsy of an itchy papule of Fig. 2. Higher magnificat. case 1 showing minimal infiltrate mar the blood vessel site of case I, showing inf. otherwise a bland dermis.   vessel with eosinophils prea

Widal test: Negative, VDRL: Negative, LE cells: Negative, Rheumatoid factor : Negative, Sputum AFB : Negative

Entamoeba hystolitica haemagglutination: Negative

Urine Examination: Normal, Stool: Normal, ANF test: Positive, Anti DNA: Negative

X'ray chest done showed thickened left pleura and infiltration of left apex.

Isotope liver scan showed hepatomegaly Isotope bone scan showed no abnormality

Biopsy was done of the axillary lymph node showed normal lymph node architecture.

Skin biopsy: Eosinophilic infiltration of the small vessels. Immunofluoroscence microscopy was negative. Bone marrow biopsy: Myeloid: hyperplasia with prepondrance of eosinophilic cell line. No evidence of malignancy.

Discussion:

Patient admitted, with pyrexia of unkown origin, later thought to be Koch's but not responding to Anti Koch's treatment. Because of the lymph nodes and hepatomegaly Hodgkins disease was considered as another possibility. This was ruled out by the biopsy of Axillary Lymph node. The skin biopsy performed revealed eosinophilic infiltration followed by bone marrow biopsy showing eosinophilic infiltration. The series of eosinophilic counts showed eosinophilia and hence he was treated as a case of Hypereosinophilic syndrome. With Prednisone 60 mg/daily he responded quite well and the cell count came back to normal.

Case Report No. 2

31 year old Mrs. K. presented (Date of Admission 20.2.91) with history of itchy skin lesions which started 7 years back. She was diagnosed with Dermatitis Herpetiformis in the city of her origin. Her total leucocyte count then was 9,800 and eosinophils were 24 percent. She was treated with Dapsone, but there was no relief. She soon developed cervical adenitis. The submandibular gland was visibly enlarged, was biopsied, which revealed reactive non- specific hyperplasia with infiltration by eosinophils. She was given AKT. Her adenitis persisted and so did the eosinophil count which remained as 24 per cent of the total count. Two years later she developed

effort intolerance and breathlessness. The EGG and Echocardiography then revealed asymmetrical septal hypertrophy, T wave inversion in most leads with sinus tachycardia. She was reported as having cardiomyopathy. The cardiologist had entertained the possibility of Churg-Strauss syndrome in view of eosinophilia, lung symptoms and CVS abnormality. Her breathlessness was being treated as bronchial asthma. She eventually received oral cortisone which resulted in the improvement of her skin lesions and breathlessness. The skin lesions had healed as hyperpigmented macular patches. Eosinophils had returned to normal. Symptomatically she improved. Oral cortisone gradually were discontinued. 1 1/2 years before admission to the hospital she had developed recurrent diarrohea, loss of appetite, loss of weight to the tune of 12-15 kg. On investigations, she was found to have hepatomegaly. Jejunal biopsy and Bone marrow biopsy done earlier, had revealed eosinophilic infiltrates.

Physical examination

31 year old healthy lady.

TPR N/94/N, BP 136/80 mmHg, Pallor +, No icterus/ clubbing. Submandibular lymphnodes + marks of skin lesion.

On systemic examination

Per abdomen : Liver 6 cm palpable beneath costal margin, firm, non tender, nodular well defined margin.

Spleen JP no free fluid. Other system normal Probable diagnosis considered were:

1. Collagen disease
2. Churg Strauss syndrome
3. Hyper eosinophilic syndrome
4. Heavy chain disease
5. Amyloidosis

Patient was investigated.

Investigations done
    Hemato
    Hb ll gm%
    TC 8370/cmm
    DC
    N 55
    L 34
    E 5
    M 5
    B l
    (on steroids)
    ESR 73 mm Hg.
    Platelet count 80,000/cmm
    B. Chemistry
    S. Na/K+/Cl/Hco3: 139/3.9/100/26
    BUN : 10 mgm%
    S. Creatinine 0.7 mg%
    T. Protein/Alb/Glo : 5.4/2.5/2.9
    S. Cal/Po4/Alk Phos : 8.7/5.4/155
    Uric Acid : 8.3

T. Bilirubin : 0.3 mgm%

SGOT : 14 IU, S. TG/Cholsterol 194/255, Urinanalysis
Stool examination-Normal.

Rheumato HIV antibody : negative

Rheumatoid Factor : negative

ANA DNA: negative Protein electophoresis 2.7 U/ml
(25U/ml N)

Coagulation BT)

CT) Normal PT)

Bence jones protein screen: negative IgE 114/IU/ml
(0-180 lU/ml)

1. X'ray chest: Prominant bronchopulmonar
markings

2. 2 D. Echo EGG: Thickened septum.

No. SAM at rest. Good LV function
T wave decreased in most leads with sinus tachycardia.

3. Ultra sonography ABD & Pelvis: Marked
hepatomegaly with normal architecture. No focal
mass/calculus. Gall bladder, pancreas, spleen,
kidneys, para aortic region normal. No mass seen.
Urinary bladder normal.
Uterusminimalenlarged.Both ovaries prominant
3.6 cm (rt) and 3.8 (It) no mass.

4. Peritoneoscopy: Liver surface shows
nodularity-biopsy taken Peritoneum normal.
Impression infiltrative disorder.

5. Liver Biopsy: Mild fibrosis with portal inflamation. No evidence of cirrhosis and Amyloidosis.

6. Bone Marrow Biopsy: (28.2.1991) Normocellular marrow with adequate megakaryocytes, M:E ratio normal. No increase in plasma cells. No evidence of neoplasia/ granuloma.

Diagnosis

1. Collagen Disease
2 Hypereosinophilic Syndrome
3. Churg strauss synd.

Discussion:

Hypereosinophilic syndrom (HES) has been infrequently reported occurring in a female(7). This lady had multiple organ involvement with eosinophilia. The jejunal biopsy, the lymph node biopsy and the bone marrow biopsy all revealed the presence of eosinophilic infiltrates. The possibility of Churg Strauss syndrome was ruled out as none of the biopsies revealed any evidence of granulomatous angiitis. Whenever she was on oral cortisone all along her 7 years illness, her symptoms abated and the eosinophil count returned to normal limits. Whenever she was off oral cortisone, new symptoms appeared.

References:

1. Dermatologic Diseases associated with Eosinophilia; Pincus S.H., Wolff S.M.: Update Dermatology in General Medicine; Fitzpatrick et al, McGraw Hill Inc. 1983; P. 13-19 .

2. Hypereosinophilic Syndrome; Fisher Micheal, Diana E. Trusky; Fe?x<£r andfgash: Update, Dermatology Update Ed|Moschella S.L.: 1982 Editiqjn;,p.^l-90 %»; ^S'

3. Eosinophils and polymorphonuclear leucocytes: Peter F. Weller; Immunobiology Section of Third ed. Dermatology in General Medicine; McGraw Hill Inc. 1987; p. 435.

4. Dermatologic Manifestations of the Hypereosinophilic Syndrome; Kazmievowski J.A., Chusid M.J., Parillo J.E.; Arch Dermatol 1978; 114; p. 531-535.

5. Cutaneous Eosinophilic Diseases; In Dermatology in General Medicine, Third ed.; Pincus S.H.; Editors Fitzpatrick T.B., Eisen A.Z., Wolff K. et al; McGraw Hill Book Book Company, New York, 1987; p. 1336-1344.

6. The Hypereosinophilic Syndrome, Analysis of fourteen cases with review of the Literature,

Medicine (Baltimore); Chusid M.J., Dala D.C., West B.C. et al; (Baltimore) 1975; 54, p. 1-27.

7. Hypereosinophilic Syndrome in a female, S. Agarwal et al, IJDVL 1990: 56: 304-305.

Toxicity in a Serologically negative SLE

Ram H Malkani

Bulletin of the Jaslok Hospital & Research Centre, Mumbai Vol XIX No.1 July 1991.

The prevalence of ANA-negative SLE is estimated at between 4 and 13% cases of SLE. The clinical picture of this sub type of SLE is dominated by photosensitivity, oral ulceration and a malar rash. Hematological, renal and neurological symptoms are less common than in ANA positive SLE patients. Hence majority of these patients (60%) present to a dermatologist.

Case history of an ANA negative SLE patient is presented. ANA negative SLE tends to feature a mild course, with little involvement of internal organs. This patient differed by its toxicity involving internal organs:

CASE REPORT

40 year old female from Raipur presented with malar pigmentation for the last 14 months. The pigmentation started during the third month of pregnancy. Patient gave history of getting pain in the joints and lumbar region for the last 4 months. The pain gradually increased. The pain in joints was accompanied by skin rash on the head, neck, elbows, extensor aspects of the arms and distal fingers. She did not give history of—photosensitivity. She gave history of

painful ulcers in the mouth off and on. She also gave history of tiny painful ulcers distally on the fingers, though there was no history or sign of Raynaud's phenomenon. She had fever, associated with malaise, headache, nausea off and on. She had dependent oedema of feet for the last 4 months. She had hypertension and diabetes mellitus for the last 2-3 years.

She was on inderal 1 bid, Depin retard, 1 bid and Glyciphage V 2 bid.

She had three full term normal deliveries in the past giving birth to three female children of 16 years, 12 years and 10 years of age. After that a female child delivered by Caesarean section which was 8 months old.

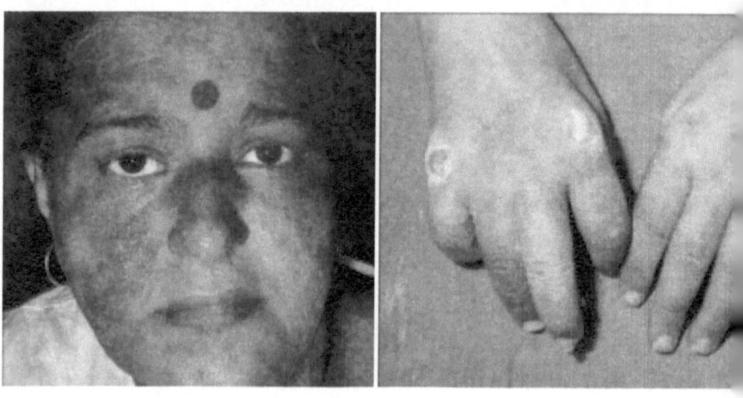

Fig1

Fig 2

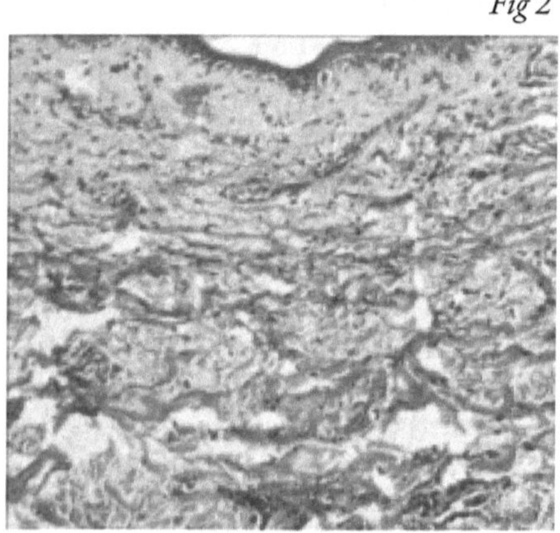

Fig 3

On examination: Patient was febrile with no cynosis, clubbing, lymphadenopathy and icterus. Skin examination revealed periorbital and malar pigmentation associated with mild erythema. (Fig. 1). She had well defined, scaly depigmented, atrophic alopecia plagues on the head.

She had erythematous, polycyclic and annular rash on the neck, V of the neck and extensor aspects of forearms.

There were vasculitic ulcers on the elbows, dorsum of the right 5th and left 5th MP joints. Right finger showed periungual ulcers. There were a few ulcers on the flexor aspects of other fingers. Palmar-erythema was present. Nails and mucosal membranes were normal. Cicatrical alopecia was evident on the scalp. RS, CVS, CNS - NAD.

INVESTIGATIONS:

On admission her hemoglobin was 10.09 mg%, WBC 3,400, ESR 62, Fasting sugar 82 mgm%, Post lunch sugar 90 mgm%, Glycoselated Hb 6.0%, RA +ve 1:20, ANF -ve, Anti DNA -ve, 24 hrs. urinary proteins l7 mgm, SGOT 375 (40), SGPT 82 (35), SGOT 765 (65), Alkaline PO4 595 (115), LDH 890 (240), Total Bilirubin 1.2 (0.15-J.O). PT-N, HBS Ag - Neg, Anti-HCV -Neg, U/S abdomen - N, T3, T4, TSH-N, C3 46 (80-180), C4 46 (15-80). ANA and LE cell phenomenon done earlier 2 months back at the place of her residence was also negative. Skin bisopsy on admission from the annular, arythematous patch showed flattened epidermis, focal vacualisation of basal cells. The dermis was myxiod and a vessel showed characteristic fibriniod necrotising vasculitis on PAS stain. (Fig. 3)

She was put on 60 mg of prednisolone per day with other supportive treatment for her hypertension and diabetes.

Investigations done 10 days later on the date of discharge read as SGOT 443 (40), SGPT 82 (35), GGT1010 (65), Alkaline PO4 425 (115), LDH 827 (240), Total Bilirubin 1,6 (0.15-1.0), Direct Bilirubin 1.0 (0.1-0.4), Haemoglobin 11.4, WBC 5,360. 4 months later while she was on 20 mg of prednisolone daily the investigations read as Haemoglobin 12.0 gm, WBC 5,900, SGOT 89 (40), SGPT 94 (35), Gamma GT 250 (65), Alkaline P04 186 (115), LDH 383 (240), Total Bilirubin 0.6 (0.15-1.0).

Another 4 months later she developed cough, breathlessness and was admitted in the ICU at her native place for LVF. She was seen by a cardiologist and diagnosed as having cardiomyopathy. She succumbed to her illness six months later.

DISCUSSION:

As a positive ANA is a major ARA criterion for SLE, patients with negative serology create a diagnostic problem. For a diagnosis of SLE 4 or more of the criteria of the American RheumatismAssociation (ARA) should be positive. The criteria are: 1) Malar rash 2) Discoid LE 3) Raynaud's phenomenon 4) Alpecia 5) Photosensitivity 6) Oral or nasopharyngeal ulcers 7) Arthritis 8) LE or ANA more than 1:64 9) False positive STS 10) Proteinuria more than 3.5 gm in 24 hours urine or biopsy proven renal disease consistent with SLE 11) Cellular urinary casts. 12) Pleuritis/pericarditis 13) Pscychoscs/convulsions 14) Cytopenia with WBC less than 4,000 per cu.mm. or platelets less than 10,000 cells per cu.mm.

The patient fulfilled criteria no. 1, 4, 5, 6, 7 and 14. Hence this patient was diagnosed as a case of ANA negative, SS-DNA negative SLE.

ANF negative SLE has similarities with patients of sub acute cutaneous LE. Both comprise around 10% of cases of LE. Both have anticyloplasmic antibodies. Anti Ro is positive in 60% and Anit La in 40%.

Subacute cutaneous LE is considered a benign subset separate from DLE and SLE. Clinically it is characterised either by nonscarring papulosquamous (%rd) or annular polycyclic rash (VSRD) usually above the waist. Diffuse non scarring alopecia and photosensitivity occur in about half the patients. Mouth ulceration, scarring DLE and alopecia are also known to occur. In subacute cutaneous LE, ANF is positive in 60% cases. About half the patients fulfill the criteria of the American Rheumatism Association for SLE with arthritis the most frequent feature. Occasional patients develop overt SLE with severe visceral disease.

In about 5-10% of patients with SLE, ANF cannot be demonstrated. There is no difference in the histology of the skin between ANA negative and positive cases. About 10% of patients eventually become ANA positive although the pattern of anticytoplamic antibodies does not alter.

Liver pathology: Since a liver biopsy was not performed it was not possible to conclude about the exact nature of pathology in the liver. Liver disease caused by SLE itself was a distinct possibility. Liver involvement in SLE is more common than previously recognised. Severe and even fatal disease can occur(5).

The prerequisities for a diagnosis of liver disease are an abnormal liver biopsy specimen and/or a two fold or greater increase in at least four determination of the following. Total bilirubin, SGOT, SGPT, LDH or alkaline phosphatase. At least two different test results had to be abnormal. Patient presented fulfilled the criteria. Patient was evaluated to determine the cause of the liver disease like drug toxicity, infection, metabolic disturbance, non hepatic causes like hemolytic anaemia, myositis etc.(5)

Review of the literature indicated that subclinical liver disease is indicated by mild elevation of enzymes in 8%. Hepatic lesions include fatty change resulting in steatosis, Granulomatous hepatitis, chronic active hepatitis (hepatic lupus as opposed to lupoid hepatitis) and cirrhosis.(6)

References

1.   K.C.NozANA-negativesystemiclupuserythematosus.   262nd SDV meeting. BritishJournal of Dermatology 1993, 129, 345- 346.

2. Maddison P.J., Provost T T, Reichlin M.Serological findings in patients with ANA negative Systemic lupus erythematosus. Medicine1981: 60: 87-94.

3. Rowell N R and Godfield M.J.D. Chapter 55"The connective tissue diseases" Rook, Wilkinson, Ebling. Textbook of Dermatology edited byChampion, Burton, Ebling. Blackwell scientificpublications 1992 P. 2186.

4. Rowell N R & Godfield MJD Chapter 55 'Theconnective tissue Disease" Rook, Wilkinson,Ebling. Textbook of Dermatology

edited byChampion, Burton, Ebling. Blackwell scientificpublications 1992 P. 2218.

5. Runyon B A, La Brecque D R, Anuras Sinn. Thespectrum of Liver Disease in Symtemic lupusErythermatosusReport of 33 Histologically-proved cases and review of the literature. TheAmerican Journal of Medicine 1980: 69: 187-195. -:

6. Green T, Champion R H, Extensive telangiectasia with chronic active hepatitis and SLE,British J. of Dermatol 1989: 121: 116

Primary systemic amyloidosis

BA Vaz[1], V Aswani[2], RH Malkani[3]

Indian J Dermatology Venereology Leprology 1993;59:93-6

Abstract

A 45-year old male had nephrotic syndrome of 2 years duration and multiple, asymptomatic, small, yellowish papules on eyelids, nasolabial folds and perioral region since 6 months. He also had progressive weakness, fatigue, breathlessness and joint pains. His voice was hoarse. Macroglossia and beaded vocal cords were present. There was a history of exsanguinating bleeding following a kidney biopsy done 6 months earlier. Proteinuria was present but Bence-Jones proteins were absent. Skin biopsy of lesional skin showed an eosinophilic, amorphous, fissured mass distending the dermal papillae and around blood vessels and

1. http://www.ijdvl.com/
   searchresult.asp?search=&author=BA+Vaz&journal=Y&but_search=Search&entries=10&pg=1&s=0

2. http://www.ijdvl.com/
   searchresult.asp?search=&author=V+Aswani&journal=Y&but_search=Search&entries=10&pg=1&s=0

3. http://www.ijdvl.com/
   searchresult.asp?search=&author=RH+Malkani&journal=Y&but_search=Search&entries=10&pg=1&s=0

appendages. Congo red stain was negative for amyloid, but crystal violet stain demonstrated amyloid in lesional as well as normal appearing skin. Electron microscopy confirmed the same. The patient deteriorated quickly and succumbed to gross haematemesis.

Introduction

Primary systemic amyloidosis is a rare disorder characterized by the multisystemic deposition of a homogeneous, hyaline amyloid material. Wilks, in 1856, was the first to lucidly describe primary systemic amyloidosis.(1)Primary systemic amyloidosis represents a plasma cell dyscrasia(2) and may be associated with multiple myeloma. Amyloid filaments have as their major protein component either an intact L chain or the amino - terminal fragment of an L chain or both.(1)

Case Report

A 45-year-old male presented with multiple small, asymptomatic periorificial facial lesions and a low, husky quality of voice of 6 months duration. Two years earlier the patient had been diagnosed as having nephrotic syndrome for which he had been on steroids on and off, without much amelioration of his condition. Six months earlier, the patient had an episode of exsanguinating retroperitoneal bleeding following kidney biopsy and necessitating transfusion of 40 units of blood. In spite of 2 exploratory laparotomies the cause of bleeding was inexplicable at that time as no bleeders were found and the patient's coagulation profile was normal. The patient gave a history of steadily increasing weakness, fatigue, breathlessness and joint pains involving mainly the small joints of both the hands since 6 months. There were no other systemic complaints or history of any chronic illness in the past.

On examination the vital parameters were normal and blood pressure 150/80 mm of Hg. Pallor and oedema feet were present. Multiple shiny, smooth, firm, skin to yellowish papules upto 0.5 cm in size were present on the eyelids, lips, nasolabial folds and periorally [Figure - 1].

A few lesions coalesced to form plaques and some were pedunculated. There was no purpura elicited with trauma. However, ecchymoses were present over sites of venipuncture. Sclerodactyly of fingers was present. The tongue was enlarged, smooth, indented by teeth and red waxy papules studded its surface [Figure - 2]. Indirect laryngoscopy revealed similar lesions on the vocal cords, giving them a beaded appearance. There was free fluid found per abdomen. Liver and spleen were not palpable and other systems were normal. A presumptive diagnosis of primary systemic amyloidosis was entertained.

The patient's haemoglobin was low. Urine showed 3+ albumin and casts. Bence-Jones proteins were absent. Serum protein and lipoprotein electrophoresis were normal. Stool showed the presence of occult blood in 3 consecutive samples. RA test, ANF and anti ds DNA were negative. ECG showed sinus tachycardia. Abdominal ultrasound showed no enlargement of kidney, liver or spleen. Kidney biopsy (done 6 months earlier) had shown a minimal lesion glomerulopathy with negative immunofluorescence and negative staining for amyloid. Skin biopsy taken from lesional skin showed the presence of an eosinophilic, amorphous, fissured mass distending the dermal papilla [Figure - 3]. Similar material was also noted around blood vessels and appendages from lesional skin as well as from a biopsy taken from apparently normal skin of forearm. This material was weakly PAS positive, but staining with Congo red failed to show apple green birefringence on repeated sections. However a crystal violet stain showed a positive eosinophilic staining of the amyloid. Electron microscopy showed the presence of straight, non-branching, non-anastomosing, often irregularly arranged filaments, suggestive of amyloid filaments [Figure - 4].

The patient was on treatment for nephrotic syndrome with salt restricted diet, diuretics, prednisolone and azathioprine. While his investigations were on, his condition steadily deteriorated. He developed severe muscle weakness, giddiness and later haematemesis to which he succumbed.

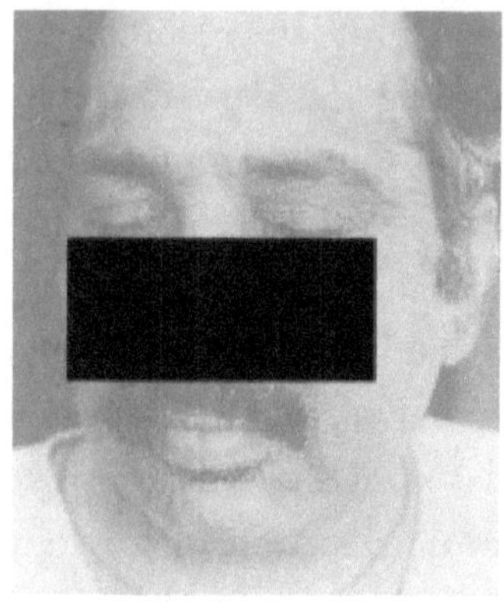

Fig 1 Waxy papules seen around eyes mouth and in nasolabial grooves

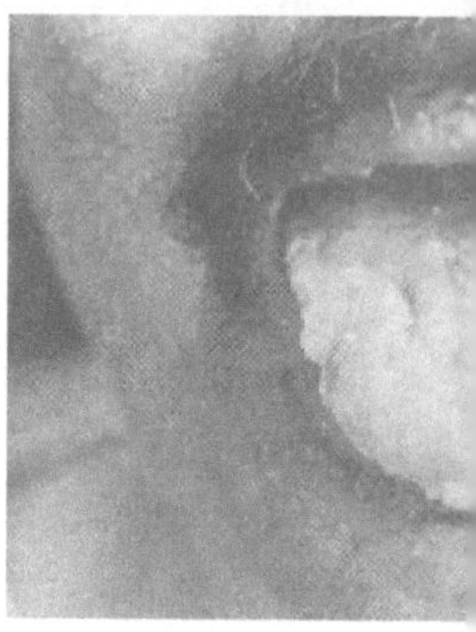

Fig 2 Papules on the lips ar the enlarged tongue

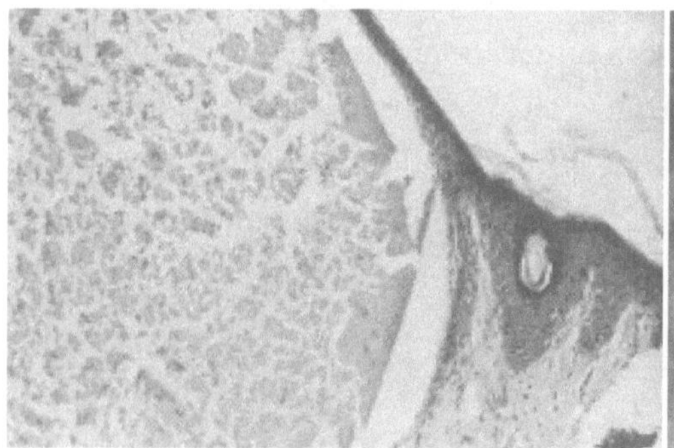

Fig 3 Amotphous eosinophilic amyloid material distending a dermal papilla (H & E x100)

Fig 4 Straight non-branci amyloid filaments (electron

Comments

With the clinical presentation of classical mucocutaneous lesions, nephrotic syndrome and post renal biopsy bleeding, a diagnosis of primary systemic amyloidosis was entertained. Bleeding or haematuria following renal biopsy has been known to occur more frequently in patients with amyloidosis as compared to patients without amyloidosis.

Widespread loss of vascular integrity because of infiltration with amyloid along with other factors like deficiency of vitamin K, factor X, increased antithrombin activity and increased fibrinolysis, all contribute to the bleeding.

Involvement of the kidneys is extremely common in patients with amyloidosis. Amyloid is first deposited in the mesangium of the glomerulus and later extends along the basement membrane. The degree of proteinuria in the nephrotic syndrome does not correlate well with the extent of amyloid deposition in the kidneys.(3) This may explain why amyloid was not demonstrated on a kidney biopsy done 6 months earlier, even though the patient had gross proteinuria.

Hoarseness or change of voice to a weak, high pitched or deep husky sound often alerts the physician to the possibility of amyloidosis. Macroglossia can be extremely impressive, however it can be sometimes difficult to decide whether the tongue is enlarged or not. Increased firmness of the tongue, enlargement of the submandibular structures and dental indentations are helpful in determining the presence of macroglossia.

The straightforward confirmation of the evident clinical diagnosis by histopathology proved difficult as repeated congo red stains failed to show the classical green birefringence. The negative congo red test could have been due to technical errors, too thin sections or excess formalin fixation which is known to alter the staining properties of amyloid. For a better positivity yield, staining of frozen fixed material, rectal and subcutaneous fat biopsy and a battery of different stains are recommended.(4)Crystal violet, a metachromatic stain and electron microscopy which is the most specific diagnostic method, helped in establishing the diagnosis in this patient.

Kyle and Greipp have seen several cases in whom the results of staining of tissue with congo red or the metachromatic stains were negative, yet electron microscopy revealed the typical amyloid fibrils. A third class of stains, the cotton dyes, Pagoda Red, RIT Scarlet No. 5 and RIT Cardinal Red No. 9 which are simple, bright, long lasting and specific for amyloid, can also be used.(5)

This patient survived for 2 years following onset of symptoms. The median survival of patients with nephrotic syndrome has been reported to be around 17 months. Melphalan has been used with occasional success in some patients with nephrotic syndrome. Other drugs like prednisolone, colchicine and DMSC have been tried. The unsatisfactory nature of the available treatment modalities is reflected in the poor prognosis of patients.

Acknowledgement

We express our thanks to Dr Vanaja Shetty of Foundation for Medical Research, Worli, Bombay-400 018 for electron microscopic studies.

References

1. Kyle RA, Greipp PR. Amyloidosis (AL) clinical and laboratory features in 229 cases. Mayo Clin Proc 1983; 58:665 - 83.

2. Buxbaum JN, Hurley ME, Chuba J, et al. Amyloidosis of the AL type. Am J Med 1979; 67:867 - 78.

3. Watanabe T, Soniter T. Morphological and clinical features or renal amyloidosis. Virchows Arch (Pathol Anat) 1975; 366:125 - 35. (quoted by 1)

4. Lever WF, Schaumberg-Lever G. Metabolic Diseases. In : Histopathology of the skin, 6th edn. Philadelphia : J B Lippincott, 1983;407 - 11.

5. Yanagihara M, Mehregan AH, Mehregan DR. Staining of amyloid with cotton dyes. Arch Dermatol 1984; 120:1184 - 5.

Bullous systemic lupus erythematosus

V Aswani, B Vaz, S Shah, RH Malkani

The Indian Journal of Dermatology, Venereology and Leprology (IJDVL)
1993, 59 : 97-100

Abstract

Bullous systemic lupus erythematosus (BSLE) is a rare variant of systemic lupus erythematosus (SLE) which histologically resembles dermatitis herpetiformis (DH) and responds dramatically to dapsone. We report a case of bullous SLE.

Introduction

Cutaneous manifestations of SLE occur in 76% of patients during the course of their disease, but blistering lesions are relatively uncommon. [1] Vesiculobullous lesions may be SLE specific or SLE nonspecific. BSLE is an example of the former. We recently followed up a patient with BSLE.

Case Report

A 36-year-old female presented with joint pains, red raised and fluid filled lesions on the face, neck, trunk and extremities. The lesions used to last for few days then burst to form raw, oozing areas, which used to become crusted.

"

The lesions did not spread after rupture, and healed with scarring, hypo and hyperpigmentation. Since 9 months patient also gave a history of redness of the face on exposure to sunlight, oral lesions and diffuse hair loss. One week before her admission she noted tiny, flat, red lesions on the upper and lower limbs distally. She developed redness of right eye with swelling of the right eyelids, just prior to admission.

The patient had slight erythema with hyperpigmentation on the butterfly area of the face and diffuse nonscarring alopecia. Patient had erythematous papules, plaques on the face, neck and trunk. Discrete, tense vesicles and bullae containing clear fluid were present on normal appearing, erythematous and urticarial skin on the face, neck, trunk and proximal extremities. Bulla spreading and Nikolsky's signs were negative. Raw oozing and crusted lesions were also present. Atrophic patches, hypo and hyperpigmented areas were also present. Carpet tack sign was positive. Purpuric lesions were present on the upper and lower limbs distally. Superficial ulcers were seen on the palate. Systemic examination did not reveal any abnormality.

A complete blood count showed a haemoglobin of 8.7 gm%, PCV 29; leukocyte count of 2450 cells/cmm with - 60 neutrophils, 35 lymphocytes, 1 eosinophil, 3 monocytes. ESR was 30mm/h. Serum iron was 22.5 microgm% (60-160 microgm) and transferrin saturation was 13.3% (15-30%) TIBC and s. electrolytes were normal. Total proteins were 4.7 gm. (6-8 gm), with albumin of 2.0 gm (3.5-5 gm). Total bilirubin, alkaline phosphatase, SGOT/PT were normal. Urinalysis showed 1+albumin with occasional erythrocytes per high power field (hpf), 4-6 leukocytes/hpf and few granular casts. Stool examination and X-ray chest were normal. Elisa test for HIV was normal. Antinuclear antibody (ANA) was negative, direct immunofluorescence of perilesional skin was negative. Anti dsDNA antibody was present (128u/ml). Coombs test, both direct and indirect; were negative.

Skin biopsy of a vesicular lesion showed a subepidermal blister, with neutrophils and fibrinous material in the blister cavity, epidermal necrolysis, neutrophilic papillary microabscesses, a band like infiltrate beneath the blister consisting of neutrophils and lymphohistiocytic infiltrate, oedema of the upper dermis with extravasated erythrocytes and sparse lymphohistiocytic infiltrate in the mid and lower dermis. [Figure - 1][Figure - 2].

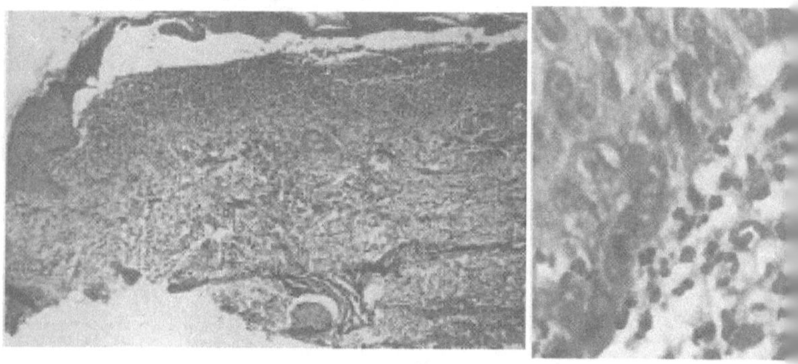

Fig 1 Skin biopsy of vesicular lesion showing subepidermal blister, epidermal necrolysis, a bandlike infiltrate beneath the blister, oedema of the upper dermis with extravasated RBCs (H&E x20)

Fig 2 Histopathology show microabscess with ear formation, oedema of the in the papillary dermis (H

Repeat skin biopsy from an erythematous plaque from the inter scapular region, 5 days after the patient was put on steroids and immunosuppressive therapy showed a thinned out epidermis with flattening of rete pegs, a clear zone in the upper dermis, bandlike infiltrate beneath this zone, with oedema of the upper dermis, neutrophilic papillary microabscesses, dilated blood vessels in the upper dermis with swollen endothelial cells surrounded by predominantly neutrophilic infiltrate. Mixed cell infiltrate was also seen in the lower dermis and around the appendages. A PAS stain showed the thickened basement membrane zone (BMZ) and fibrinoid material in the upper oedematous dermis [Figure - 3].

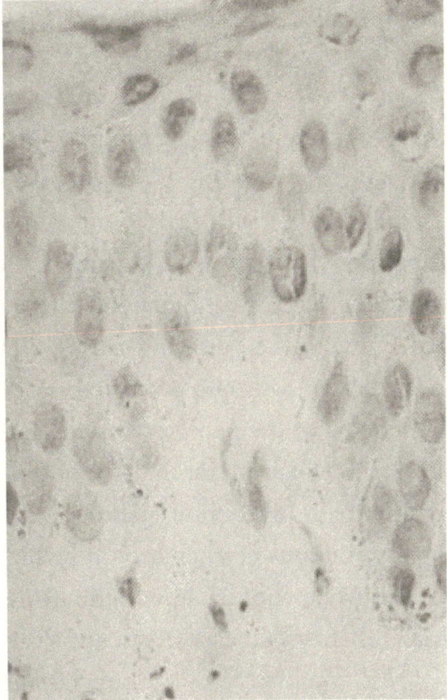

Fig 3 PAS stain highlighting the thickened BMZ and fibroid material in the upper oedematous dermis (PAS x450)

Patient was put on prednisolone 60 mg as single dose in the morning, azathioprine 10 mg/d, erythromycin 1 gm/d, ranitidine 150 mg bid, hydroxyzine hydrochloride 10 mg tid, haematinics and steroid for topical use. Prednisolone was tapered to 40 mg/d at the rate of 10 mg/ week and then at the rate of 5 mg/week. At the time of first follow-up after 1 month patient was free of all lesions, which had healed with scarring and dyspigmentation, patient complained of malar rash on exposure to sunlight and was put on chloroquine phosphate 250mg/d and a sunscreen cream for external use. A complete blood count showed haemoglobin 10.9 gm, leukocyte count of 7,300; neutrophils 59, lymphocytes 31, ESR 58, urinalysis was normal and Anti dsDNA was negative.

At the end of 6 months patient was on prednisolone 5mg/d, azthioprine 100 mg/d, chloroquine 125mg/d and a sunscreen and was free of all skin lesions.

The occurrence of bullous skin lesions in patients with SLE is a well recognized albeit rare phenomenon. Blisters can occur in a case of SLE due to the following causes : (1) They can occur due to extensive hydropic degeneration of the basal cell layer and oedema of the papillary dermis. (2) Bullous lesions occur in BSLE, which is a rare variant of SLE with a DH like histopathology. (3) Bullous pemphigoid, DH, bullous drug reaction, bullous erythema multiforme, epidermolysis bullosa acquisita, linear IgA dermatosis, porphyria cutanea tarda and leukocytoclastic vasculitis can occur in a case of SLE. [1,2] Bullous SLE is a rare variant of SLE with DH like histopathology. Clinically the bullous lesions are predominantly on the face, neck, upper trunk but may be more widespread as seen in our case. The patient may initially present with lesions resembling erythema multiforme.[3] Glomerular nephritis is common, associated with hypocomplementaemia and anti-DNA antibodies. Direct immunofluorescence shows linear deposition of IgG, IgM, IgA and to a lesser extent C3 at the basement membrane resembling bullous, pemphigoid and unlike the IgA seen in the dermal papillae in DH. Circulating antibodies may be absent. A recent study using immunochemical and immuno ultrastructural analysis has demonstrated circulating IgG autoantibodies that are indistinguishable from those found in epidermolysis bullosa acquisita.[3,4] lmmunoelectron microscopy has shown that the immune deposits are predominantly beneath the lamina densa, with globular aggregates also found slightly deeper in the dermis in some areas, subendothelial deposits are frequently seen in superficial dermal blood vessels. [5]

BSLE may or may not be associated with exacerbation of systemic LE. In the former group cutaneous eruption resolves with the treatment and resolution of their SLE. [6] Patients of bullous SLE may respond to high dose steroid therapy and/or immunosuppressive drugs, but the response to dapsone is dramatic. This patient was not given dapsone because her haemoglobin was 8.7 gm%. Dapsone can rarely exacerbate the disease. [3]

Histopathologically BSLE like picture is seen in

(1) DH and DH like drug eruption. The presence of mucin among the collagen bundles in the dermis, the depth of the infiltrate and the

thickened BMZ in BSLE differentiates it from DH and DH like drug eruption.

(2) In bullous pemphigoid the predominant cell is usually the eosinophil. The absence of mucin and thickened BMZ differentiates it from BSLE.

(3) Cicatricial pemphigoid is also characterised by a subepidermal blister with neutrophils in the blister fluid and the dermal papillae, but the absence of mucin and thickened BMZ, and clinical features help in differentiating this entity from BSLE.

(4) Leukocytoclastic vasculitis (LCCV) and septic vasculitis have a histopathologic picture similar to BSLE, but in LCCV the infiltrate invades the walls of the blood vessels while in BSLE it is perivascular. Clinically, generalised vesicles and bullae can occur in LCCV, but they usually become purpuric. In septic vasculitis thrombi are seen inside the blood vessels.

(5) In chronic bullous disease of childhood the histopathologic picture closely resembles that of DH and the absence of mucin, thickened BMZ, and the depth of the infiltrate helps in differentiating it from BSLE.

Camisa and Sharma proposed criteria for diagnosis of BSLE; [7]

(1) A diagnosis of SLE based on ARA criteria. (2) Vesicles and bullae arising on, but not limited to, sun exposed skin, (3) Routine histopathologic findings compatible with DH. (4) Indirect IF negative for circulating BMZ antibodies. This has now been revised as follows Negative or positive indirect IF for circulating BMZ antibodies, using separated human skin as substrate.[1] (5) Direct IF revealing IgG and/or IgM and often IgA at dermoepidermal junction.

References

1. Camisa C, Columbus OH. Vesiculobullous SLE. J Am Acad Dermatol 1988, 18:93 - 100.Back to cited text no. 1

2. Ackerman AB. Histologic diagnosis of inflammatory skin disease. Philadelphia: Lea and Febiger; 1978:629 - 31.Back to cited text no. 2

3. Barton DD, Fine J-D, Gammon WR, et al. Bullous systemic lupus erythematosus: unusual clinical course and detectable circulating autoantibodies to the epidermolysis bullosa acquisita antigen. J Am Acad Dermatol 1986;15:369 - 73.Back to cited text no. 3

4. Rappersberger K, T Schachler E, Tani M, et al. Bullous disease in systemic lupus erythematosus.

J Am Acad Dermatol 1989;21:745 - 52.Back to cited text no. 4

5. Olansky AJ, Briggaman RA, Gamman WR, et al. Bullous systemic lupus erythematosus. J Am Acad Dermatol 1982; 7:511 - 20.Back to cited text no. 5

6. Hall RP, Lawley TJ, Smith HR, et al. Bullous eruption of systemic lupus erythematosus. Ann Intern Med 1982;97:165-70.Back to cited text no. 6

7. Camisa C, Sharma HM. Vesiculobullous systemic lupus erythematosus. J Am Acad Dermatol 1983;9:924 - 33.Back to cited text no. 7

Glucagonoma syndrome

VL Aswani, RH Malkani

Indian J Dermatol Venereol Leprol
1996;62:246-9

Introduction

Changes in the skin can provide clues to the presence of internal malignant neoplasms. When cutaneous signs or symptoms antedate other manifestations of a malignancy, awareness of the relationship between dermatosis and neoplasm may lead to early diagnosis and possible cure. Necrolytic migratory erythema (NME) is a distinctive eruption associated with glucagon secreting islet cell tumour of the pancreas (glucagonoma).

The earliest report of a case of this type was by Becker et al in 1942.[1] Wilkinson in 1973 coined the term NME,[2] and Mallinson et al in 1974[3] published the first series of 9 patients and established the glucagonoma syndrome as a distinct entity.

Case Report

A 38-year-old married businessman from Surat presented to us in August 1994 with reddish scaly, itchy skin rash and skin lesions resembling chemical burns for 2 years on the genitals, perineum, buttocks, thighs and legs with variable periods of waxing and waning. There was history of fluid filled lesions on the legs off and on. One year prior to presentation progressive weight loss and weakness began and there was history of oedema of the feet on dependency off and on. The rash used to respond to systemic steroid therapy.

There was no history of fever, malaise, headache, joint pains, nausea, vomiting, diarrhoea or jaundice, oral cavity involvement, drug ingestion or previous skin diseases. His family history was non-contributory.

The patient was averagely built, afebrile, but looked chronically ill. His pulse and blood pressure were normal. He had pallor. An eruption consisting of erythematous erosions with peripheral scales was seen on the legs extending onto the dorsum of the feet and toes. Occasional intact flaccid bullae could be identified on the legs. The lesions resembled chemical burns [Figure - 1]. Annular, erythematous, scaly lesions, crusts, scaly papules were seen on the buttocks, thighs, back and extensor aspect of the forearms. Crusting was seen on the shaft of the penis. The lesions healed with hyperpigmentation. Hair, nails and mucous membranes were normal. Investigation disclosed the following laboratory values: Hb was 12.1 gm% (normocytic, normochromic); ESR 40 mm in 1st hour; CBC 4400/mm3, N-57, L-40, E-2. Platelet count was normal, blood sugar fasting was 90 mg% and after 75 gm of glucose was 188mg%, S amylase was elevated to 896. Serum iron, TIBC, and transferrin saturation were normal. ANF, thyroid function tests, S cholesterol, LDH, CPK, uric acid, serum calcium, BT, CT, PT, RFT, LFT were normal. HBsAg and Elisa test for HIV I and II were negative. Urinalysis was normal. Stool examination revealed occult blood and ova of Entamoeba histolytica.

Skin biopsy specimen showed hyperkeratosis, necrolysis of the upper stratum malphighii resulting in the formation of upper epidermal blister [Figure - 2]. The necrolytic epidemal cells appeared pale with pyknotic nuclei [Figure - 3]. These changes occurred in the midst of psoriasiform hyperplasia with occasional spongiosis. There were no acantholytic cells. Sparse upper dermal lymphocytic infiltrate was seen.

USG showed focal hypoechoic lesion in the region of the head of the pancreas measuring 5 x 3.5 x 5 cm. A speck of calcification was seen within the mass. CT scan showed soft tissue mass in the head of the pancreas with dilatation of the pancreatic duct. A small calculus was also seen.

The patient underwent Whipple's pancreaticoduodenectomy. The skin lesions disappeared few days after the operation. Histopathology confirmed the diagnosis of malignant islet cell tumour of the pancreas. A mesentric nodule revealed a metastatic islet cell tumour. Subsequently the patient received radiotherapy and chemotherapy.

Discussion

The pancreas is composed of two major types of tissues (1) the acini, which secrete digestive juices and (2)Islets of Langerhans More Details, which secrete insulin and glucagon directly into the blood. The islets contain two major types of cells, the alpha and beta cells. The beta cells produce insulin and glucagon is secreted by the alpha cells. Glucagon causes glycogenolysis and gluconeogenesis.

NME is a peculiar cutaneous reaction with a prolonged fluctuating course characterised by dermatitis, glucose intolerance and hyperglucagonaemia caused by an alpha cell tumour of the pancreas. Glucagonomas occur in the middle age or in the elderly, and are slightly more common in females.

The major diagnostic criteria for diagnosis of glucagonoma syndrome are:

(1) Weight loss, often profound weakness

(2) NME

(3) Glossitis, stomatitis, angular cheilitis

(4) Histopathology showing subcorneal and midepidermal clefts with fusiform keratinocytes with pyknotic nuclei

(5) Diabetes mellitus

(6) Elevated plasma glucagon level

(7) Alpha cell tumour of pancreatic islets with or without metastasis. Glucagonoma may be a rare component of multiple endocrine neoplasia (MEN) either type I or II.

Out of all the features of the syndrome the cutaneous component, necrolytic migratory erythema, appears most often. Cutaneous lesions often precede the diagnosis of the syndrome for long periods, with a mean of 6-8 years and a maximum of 18 years. Characteristically the skin lesion starts as an erythematous area typically at periorificial or intertriginous areas such as groin, buttocks, thighs or perineum and then spreads laterally. The lesions subsequently become raised with superficial central blistering which breaks down to leave an eroded area that crusts. The lesion tends to heal in the centre with peripheral spread. This entire sequence takes 1 to 2 weeks, and while new lesions are developing, others are healing. In a few cases rash has had the appearance of eczema craquele, or may resemble chemical burns. Drier lesions may show a collarette of scale or an entire erythematous plaque may be surmounted by scale, giving a psoriasiform appearance. Perioral and paranasal crusting is almost invariably present at sometime. Thinning of nails with distal friability, decrease in hair density, atrophic glossitis, stomatitis, and angular cheilitis are frequently associated findings. Typically the skin lesions wax and wane, responding poorly to therapy of any type, yet regressing without apparent cause.

Mallinson et al have suggested that glucagon induced hypoaminoacidaemia may be reseponsible for producing the skin lesions through deprivation, so that epidermal proteins cannot be made.[3]

Glucose intolerance with or without frank diabetes occurs in 83-90% of cases. Tumour resection and normalisation of blood glucagon may not result in normalisation of glucose intolerance.[4] The blood glucose returned to normal in our case after the operation.

Weight loss without noticeable anorexia may be a unique feature of glucagonoma. It is seen even in patients with small tumours without metastatic spread and has been attributed to the known catabolic effects of glucagon. Anaemia occurs in 44-85% of cases, is usually of the normocytic normochromic type. Serum iron is normal as was in our case. Anaemia may be due to glucagon excess, because prolonged treatment with a long acting glucagon preparation decreases erythropoiesis in animals. ESR is always elevated. Plasma glucagon levels are elevated. A plasma glucagon concentration of 1000 pg/ml is diagnostic of glucagonoma. Due to nonavailability, it could not be done in our patient. A normal level of plasma glucagon may be able to exclude pancreatic tumour in patients with NME. Two patients have been described[5] with NME without glucagonoma. Both had normal glucagon levels with small intestinal villous strophy and diarrhoea. Cases have also been described with NME without glucagonomas, but with cirrhosis and chronic pancreatitis.

Skin biopsy reveals irregular acanthosis, spongiosis, and the characteristic, well demarcated necrolysis (sudden death) of the outer cell layers in the stratum malphighii. Later, clefts and separation occur at the site without acantholysis. Karatinocytes appear fusiform with pyknotic nuclei. Direct immunofluorescence is negative.

The initial procedure of choice for localisation of the tumour is CT scan as was done in our case. For some patients with small tumours, CT or USG may not localize the tumour, and then selective angiography is the procedure of choice.

Since glucagonomas are generally malignant and it is not possible to predict in a given patient when metastasis may develop, surgical resection should be considered in all patients if feasible. Approximately 50-80% of patients have metastasis at the time of diagnosis. To improve the metabolic status before surgery, blood transfusion for severe anaemia and parenteral amino acids to correct hypoaminoacidemia and thereby the skin rash, is recommended. In cases with hepatic metastasis, at the time of diagnosis, streptozocin has proved beneficial in some cases. Successful treatment with dacarbazine has been reported.[6] Octreotide has also been used to improve the skin rash and symptoms of weight loss, abdominal pain and diarrhoea. Octreotide is a synthetic analogue of somatostatin (growth hormone inhibitor). Somatostatin inhibits the secretion of both insulin and glucagon. Streptozocin, dacarbazine and octreotide can thus be used as palliative agents in this condition. Radiotherapy and other chemotherapeutic agents, as used in our case following surgery, have improved the prognosis in these patients.

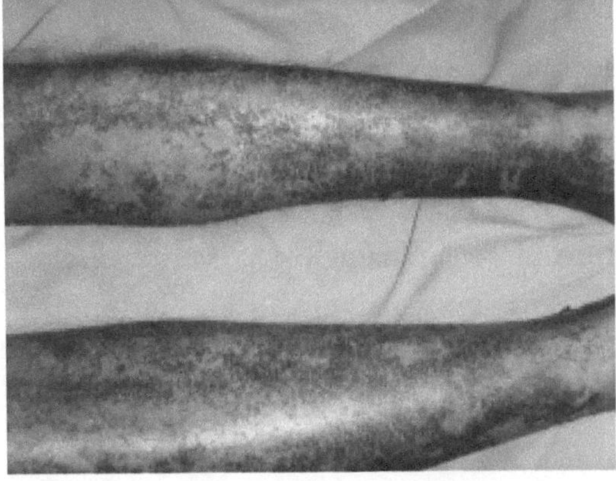

Acknowledgement

The authors are thankful to Dr V N Shrikhande, Hon Professor and Head of General Surgery, Bombay Hospital for surgical management of the patient.

References

1. Kahan R, et al. Necrolytic migratory erythema: distinctive dermatosis of the glucagonoma syndrome. Arch Dermatol 1977;113:792-7.

2. Wilkinson DS. Necrolytic migratory erythema with carcinoma of the pancreas. Trans St John's Hosp Dermatol Soc 1973;59:244-50.Back to cited text no. 2[PUBMED]

3. Mallinson CN, et al. Glucagonoma syndrome. Lancet 1974;ii:1-5.

4. Leichter SB. Clinical and metabolic aspects of glucagonoma. Medicine 1980;59:100.

5. Goodenberger DM, et al. Necrolytic migratory erythema without glucagonoma. Arch Dermatol 1979;115:1429-32

6. Weismann K, Graham RM. Systemic disease and the skin. In: Champion RH, Burton JL, Ebling FJG, editors. Textbook of dermatology. Oxford: Blackwell, 1992:2430-2.

Well's Syndrome

Ajay Chaudhary, Vijay Aswani, Ram Malkani

Indian Journal Dermatology Venereology Leprology; 1997;63:117-9

Introduction

Wells' syndrome or eosinophilic celluitis is a rare, recurrent inflammatory dermatosis of uncertain pathogenesis. It was described by Wells in 1971 as "recurrent granulomatous dermatitis with eosinophilia.[1][2] Wells reported 4 patients with distinctive cutaneous lesions, initially resembling bacterial cellulitis and characterised histopatholgically by dermal eosinophilia, phagocyte histiocytes and presence of "flame figures".

The term "eosinophilic cellulites" was introduced by Wells and Smith in 1971.[2] The observation of similar histopathologic features in a variety of conditions associated with tissue eosinophilia has led some to question the existence of Wells' syndrome as a distinct entity.[3] Wells' syndrome has been described both in adults and children.[2] Associated disorders and potential precipitating factors include insect bites,[3] onchocerciasis, varicella, mumps, atopic diathesis, fungal infections,[2] drug reactions and myeloproliferative disorders.[1][2]

Case Report

A previously healthy 14-year-old female was stung by an unknown insect on her left foot. Within few days, a painful red, infiltrated, blistering plaque developed at the site of the sting. Treatment with oral antibiotics was ineffective. The patient was then subjected to a skin biopay. A biopsy specimen from an erythematous papule on the dorsum of the left foot revealed that the epidermis was mildly hyperplastic and and a slight degree of spongiosis was present. Dermis was diffusely infiltrated by eosinophils both perivascular and interstitial. Collagen bundles incrusted with eosinophilic granules characteristic of "flame figures" were seen. Few lymphocytes were also observed around the dermal vessels.

The patient initially was treated with systemic steroids. The patient initially did respond to steroids, but on discontinuing them, the lesions started to increase in size. Later the patient was treated with antihistaminics along with 10 mg of dapsone. The lesions became nonindurated and flat within 10 days of starting treatment. By the 20th day, only postinflammatory hyperpigmentation was seen.

Discussion

Wells described a clinical and a histopathologic disorder characterised by recurrent granulomatous dermatitis with eosinophilis. Clinical course consists of 2 stages, first or the cellulitic stage being characterised by localised erythema and oedema of the skin, sometimes with blistering and the second or the granulomatous stage charaterised by a gradual resolution of erythema from the centre of the lesions, which remains oedematous and slate colored for several weeks.

Histopathologically, acute stage was characerised by dermal oedema and masses of leucocytes mainly eosinophils. The subacute stage demonstrated dermal eosinophils and histiocytes around angular, focal, fibrinoid masses. The "flame figures" were composed of granules, eosinophilic material adherent to collagen and surrounded by granulomatous inflammation. The late stage reveals resolution of lesions characerised by histiocytic necrobiosis and persistence of "flame figures".

Some authors do not believe that Wells' syndrome is a distinct clinical entity, but rather consider it a histopathologic reaction pattern common to multiple disorders characterised by tissue eosinophilia.[3] Others emphasize that the diagnosis should be reserved for cases with typical features, characerictic histopathology and recurrent course. The "flame figures" can also be found in diverse other diseases including insect bite reactions, dermatophyte id reactions, pemphigoid and Churg Strauss syndrome.[1]

The pathogenesis of Wells' syndrome is unknown. An abnormal or dysregulated eosinophil response appears to be implicated.[4] The "flame figures" are composed of eosinophilic major basic protein deposited on the collagen bundles.[5] Wells' syndrome is known to respond spontaneously. Although systemic steroids appear to be the only therapeutic modality of benefit in Wells' syndrome, antihistaminics and dapsone have been found to be useful.

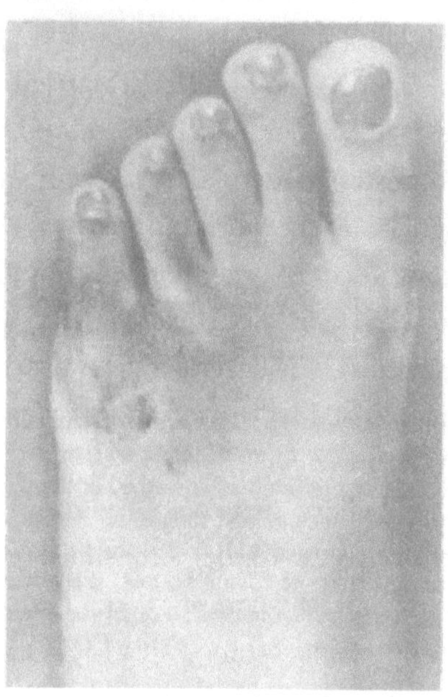

Fig 1 Showing the plaque on the left foot

Fig 2 Showing the characte[r]istic infiltrate and 'flame figures'.

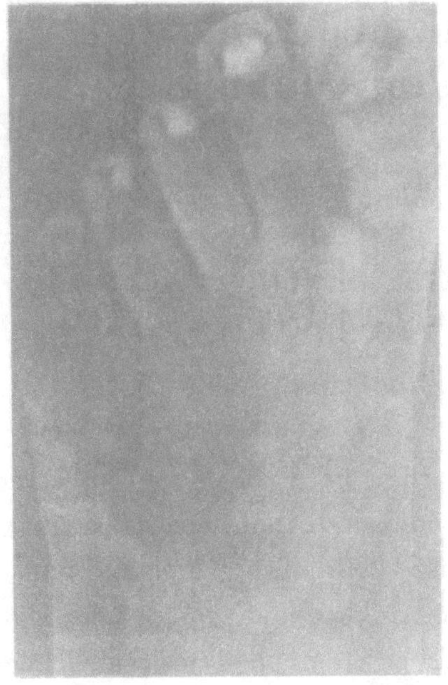

Fig 3 Showing post-inflammatory hyperpigmentation on day 20 of treatment

Generalized umbilicated granuloma annulare

Ajay Chaudhary, Ram Malkani, Vijay Aswani

Indian J Dermatol Venereol Leprol
1998;64:305-6

Introduction

Granuloma annulare has been described in several morphologic forms i.e annular disseminated, subcutaneous, papular and perforating.[1] Although granuloma annulare is primarily a disease of children and young adults, it has been reported in virtually all age groups. Females are affected twice as often as males, and females are affected twice as often as males, and familial occurrence is rare.[2] No associated systemic sequelae are present, and laboratory evaluation is usually normal. Disseminated granuloma annulare is classified separately form the localised form because of the possible association with diabetes, a later age of onset, and rare spontaneous resolution.[3]

Therapy is usually disappointing. Various forms of therapies that have been reported to have a variable response are topical and intralesional steroids, dapsone, retinoids, niacinamide, chloroquine, colchicine, cryotherapy, electrodessication and X-ray therapy.[4] We have recently seen a patient with generalised umbilicated granuloma annulare and believe it to represent a distinct clinico-pathologic entity.

Case Report

A 58-year-old man presented with recurrent episodes of progressive, asymptomatic papular eruption since 7 years. The patient was in good health and denied any recent illness or ingestion of medications. There was no history of diabetes mellitus. On examination the eruption consisted of scattered, erythematous, dome shaped umbilicated papules ranging in size from 0.5 to 1.0 cm. Some papules persisted to increase in size while some regressed spontaneously to leave behind pigmentation.

Initial laboratory examination revealed the following normal or negative results; complete blood cell count, erythrocyte sedimentation rate, liver and renal function tests, urinalysis and chest X-ray. Histopathological examination of the lesion revealed an ill-defined palisading granuloma around the superficial plexus and in the papillary dermis and a central focus of degenerated collagen in the deep dermis inflammatory infiltrate composed of histiocytes, eosinophils and lymphocytes was seen surrounding the necrobiotic collagen [Figure - 1]. Careful serial sectioning failed to show any evidence of epidermal perforation, although there was epidermal thinning, loss of granular layer and parakeratosis.

The patient was treated with long term dapsone, colchicine along with topical steroids which resulted in waxing and waning of the disease process but never total resolution.

Discussion

Our case presented with a distinctive clinical pattern of asymptomatic, flesh-colored, firm papules with a central umbilication distributed over the extremities and the trunk. Histopathologicaily, the palisading granulomas with necrobiotic collagen and a mixed inflammatory infiltrate were distinctive and compatible with granuloma annulare. Epidermal thinning and parakeratosis were present directly over the focal collagen necrobiosis. However, deep serial sectioning through the blocks to look for transepidermal elimination of degenerated collagen failed to reveal any true perforation. Some authors have noted that, if serial histologic sections are not carefully cut, the actual perforation may be missed. However, even with multiple sections, transepidermal elimination has not always been documented.[1]

We propose that there is a spectrum from papular to perforating granuloma annulare, with perforating lesions representing a minority of cases.

Thus, we present this case of generalised papular form of granuloma annulare; the most striking feature of the disorder being central umbilication of papules, probably representing focal collagen degeneration. When this material is eliminated through the epidermis, a true perforating disorder ensues. In most cases, how ever, the necrobiotic material is not extruded and histopathologically, no perforation can be documented. Thus, we propose the term" generalised umbilicated granuloma annulare " as a more appropriate description for the disorder.

We present this case to alert clinician to the distinctive form of granuloma annulare that may be difficult to identify both clinically and histopathologically.

References

1. Cunliffe W J. Necrobiotic disorders, Champion R H, burton J L, Ebling F J G, Eds. Textbook of Dermatology, 5th Edition, 2027-2040.

2. Friedman S J, Winkelmann R K. Familial granuloma annulare. J Am Acad Dermatol 1987;16:600-605.

3. Dabski K, Winkelmann RK. Generalised granuloma annulare: clinical and laboratory finding in 100 patients J Am Acad Dermatol 1989;290:39-47.

4. Samlaska CP, Generalised papular granuloma annulare. J Am Acad Dermatol 1992;27:319-322.

Angiolymphoid hyperplasia with eosinophilia

Ram H. Malkani, Sharmila Nayak

Skin sight issue 3 1999 p. 10-11.

The publication made with educational grant from Books Piramal Health Care Ltd.

A 35 year old female presented with multiple itchy lesions behind the right ear for 4 months duration. There was a history of bleeding from the lesions which was often caused by scratching. There was no history of preceeding trauma, insect bite, allergic contact dermatitis or any major illness in the past. There was no history of similar lesions elsewhere on the body.

Cutaneous examination revealed multiple, small, discrete, soft, erythematous papular lesions with well defined margins over the right post auricular region. There was ho enlargement of pre or postauricular lymph nodes.

On investigation: There was no peripheral blood eosinophilia and serum IgE level was raised (1050.8).

The skin biopsy revealed moderate irregular hyperplasia of epidermis and a moderately dense lymphocytic infiltrate in the upper and mid reticular dermis which was situated predominantly around irregularly shaped vascular spaces. Some of the elongated vascular spaces were lined with prominent histiocytoid endothelial cells.

A diagnosis of pseudopyogenic granuloma (PPG) was made based on the clinical and histopathological findings.

The patient was treated with liquid nitrogen after which there was a considerable flattening of the lesions.

Discussion

An angiolymphoid hyperplasia with eosinophilia (ALHE) is considered as a reactive condition rather than a neoplasm. The dermal form is known as Pseudopyogenic granuloma, whereas, the subcutaneous form is known as Kimura's disease. Previously, ALHE was considered as a late stage of Kimura's disease (KD) and these terms were used synonymously, but now, both are considered as two different clinicopathologic entities.

The aetiology of PPG is obscure, but possibly trauma, low grade infection, nervous factors and the patients' hormonal status play some part in the aetiology.

The features common to both ALHE and KD include a male predominance, predilection for head and neck, a tendency to recur, and lymphoid and eosinophilic infiltrates. However, ALHE occurs in older patients, has a shorter duration and consists of multiple, small, dermal papular or nodular eruptions and it is less frequently associated with peripheral blood eosinophilia. On the other band, KD is usually seen in younger individuals, has a longer duration and occurs as a deeply seated large soft tissue mass without any significant change in the overlying skin. It is associated with lymphadenopathy, peripheral blood eosinophilia and increased serum IgE levels.

Features common to Kimuras disease and ALHE

- Male predominance
- Predilection for Head and Neck
- Tendency to recur
- Lymphoid and eosinophili infiltrates

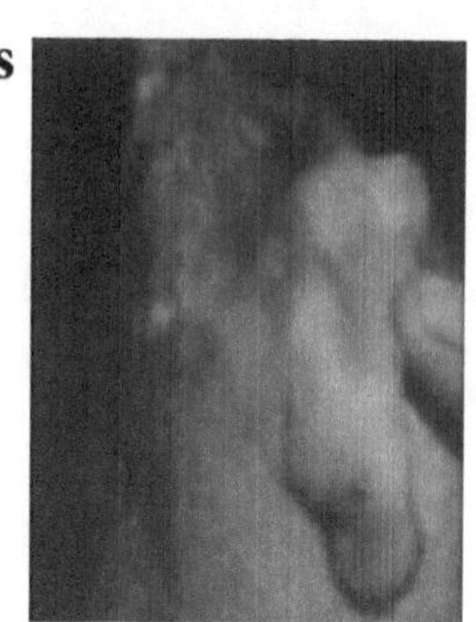

Histopathological studies show that ALHE affects the thick walled blood vessels which have "histiocytoid" on epitheloid" endothelial cells. Whereas in KD the thin walled blood vessels are involved and lymphoid follicles with active germinal centres are seen. "Eosinophilic folliculolysis" is seen only in KD. IgE deposits may be found in the germinal centres.

Among the differential diagnosis ordinary pyogenic granuloma and pyogenic granuloma with multiple recurrent satellites should also be considered.

Therapeutic modalities include surgery, radiotherapy and cryotherapy. There may even be spontaneous regression of smaller lesions within 3-6 months.

In our case, the diagnosis of pseudopyogenic granuloma was made on the basis of clinical and histopathological findings, the unusual feature being raised serum IgE level

References

1. Angiolymphoid hyperplasia with eosinophilea. Text book of Dermatology 5th ed. Champion R. S. Burton J. L., Vol No. 4. P2685.

2. Kimura's disease. J Am Aca Dram, vol. 38 no. 2 part 1, Feb 1998.

3. Inflammatory angiomatous nodules with abnormal blood vessels occurring about ears and scalp (pseudo or atypical pyogenic granuloma). Wilson Jones E,of Bleehem. British Journal Dermatology 1969, 81, 804.

4. Dermal ALHE vs. pseudopyogenic granuloma-Ezzat Kandil. British Journal of Dermatology, 1970, 83 P405.

Pseudo-Kaposi's Sarcoma (Acroangiodermatitis) - A case report

Maithili Shrikhande, Ram Malkani

Bulletin of The Jaslok Hospital and Research CentrE, Vol. XXV No. 1 2000

Introduction

Venous stasis of the lower limbs is a common clinical condition. Skin changes suggestive of stasis induced dermatitis in the form of pruritus, hyperpigmentation etc. are routinely encountered in these cases. We present a rare but known skin manifestation in association with venous stasis called "Pseudo-Kaposi's sarcoma" or "Acroangiodermatitis".

Case Report

A 45-year old housewife, a resident of Baroda, presented with a non healing painful ulcer with an overlying crust over the left lower limb of 3 months duration. She had also noticed a reddish discolouration of the skin over both the lower limbs since 2 years that was gradually increasing in size and number. There was history of intermittent oedema feet. There was no history of diabetes mellitus, hypertension, ischaemic heart disease or any other significant constitutional symptoms. She was referred to us by a dermatologist from Baroda.

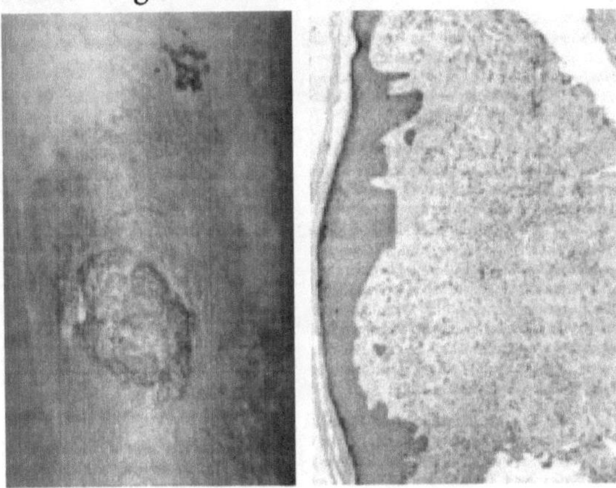

Fig 1 Ulcer with overlying crust over anterior aspect of left lower leg with surrounding reddish-brown discolouration of skin

Fig 2 Histology of Pseudo-Kaposi's sarcoma showing normal overlying epidermis with proliferation of dermal capillaries and fibroblasts, fibrosis, extravasated RBC's and hemosiderin deposition.

On examination, she had an ulcer over the anterior aspect of the left lower leg of approximately 4 cm X 3 cm size. It was covered with a thick yellowish-brown crust that was adherent. The skin around the ulcer showed presence of reddish-brown nonblanching macules and plaques. Similar reddish- brown macules were also present on the anterior aspect of the right lower limb. There was no clinical evidence of varicose veins apart from pitting oedema up to the ankles on both feet.

The blood investigations, which comprised of a complete blood count, renal and liver function tests, blood sugar, antinuclear antibodies, a thyroid profile and tests for HIV and Australia antigen (HBsAg) revealed no abnormality. A punch biopsy taken from a reddish-brown plaque adjacent to the ulcer was reported as a regenerated overlying epidermis over a well vascularised dermis. No indication as regards the ulcer etiology could be ascertained.

A repeat punch biopsy was taken from the reddish-brown plaque and sent for a dermatopathologist's opinion. It showed evidence of a dermal pathology. There were multiple, proliferated and dilated blood vessels within the upper and mid dermis. Additionally, fibroblasts and fibrosis along with extravasated red blood cells (RBC's) and hemosiderin deposits were noted in the dermis. Based on these characteristic histopathologial findings, a clinical diagnosis of acroangiodermatitis (Pseudo-Kaposi's sarcoma) was reached.

Although the doppler studies of this patient did not suggest a deep venous thrombosis, further detailed studies to look for venous incompetence have been asked for. She was treated along the lines of a stasis (venous) ulcer with antibiotics, rest, leg elevation and elastocrepe bandaging. The ulcer healed within 6 weeks.

Discussion

Acroangiodermatitis was a term coined by Mali et al in 1965, wherein he presented a review of 18 cases studied over a 5-year period . He observed that the incidence was more in females than males and that the onset of lesions was around the age of 30-40 years. Earhart named it Pseudo-Kaposi's sarcoma owing to its clinical and histological resemblance with Kaposi's sarcoma, a vascular malignancy. Clinically, the lesions comprise of violaceous or reddish-brown macules, plaques and/or nodules on the dorsum of toes, feet and/or legs at sites devoid of any direct pressure from within or from without . The lesions may undergo painful ulcerations.

There are two types of disorders that may present as Pseudo-Kaposi's sacroma . They have been summarized in the table below.

"Stewart-Bluefarb" type	"Mali" type (Acroangio-dermatitis)
Associated with Klippel-Trenaunay -Weber syndrome i.e. a congenital syndrome comprising of a venous malformation/AV fistulas	Associated with long standing venous stasis
Early onset in life	Onset later in life
Unilateral	Usually bilateral

The case presented here conforms to the "Mali" variety of Pseudo-Kaposi's sarcoma.

The histologic findings of this angiopathy resemble Kaposi's sarcoma with fibroblastic and neovascular proliferation, extravasated RBC's and hemosidering deposits. However, the classic vascular slit pattern, atypicality of endothelial cell nuclei and spindle cells seen in Kaposi's sarcoma, are absent in Pseudo-Kaposis's sarcoma. Unlike stasis dermatitis, acroangiodermatitis is usually associated with minimal epidermal changes and eosinophils in the inflammatory infiltrate of the dermis(5).

In case of any clinical and/or histological diagnostic dilemma between Kaposi and pseudo-Kaposi sarcoma, immunolabelling with CD34 antigen serves as an important diagnostic marker of Kaposi's sarcoma cells . In chronic venous insufficiency, the insufficiency of the calf muscle pump results in an elevated capillary pressure. Mercury gauge plethysmography studies have concluded that patients with Pseudo-Kaposi's sarcoma present an insufficiency, not only of the muscular pump of the calf but also of the venous pump of the foot . The long standing oedema and relatively high oxygen saturation of the affected tissue results in proliferation of fibroblasts, collagen and smaller vessels .

This case has been reported for its rare occurrence and its clinical and histological resemblance with the vascular malignancy, Kaposi's sarcoma. Kaposi's sarcoma, a malignancy of vascular origin is either seen sporadically in elderly males or endemically in children and adults in some African countries or is associated with non-HIV related immunosupression e.g. transplant patients or with late stages of HIV disease.

In view of India's increasing incidence of HIV infection, it is important to differentiate this benign condition of Pseudo-Kaposi's sarcoma from Kaposi's sarcoma.

References

1.	MaliJWH,KuiperJP,EarnersAA: Acroangiodermatitis of the foot. Arch Dermatol 1965;92: 515-518.

2. Earhart RN, Aeling JA, Nuss DD et al: Pseudo Kaposi Sarcoma. Arch Dermatol 1974;110: 907-910.

3. Bluefarb SM, Adams LA: Arteriovenous malformation with acroangiodermatitis. Arch Dermatol 1967;96: 176-181.

4. Walter F. Lever, Gundula Schaumberg-Lever.Tumors of vascular tissue. pp689-721. In:Histopathology of the Skin. Walter F. Lever, Gundula Schaumberg-Lever (Eds); Lippincott Company, 7th edition, 1990, Philadelphia, USA.

5. Rao B, Unis M, Poulos E: Acroangiodermatitis: a study often cases. In J Dermatol 1994; 33 (3):179-183.

6. Kanitakis J, Narvaez D, Claudy A: Expression of the CD34 antigen dishtinguishes Kaposi's sarcoma from pseudo-Kaposi's sarcoma (acroangiodermatitis).BrJDermatol 1996;134(1): 44-46.

7. Collard JJ. Kuiper JP, Brakkee AJ: Action of the venous pump of the foot in patients with acroangiodermatitis. Philebiologie1978;31(3):249-256.

Livedoid Vasculitis

Vijay Aswani, Ram Malkani

Bulletin of The Jaslok Hospital And Research Centre Vol. XXV No. 4 2001 p 11

Introduction

Livedoid vasculitis is a chronic, recurrent, hyalinising vasculopathy of the small blood vessels of the legs. The ulcers that may result from it heal with small stellate white scars called atrophic blanche.

The initial lesions consist of petechiae, purpuric papules, haemorrhagic bullae. Some lesions heal without further progression, whereas others become necrotic and coalesce to form angular ulcers, Healing, which takes place over several weeks or months, leaves a white depressed scar with small telangiectasia at the margins. The pain associated with this syndrome is more diffuse, and more severe, than the appearance of the lesions could suggest.

We report a case of livedoid vasculitis, with excruciatingly painful, large ulcers, on the lower extremities, in a female.

Case Report

A 58 years old housewife presented to us on 23rd June 1999 with exquisitely painful ulcers on the legs, ankles, and dorsum of feet since 6 years, associated with ankle edema. Varicose veins were present in both the legs, since seven years.

She had no history of connective tissue disorder, dysproteinaemia, thrombophlebitis, Raynauds phenomenon or intermittent claudication. There was no history of blunt trauma, contact allergies or hypertension. She did not give history of summer or winter exacerbation. On physical examination patient was found to have multiple, well defind ulcers, on the legs, ankles and dorsa of feet ranging in size from few mms to 5 cms, some covered with yellow slough, and some with haemorrhagic crust, surrounded by erythematous, hyperpigmented border (Fig.1).

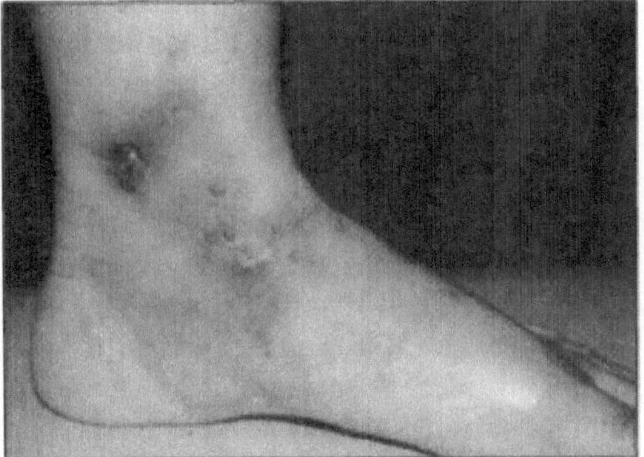

Her Hb was 11.3 gms%, CBC was normal, ESR was 45 mm at the end of 1 hr.

Her platelet count, blood sugar, BUN and Urine examination were normal, ASO Titre was 100. Her Serum bilirubin, SGOT, GGT were normal, but SGPT was 92 mm on 23/6/1999 which came down to 30 mm 4/8/99. Her VDRL and LDH isoenzymes were normal.

Her ANA, cryoglobulins, Cardiolipin antibody, PTT, Serum Protein electrophoresis, were all normal, as well as her serum calcium and phosphorous.

Her pus swab revealed MRSA and E.coli, AFB were not seen. Doppler did not reveal any DVT.

Skin biopsy taken from an erythematous plaque around an ulcer, showed a partially necrotic, superficial epidermis, acanthosis, spongiosis, and a superficial perivascular lymphohistiocytic infiltrate.

A blood vessel in the deeper dermis was occluded and infiltrated by eosinophilic fibrinoid material and surrounded by a lymphohistiocytic infiltrate.

The patient was put on Tab. Aspirin 1/2 tablet OD, Tab. Dipyridamole 25 mg BID, Tab. Stnazolol 4 mg BID. Along with antibiotics and painkillers, cleaning and dressing of the ulcers was done daily. The small ulcers had healed at the end of two weeks, while the large ulcers healed at the end of three months.

Discussion

Livedoid Vasculitis, originally defind by Feldaker et al, is an uncommon condition occurring principally on the lower legs and ankles of women. It is associated with varicose veins in some patients, and it was found in 21 of 81 patients attending a surgical clinic with symptoms of venous insufficiency. Rarely, lesions occur on the dorsum of the hand, or elsewhere on the limbs. In an early lesion, in the absence of ulceration the condition is often symptomless .

Recurrent ulceration and healing often produce scars with a reticular pattern. This latter condition is often referred to as Atrophic Blanche.

Atrophic Blanche is classified into :

1. Idiopathic Atrophic Blanche. Patients may show purpuric macules, haemorrhagic bullae, progressing to form ulcers, that heal with characteristic scars, or only show scars without any evidence of inflammation or ulceration.

2. Idiopathic Atrophic blanche associated with Idiopathic Livedo reticularis. One third patients in this group have Raynaud's phenomenon as, and may have hypertension.

3. Atrophie blanche as a manifestation of systemic disease. Eg. LE, Periarteritis nodosa, Raynaud's phenomenon.

Histologically striking feature is the eosinophilic fibrinoid material in the wall and lumen of blood vessels in the middle and deep dermis. This is a vasculo occlusive disorder, unlike LCCV- Leucocytoclastic vasculitis, which result from circulating antigenantibody complexes.

No single form of therapy has been consistently effective for the treatment of Atrophie blanche, but drugs that inhibit platelet thrombus formation eg. Aspirin, or stimulate endogenous fibrinolytic activity eg. phenformin, arrest the disease in most patients.

References

1. Feldaker M, Mines EA, Kierland RR:Livedo reticularis with summer ulcerations.ArchDermatol 1055; 72: 31-42.

2. Frain Bell W. Atrophie blanche.Trans St. John's Hospt Dematol Soc 1959; 42-59-65.

3. Milstone LM, et al: Classification and therapy of atrophie blanche. Arch Dermatol 1983, 119:963.

Primary Systemic Amyloidosis

Maithili Kamat, Ram Malkani

Paper presented at the clinical meeting held at the Jaslok Hospital & Research Centre on Nov '15, 2002

REFLECTIONS

*The patient presented with purpura on the tongue, face, feet. He would develop purpura on coughing, which reflected the blood vessel wall was fragile because of deposition of amyloid on the walls of the arterioles, capillaries. The diagnosis of Systemic Amyloidosis was obvious on clinical presentation. A search was made to confirm the existence of Multiple Myeloma, as it was a case of **Primary Systemic Amyloidosis, and** was not successful. Patient belonged to another city and was lost to follow up.*

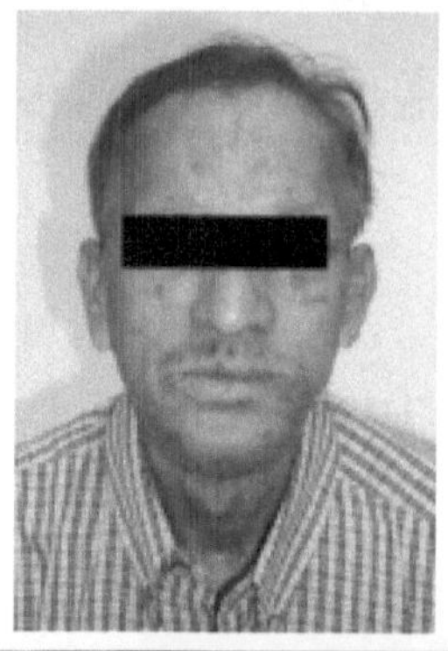

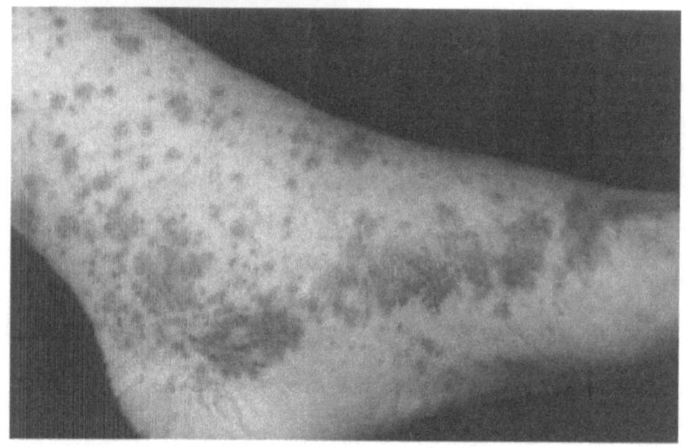

Echymoses

History

- 65 yr old male patient presented with

- C/C:

- Asymptomatic red lesions around the eyes off
and on since 1 yr

- Similar lesions on rest of the face and neck

- Reddish patches & nodules on tongue off & on; inability to eat spicy food

- Lesions appeared spontaneously or on minor trauma

Investigations

CBC / ESR: WNL
Platelet Count: adequate
Renal / Liver / Lipid profile: WNL
BS(random): WNL
ECG / 2D Echo: NAD
Urine for Bence Jones proteins: Absent
S.Immunoelectrophoresis: Normal
USG (abdo): s/o suspicious slight echotexture of liver

Diagnosis

- Systemic amyloidosis
- - ? primary
- - ? multiple myeloma associated

AMYLOID & SKIN – CLASSIFICATION

SYSTEMIC AMYLOIDOSIS

PRIMARY / MYELOMA ASSOCIATED	SECONDARY
(underlying plasma cell dyscrasia)	- Rheumatoid arthritis (14 - 26%) - Reiter's syndrome - Ankylosing spondylitis - Tuberculosis - CTD's - Behcet's syndrome - Leprosy - Drug abuse

Addison`s pigmentation

Vijay Aswani, Ram Malkani

Presented at the clinical meeting held at the Jaslok Hospital & Research Centre on Nov' 21 -2003

Reflections

Patient had classical clinical presentation of Addison's disease. In this patient, it turned out to be Addisonian pigmentation, as his serum cortisol levels were normal. On skin biopsy clofozamine deposits were seen in the dermis.

- The cutaneous manifestations include darkening of the skin especially in sun exposed areas

- Hyperpigmentation of the palmar creases, frictional surfaces, vermilion border, recent scars, genital skin, and oral mucosa

- Case History

- 24 year old male, a case of tuberculous meningitis, on primary & secondary line of drugs including clofazimine, presented with diffuse brownish pigmentation on the face, neck, proximal & distal inter phalangeal joints.

- Increased pigmentation of palmar & flexural creases of the fingers.

A 24 year old, male presented with

- Increased pigmentation over the knuckles, dorsum of the fingers and face since 4 months.

- K/C/O Tuberculous meningitis, diagnosed 2 ½ years ago, still on medication for the same.

- On oral steroids (Prednisolone) since June 2002.

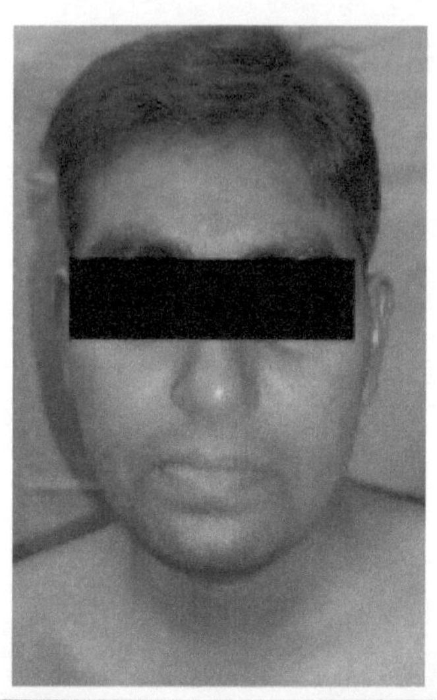

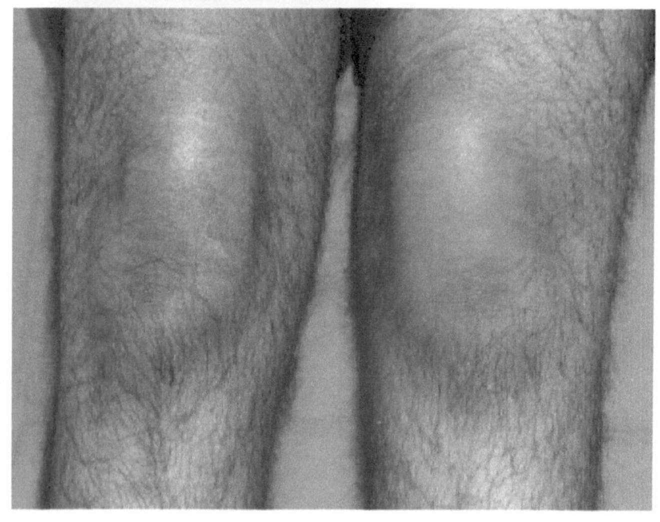

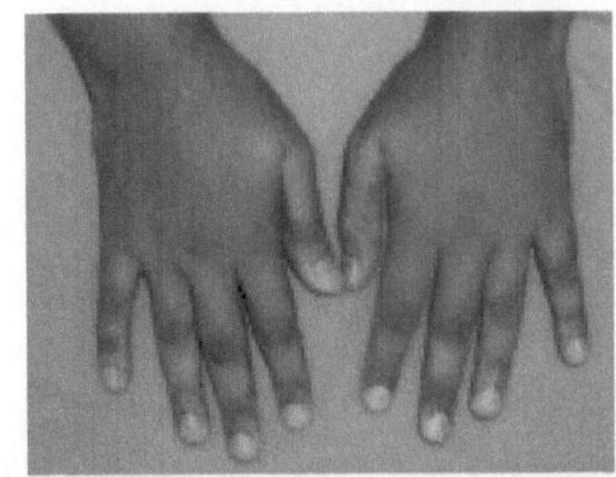

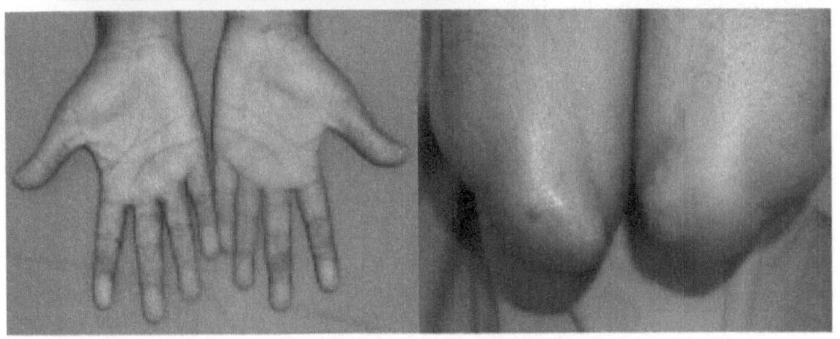

INVESTIGATIONS

- HB - WNL S.VIT – B12 level -> 1200pg/ml
- CBC - WNL(174–878)
- LFT - WNL S.FOLATE level - 14.4 μgm/ml
- RFT - WNL (3–17.0)
- TFT - WNL S.ACTH - 22.5pg/ml (0-46)
- Urine - WNL
- Serum Cortisol – 7.7 μgm/ml(8 to 25) (9.15 a.m.)

0.2 μgm/ml(1 to 17) (4.00 p.m.)

FINAL DIAGNOSIS

CLOFOZIMINE INDUCED ADDISONIAN PIGMENTATION

CAUSES OF ADDISONIAN PIGMENTATION

1. ADDISON'S DISEASE
2. NUTRITIONAL – FOLATE DEFICIENCY
3. – VIT B12 DEFICIENCY
4. PITUITARY DYSFUNCTION
5. DRUGS- ZIDOVUDINE, CLOFOZIMINE & BLEOMYCIN

Acute Graft - Versus Host Disease manifesting as skin lesions in a post allogenic stem cell transplantion in Chronic Myeloid Leukemia

Namita Talsania, M.M. Basade, Ram Malkani

Bulletin of the Jaslok Hospital & Research Centre, Vol XXVII No 4 April 2003; p 12

Introduction

Graft Versus host disease (GVHD) is the consequence of immunocompetent donor T cells targeting recipient tissues that possess the antigens absent from the donor. We report a case of acute GVHD presenting as a generalised maculopapular rash in a post allogenic stem cell transplantation in Chronic myeloid leukemia (CML).

Case Summary

A 32 years old female, hailing from Bangladesh presented to us in December 2000 with complaints of fever since 2 months loss of weight and appetite since 1 ½ months. Patient was initially well. Patient was investigated in Bangladesh a month before presenting to us for the same. Bone marrow Aspiration was suggestive of CML. USG of the abdomen revealed moderate splenomegaly. The patient was referred to us for further evaluation and management.

At Jaslok Hospital patient was investigated. A repeat Bone marrow aspiration was done which was suggestive of CML in chronic phase. Patient was given option of treatment and was chosen for allogenic stem cell transplant. HLA matching of the siblings were done. One of the brother was taken up as a donor for the stem cells as he was fully matched. Patient was started on chemotherapy with Salvin protocol in March 2001, which consisted of Fludarabine, antithymocytic globulin, methyl prednisolone. At the same time, donor was given Inj. Grastim (G-CSF) 600 microgram per day and on 4th day his peripheral blood stem cells were harvested. The total mononuclear blood stem cells dose was 7x10 per kg (CD34 + cells were 0.75%). Patient was given cyclosporine as immunosuppressive agent Patient recovered without requiring any blood component support. Stem cell reinfusion was done on 19th March 2001. In mid April 2001 a repeat bone marrow done showed normal marrow 98% of the cells as donor cells 2% as Philadelphia +ve. In mid May 2001 Bone marrow aspiration done showed all the cells were of the donor. Patient was kept on immunosupressants and discharged. She was asked to taper off Cyclosprine over 6 weeks period.

Patient presented to us +95 days post transplant with history of maculopapular rash, fever, generalized bodyache and erosive oral lesion for 15 days. Maculopapular lesion started on the palms which spread over to the limbs, trunk and face becoming generalized soon.

The lesions on the palm were more prominent. The lesions were associated with severe itching. The fever was noted after the rash. Fever was continuous low grade. There was severe edema on the face and palms.

Patient was investigated and treatment was started immediately considering acute GVHD as the diagnosis.

Following investigations were done: Blood investigation showed WBC 3890, Hb-11.3, platelets 1,60,000. Liver function test was deranged total bilirubin -2.5, direct bilirubin- 1.6, SGOT-95, SGPT-133, GGT-446. USG of the abdomen showed mild splenomegaly. Liver normal in appearance and morphology. Portal vein and bile ducts normal. Urine examination showed bile pigment +ve, RBC-1-2, pus cells 2-3, faint trace of albumin, amorphous urate crystals in large number.

Examination

Local: There were 2 type of skin lesions affecting almost the whole body with greater density on the palms. There were desquamating erythematous lesion on the forehead and scalp. The lesion on the forearm were exfoliated. The second type of lesions were more in number, were maculopapular confluent rash affecting the whole body. The lesions on the palm were papulonodular type.

Systemic: There was mild icterus, oedema on the face and dorsal aspect of the wrist. There were erosive oral lesions. Rest of the system were normal.

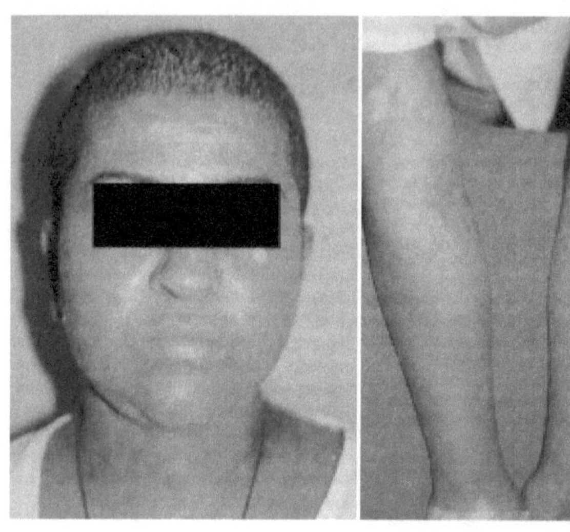

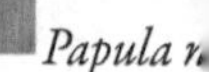

Desqumating erythematous lesion involving the face and the scalp   *Erythematous maculopapular rash involving the forearms*   *Papula r*

In view of acute GVHD patient was started on following medications. Inj Cefrom, Inj Tobraneg, Inj Forcan Inj Cyclosporin (60mg) 12 hrly. Inj Methyl prednisolone (500 mg) 6 hrly, Tab. Zovivax (400 mg) 5 times a day. Dexona eye drops.

Discussion

GVHD develops when immunocompetent lymphoid T-cells which are histoincompatible are given to an immunodeficient patient. If the recipient is normal because of the differences in histocompability donor lymhocytes would ordinarily be destroyed, but if recipient is immunodeficient, the cells, instead of being destroyed, proliferate and attack the recipients (host) tissue producing a reaction involving the skin, gastrointestinal tract and liver.

GVHD chiefly occurs in patient receiving bone marrow transplant for leukemia, and aplastic anaemia. The specific antigens which induce GVHD are Human leucocyte antigens.

Graft versus host reactions (GVHR) is the term that denotes the specific immunological phenomena induced by the graft of competent foreign lymphoid cells in a recipient incapable of rejecting them. The recipient must possess antigens absent in the donor against which the grafted cells react. GVHR occur in patients even after successful marrow grafting for various disorders including immunodeficiency diseases, aplastic anemia, acute leukemia and radiation exposure despite careful histocompatibility matching. The antigen which are disparate between the patient and donor serve as a target for GVHD in HLA identical sibling transplants are referred to as minor histoincompatibility. In our case to there was minor histoincompatibility.

Among the manifestations of GVHD it is customary to distinguish between early or acute lesions (before 100th day) and chronic or late manifestations (after 100th day). The acute form develops usually within 100 days of post transplant period. The acute form appears to be caused by cytotoxic cells that have lost the controlling influence of regulating suppressor cells. In acute GVHD tissues most susceptible are the epithelium of the skin, mucous membrane, intestines and liver. In gastrointestinal GVHD predominantly involves the distal small bowel and colon. It is clinically associated with cramping abdominal pain and watery diarrhoea. Hepatic involvement is characterized by a rise in alkaline phosphates and total bilirubin often in association with a mild to moderate increase in liver transaminases. Our patient had hepatic involvement with raised liver enzymes. It is not clear why some organs are spared from damage in systemic immune response. In addition to the affected end organs, florid acute GVHD is associated with immunosuppression and susceptibility to infection. Reduction in the incidence and grade of GVHD is associated with higher rates of tumor relapse.

The observation that there is increased risk of leukemic relapse after T-cell depletion of the allograft as well as the observation that relapse was less likely in patient with a history of acute or chronic (GVHD, lent credence to the concept that a donor immune mediated antimalignant effect called Graft- Versus-leukemia (GVL) effect. The most compelling evidence for the GVL effect is seen in patient with relapsed CML, after transplant who are successfully induced back to complete remission following the infusion of donor lymphocytes. The efficacy of donor lymphocyte infusion (DLI) for the treatment of relapsed leukemia is disease-dependant with remission induction occurring in a substantially higher percentage of the patient with chronic phase CML than in patient with advanced CML or other acute leukemia. The major complication associated with DLI is acute and chronic GVHD(6).

CD4+ T helper cells appear to play a particularly important role in the GVL effect in CML, CD4+ T cells are cytolytic to CML cells. Donor T cells are principle mediators of GVHD in an HLA- mismatched setting, CD8+ T cells may target major histocompatibility (MHC) class-I mismatched antigen, whilse CD4+ T cells are responsible for the recognition and targeting of MHC class-II mismatched antigens. The antigen that are disparate between the patient and the donor serve as a target for GVHD in HLA identical sibling transplant.

The usual methods for bone marrow transplantation: The ideal donor is a related subject, compatible for the ABO blood groups as well as being HLA identical. These latter groups are dependent upon the major histocompatibility compex (MHC). This complex is divided into A, B, and C loci whose products are detected by serological methods (SD), and another locus, D, differentiated by mixed lymphocyte culture. When dealing with marrow transplantation, identical serological groups A and B and the absence of reactivity between donor and recipient lymphocytes in mixed lymphocyte culture (testifying to D identity) are verified. The existence of identical A, B and D loci in related subjects assures, in principle, that all the major histocompatibility genes, contained in humans wholly on the 6th chromosome, are identical(7).

Matched related allogenic stem cell transplant: The transplant related mortality range between 10 to 40% but can be as high as 68%. Younger patient do better, older patient do worse mainly because of an increased related mortality. Largest effect of treatment is achieved in chronic phase of CML. Anti-CML chemotherapy before transplant influences posttransplant outcome. Acute GVHD occurs in 8 to 63% of patient while chronic GVHD in 75%. T-cell related transfusion improved tolerance and decrease treatment related mortality. The incidence of relapse post transplant is lowest in chronic phase and highest in blastic phase.

Matched unrelated donor (MUD): The transplantation involved donors who are chosen on the basis of molecular HLA typing. Matching at the HLA- DRB 1 locus was the most significant factor, influencing overall survival, disease free survival and treatment related mortality. T cell depletion of MUD allograft is associated with a decrease in severe acute of chronic GVHD although there appears to be no beneficial effect in survival. There is some evidence, however, that survival may be better in the recipients of MUD transplants containing higher stem cell doses. This observation has stimulated interest in the develop of transplant that use higher total CD34+ cells doses for instance, through the use of granulocyte colony-stimulating factor .

Mismatched related donor: The availability of haploidentical (half matched related donors) has led to the use of mismatched family members as an alternative source of stem cells for those patients who lack an HLA identical sibling. The number of mismatched MHC antigens in the patient is conventionally used to define the degree of mismatch may range from 3 (haploidentical) to zero antigen, depending on the number of phenotypically shared antigen coming from the mismatched haplotyope. T cell depletion, is associated with a significant decrease in incidence of severe GVHD, although the incidence of graft rejection is increased.

Cutaneous manifestations of GVHD:

The skin rash begins initially as itching, pain on pressure and erythema on the post auricular region, face, neck and shoulders and spreads on to the trunk and limbs and may develop diffuse maculopapular erythema with lichenoid papules or bullae. Rarely a severe toxic epidermal necrolysis like rash or exfoliative erythroderma can develop outcome of which is fatal. A distinctive follicular pattern may develop. Acral involvement, characterized by an erythematous rash of the palms and soles and violaceous discoloration of the ears. Rash may sometimes be a scarlantini form with confluent sheets of erythema that desqumate and leave areas of hyperpigmentation. Even the clinical picture suggestive of varicella form may be present.

Treatment

Reintroduction of immunosuppression agents like Cyclosporine, Methotrexate, Steroids, Azathioprine.

References

1) IADVL. Texbook and Atlas of dermatology and venerology. Volume-2, 2nd edition. Editor in chief. R.G. Valia, assistant- editor Ammet. R. Valia.

2) Texbook of Dermatology, 4th edition. Edited by Arthur Rook/D.S. Wilkinson. F.J.G. Ebling/ R.H. Champion J.L. Burton. Volumes 1 and 2. Blackwell Scientific Publications.

3) Cancer Principles and Practice of Oncology. Vicent Y. Devita, Jr Saumet Hellman Steven. A. Rosenberg, Lippincott Williams and Wilkins.

4) Harrison's Principle of internal Medicine, 14th edition. Fauci, Braunwald, Isselbacher, Wilson, Martin, kapsen, Hauser, Longo. International edition.

5) Schweiz Med Wochenichr 1996 March 2:126(9):339-47. Itinph, Lautenschlagers, Orto B, Rufli T, Gratwohl A, department fur Dermatologie, Universiat Sklinik Base.

6) Cancer principles and practice of Oncology, Vincent T. Devita, Jr., MD. Samuel Hellman, MD. Steven. A. Rosenber MD, Ph.D.

7) Graft versus host reactions. F.C. Roujeau, J.Revuz, R. Touraine.

Reversal of nail changes after liver transplantation in a child

Vidhyachandra Gandhi, Aabha Nagral, Sujith Philip, Ram H. Malkani, Rujuta Pimputkar

Indian J Gastroenterol 2009(July–August):28(4):154–156 DOI: 10.1007/s12664-009-0054-8

Abstract

We report a 6-year-old girl who received a left-lobe live-related liver transplant for decompensated liver disease after a failed Kasai's surgery for biliary atresia. Preoperatively, her nails were white, dystrophic, brittle with severe onycholysis, clubbing and watch-glass deformities. Nail scrapings were negative for fungus. Five months after transplantation, her nails had become near normal. There is only one such documented case in literature on reversal of nail changes in an adult.

Introduction

Liver cirrhosis is associated with various extrahepatic manifestations including nail changes. Data on reversal of nail changes in patients with liver cirrhosis are limited. We report here a child with liver cirrhosis and who had marked nail changes that reversed after liver transplant.

Case Report

A 6-year-old girl had undergone Kasai's surgery for biliary atresia at the age of 3 months. She presented with pruritus, recurrent ascites, failure to thrive and recurrent episodes of cholangitis due to secondary biliary cirrhosis. On examination, she was severely malnourished, had deep icterus and moderate ascites, liver palpable 3 cm and spleen palpable 4 cm below the costal margin. Her Pediatric End Stage Liver Disease (PELD) score was 36 and Child-Pugh Score was 13. She was subjected to a leftlobe living related liver transplantation from her mother. Preoperatively, finger nails were dystrophic (discolored and distorted) and brittle (Fig. 1A). Nails in both hands and both feet had severe onycholysis (Figs. 1A, 2A), grade 3 clubbing (predominantly in the ring finger) (Fig. 1A) and watchglass deformity (predominantly in the little finger of the left hand and second toe of left foot) (Figs. 1A, 2A). Also, the nails were white (leuconychia) (Fig. 1B). Nail scrapings were negative for fungus.

The nail abnormalities started regressing from the first month after transplantation. The leuconychia became more prominent as the dystrophic changes reversed. By 5 months, the appearance of nails had returned to near normal (Figs. 1B, 2B).

Discussion

There has been only one report (image) in literature mentioning reversal of nail changes after liver transplantation in adults.[1] We believe that the present case is the first detailed documentation of reversal of nail changes after liver transplantation in a child. Nail changes in cirrhosis include changes in the nail plate and nail color. The nail plate changes include clubbing, watchglass deformity, onycholysis, Beau's lines[2] (horizontal deep grooved lines caused by any disease severe enough to disrupt normal nail growth) and brittleness. Our patient showed all the nail plate changes except Beau's lines. Clubbing is due to peripheral vasodilatation and opening up of arteriovenous fistulae in the nail beds and an increase in nail bed connective tissue.[3] The watch glass deformity (convex deformity) is a milder form of clubbing with a slightly convex surface of the nail.[3]

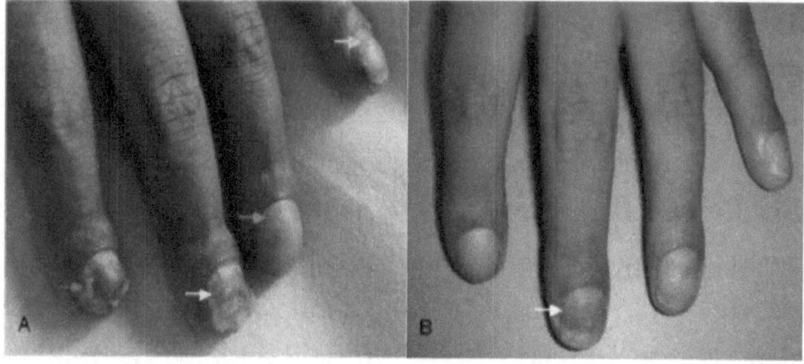

Fig. 1 Appearance of finger nails before (A) and after (B) liver transplantation. The abnormalities observed before transplantation included onycholysis (index finger; red arrow), discolouration and distortion (dystrophy) (middle finger; yellow arrow), clubbing (ring finger; blue arrow), and watch glass deformity (little finger; green arrow). After transplantation, the abnormalities reversed, though a white nail (Terry's nail; white arrow) persists in the middle finger

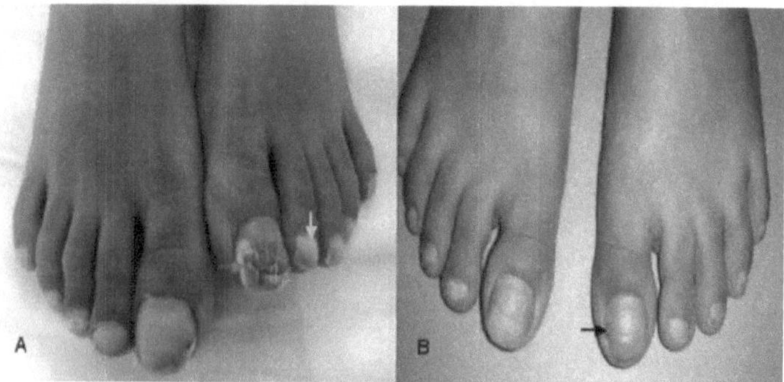

Fig. 2 Appearance of toe nails before (A) and after (B) liver transplantation. The abnormalities observed before transplantation included onycholysis (great toe, red arrow) and watch glass deformity of second toe (green arrow). After transplantation, the abnormalities reversed; the black arrow points to a new nail on the great toe that is replacing the old nail

Our patient had a significant regression of clubbing after liver transplant. Onycholysis occurs when the nail plate is separated from the nail bed resulting in white discoloration of the affected area. It can be caused by systemic disorders, local infection or trauma.[4] In our patient the nail scrapings were negative for fungus. Though onycholysis is not described in liver disease, it could have occurred in our patient secondary to increased brittleness and unnoticed trauma. However, it reversed after transplant, suggesting that onycholysis may be a manifestation of liver disease.

The nail color changes described are white nails or leuconychia (Terry's nails), Muehrcke's bands and red lunulae. Terry's nails were initially attributed to hypoalbuminemia, but are now believed to be due to an abnormal ratio of estrogen to androgens, abnormal steroid metabolism and increased digital blood flow. Muehrcke's lines are paired narrow white bands that extend all the way across the nail. These occur in patients with hypoalbuminemic states.[6] Red lunulae are attributed to either increased arteriolar blood flow or changes in the optical properties of the overlying nail making the normal blood vessels become more prominent.[7]

Overall, the nail changes in patients with liver cirrhosis are secondary to disturbances in hormone metabolism, altered digital blood flow, hypoalbuminemia and soft tissue overgrowth in the nail bed. Liver cirrhosis is associated with various extrahepatic manifestations. Some of these, though not specific to liver disease, reverse after liver transplantation possibly because etiopathogenetic factors underlying these cease to exist.[8] We believe that this is also the reason for reversal of nail changes.

References:

1. Marinho RT, Perdigoto R. Reversal of nail changes in rimary biliary cirrhosis after liver transplantation. J Hepatol 1999;30:330.

2. Noronha PA, Zubkov B. Nails and nail disorders in children and adults. Am Fam Physician 1997;55:2129–2140.

3. Smith KE, Fenske NA. Cutaneous manifestations of alcohol abuse. J Am Acad Dermatol 2000;43:1–16.

4. Fawcett RS, Linford S, Stulberg DL. Nail abnormalities: clues to systemic disease. Am Fam Physician 2004;69:1417–1424.

5. Holzberg M, Walker HK. Terry's nails: revised definition and new correlations. Lancet 1984;i:896–899.

6. Muehrcke R. The fingernails in chronic hypoalbuminemia. Br Med J 1956;1:1327–1328.

7. Wilkerson MG, Wilkin JK. Red lunulae revisited: a clinical and histopathologic examination. J Am Acad Dermatol 1989;20:453–457.

8. Stracciari A, Tempestini A, Borghi A, Guarino M. Effect of liver transplantation on neurological manifestations in Wilson disesase. Arch Neurol 2000;57:384–386.

Pigmentory purpuric dermatoses a manifestation of chronic venous insufficiency

Sneh Thadani, Ram Malkani

Presented as a poster at DERMACON 2012

Abstract

A 32 year old male complains of pigmentation and swelling of both lower limbs since 4 years. Pigmentation started around the ankle and has progressed proximally. Occasional pain on standing for long hours

On investigation

Colour Doppler

Both Saphenofemoral and saphenopopliteal junctions are competent. No evidence of any deep vein thrombosis seen. Perforators noted as follows: Incompetent perforator measuring 4.9 mm seen in right leg about 25.0 cm above medial malleolus. An incompetent perforater measuring 3.1 mm is seen in left leg about 8.0mm above medial malleolus In view of the above, we observed that Pigmentory purpuric dermatoses (PPD) can be a manifestation of chronic venous insufficiency, Since the pathology of PPD and venous insufficiency is similar, i.e. damage and breakage of vessel wall.

Case History

32 year male complains of swelling, pain and pigmentation of bilateral leg since 4 yrs which is progressive

Pigmentation of bilateral leg has been progressive increasing since 2002

Gives history of LONG STANDING

H/o increase in pain and swelling after standing for long hours, which used to come down after resting but now the swelling is constant and pain has increased. H/o of progressive pigmentation

Investigation: Colour Doppler

Both Saphenofemoral and saphenopopliteal junctions are competent. No evidence of any deep vein thrombosis seen. Perforators noted as follows: Incompetent perforator measuring 4.9mm seen in right leg about 25.0cm above medial malleolus. An incompetent perforater measuring 3.1mm is seen in left leg about 8.0mm above medial malleolus.

According to CEAP classification

He is C4aEnApPr

VCSC 12

He has

1) APCR 146 (N)
2) FACTOR 5 (N)
3) HOMOCYSTEINE LEVEL (N)
4) LIPID PROFILE
S. CHOLESTROL 159(N)
HDL. 48(N)
S. TG 51(N)

LDL 119(N)

5) VDRL NEGATIVE

6) D-DIAMER 500-1000(RAISED)

On examination:

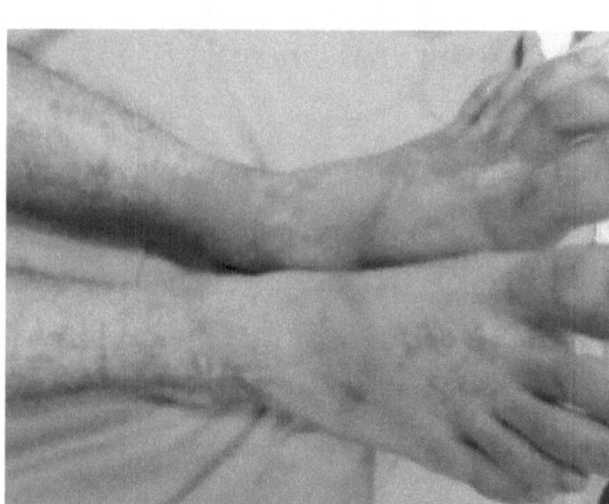

Progressive swelling and hyperpigmentation of bilateral lower limbs, extending from foot to the mid calf region. No active ulcer. Few varicosites seen. Pigmentation - hyperpigmented macules to patches over the ankle and tibial area.

Review of literature

Introduction

PIGMENTORY PURPURIC DERMATOSES (PPD)

The pigmented purpuric dermatoses are a group of disorders characterized by purpuric pigmented lesions resulting from extravasation of erythrocytes in the skin with marked hemosiderin deposition. PPD commonly occurs on the lower extremities of individuals.

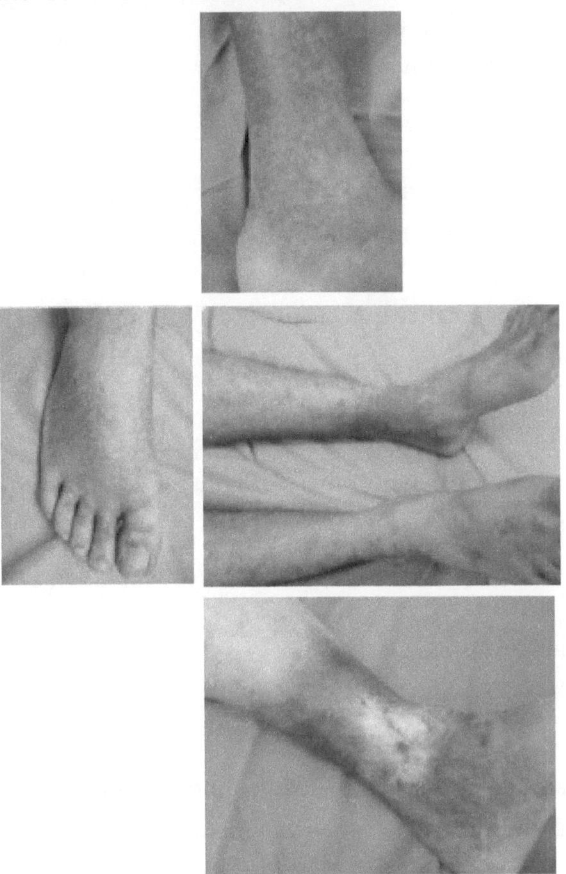

Morphology

Punctuate purpuric macules develop on the lower extremities, particularly around the ankle and on the prebital region. Widespread lesions with involvement of trunk or upper extremities may regularly occur.

Confluence of lesions produces irregularly shaped larger macules that may have a brownish color.

Pathogenesis

Several mechanism have been proposed, but no single theory has explained all of the changes

Venoushypertension

Exercise

Delayed humoral immunity

Delayed hypersensitivity

Perforator vein incompetence

Venous statis

Vascular abnormality leading to vessel wall fragility

Clinical types

Schamberg's disease

Majocchi's disease (Purpura annularis telangiectodes)

Gougerot-Blum syndrome (Pigmented purpuric lichenoid dermatitis)

Ducas and Kapetanakis pigmented purpura

Lichen aureus

Granulomatous PDD

Histology

Histologically, a perivascular T-cell lymphocytic infiltrate is centered on the superficial small blood vessels of the skin, which show signs of endothelial cell swelling and narrowing of the lumen. Extravasation of red blood cells with marked hemosiderin deposition in macrophages is also found, and a rare granulomatous variant of chronic pigmented dermatosis has been reported.

CHRONIC VENOUS INSUFFICIENCY(CVI)

Chronic venous insufficiency (CVI) is a condition that affects the venous system of the lower extremities rendering the superficial, perforator, and deep veins incompetent. This results in venous hypertension causing various pathologies including pain, swelling, edema, pigmentation and ulceration.

Pathogenesis

The underline pathology leading to CVI is a consequence of venous hypertension.

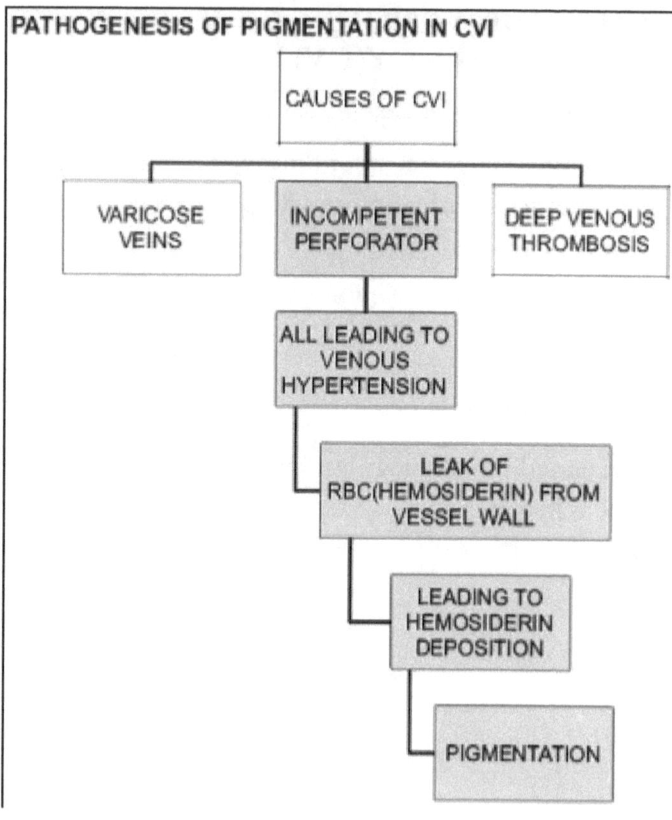

Conclusion

In the above cases, the pathophysiology of the two diseases mentioned are similar that in perforater incompetence and venous hypertension.

As we observe the cause of pigmentation in both remains the same i.e. inflammation of the vessel wall leading to their fragility and extravasations of RBC into the superficial dermis. As hemosiderin, a breakdown product of RBC, which is indigestible by macrophages .The pigmentation is persistent and progressive.

SO CAN IT BE CONCULDED THAT PIGMENTORY PURPURIC DERMATOSES CAN BE A MANIFESTATION OR A PART OF CHRONIC VENOUS INSUFFICIENCY

Reference

1 Aiba S, Tagami H. Immunohistologic studies in schamberg's disease .Evidence for cellular immune reaction in lesional skin .Arch dermatol.1988;124;1058-62.

2 Author: Darius Mehregan, MD, Associate Professor, Hermann Pinkus, Chairman of Dermatology, Department of Dermatology, Wayne State, University; Clinical Associate Professor of Pathology, University of Toledo;Dermatopathologist, Pinkus Laboratory; Consulting Staff, Department of Dermatology, J Dingell Veterans Affairs Medical Center Coauthor(s): Jennifer Michelle Heyl, MD, Resident Physician, Department of Dermatology, Wayne State University School of Medicine

3. Peter . J. Pappas, Brajesh K . Lal, Frank T. Jr, Robert W. Zickler, and Walter,

4. The Vein Book. John J. Bergan

5. S. Das. A Manual on Clinical Surgery

Erythromelalgia

Venisha B Shah, Chandni N Merchant, Ram H Malkani

Presented as Poster at the IADVL National Conference DERMACON 2013

Introduction:

Erythromelalgia (EM), a condition initially described by Mitchell a painful disorder of the extremities characterized by redness, swelling, a burning sensation, and an increase in skin temperature exacerbated by exposure to heat.(1) An early description was reported by Mitchellin 1878(2). The name is derived from 3 Greek words: erythros ("red"), melos ("limb"), and algos ("pain").

Erythromelalgia may occur either as a primary or secondary disorder .Primary erythromelalgia is an autosomal dominant disorder. It is classified as either juvenile or adult onset. Juvenile onset occurs prior to age 20 and frequently prior to age10.

Secondary erythromelalgia can result from small fiber peripheral neuropathy of any cause, essential thrombocytosis (erythromelalgia can also develop in the presence of normal platelet counts in patients with myeloproliferative disorder), hypercholesterolemia, mushroom or mercury poisoning, and some autoimmune disorders.(3) Here we present a case of erythromelalgia secondary to juvenile diabetes.

Case Report

A 34-year-old female was referred to our dermatology department for redness and burning sensation over the soles associated with episodic intense pain since the past 18 months (Figures 1 and 2).The pain was excruciating, burning in quality, and worsened with ambulation as well as being placed in a dependent position. It was triggered by prolonged standing and exposure to warmth, and was alleviated on resting the limbs along with elevation and on application of ice cold water. The patient was diagnosed as a case of juvenile diabetes mellitus at the age of eight years and is on insulin therapy. At the age of 27 she was diagnosed to have diabetic nephropathy and was on maintenance dialysis for the same. She used to have hypertensive episodes in between and was on antihypertensive medication.

The patient had symmetrical erythema, scaling, warmth and erythemotousblanching on the instep and plantar surface of both feet which supported the diagnosis of erythromelalgia. All toe and finger nails showed thickening and yellow discoloration of the nail plate. There were no sensory deficits to light touch and pin prick. Keeping in mind the secondary causes of erythromelalgia patient was thoroughly investigated. In complete blood count haemoglobin was low blood sugars were high, Renal function test showed high creatinine. Liver function test enzymes were elevated. Serum electrolytes revealed low sodium, high potassium

ANA profile was done and was weakly positive. HCV antibody was positive. She developed ascites also and ascitic fluid analysis showed high proteins, sugar 223mg/dl, albumin and counts were normal. Keeping in mindthe diagnosis of vasculitis, serum cryoglobulinsand complement levels were checked which were normal. Skin biopsy from the instep of sole showed stasis changes and ecchymoses.

In view of the above, a diagnosis of Erythromelalgia secondary to diabetic and chronic kidney disease was made. Patient was started on Gabapentin 75 mg daily which relieved the pain but erythema, burning and warmth persisted.

The patient stayed in remission for almost 8-9 months after which she presented again with similar complaints. She was started on Tab Gabapentine 75 mg daily and Tab Propranolol 10 mg thrice daily for 15 days, to which she responded with gradual decrease in the pain and redness on her soles. In her follow up tab cilastozol was also added and now patient responded well.

Discussion :

Erythromelalgia was formerly known as Mitchell's disease (after Silas Weir Mitchell), acromelalgia, red neuralgia, or erythermalgia(4) Mitchell first described erythromelalgia in the 1870s, and Smith and Allen further categorized it in 1938, proposing the term erythermalgia to emphasize the characteristic warmth.

Its distinctive triad of intense burning extremity pain associated with erythema and increased skin temperature are diagnostic(5).

Raynaud's phenomenon occurs in response to cold exposure and presents as pallor of the fingers or toes, often followed by cyanosis and rubor. Why did you start with

Raynauds? Attacks last from a few minutes to several hours are most commonly set off by exposure to cold or emotional distress and consist of pallor, sometimes followed by cyanosis and rubor of fingers and less commonly of toes, nose, and ears.(6) Our patient had persistent erythema and had history of worsening of symptoms in high temperature.

Erythromelalgia is a rare condition that has remained an enigma diagnostically and therapeutically for decades. Recent research in the U.S. found the incidence of EM (the number of people a year diagnosed with EM) to be 1.3 per 100,000. The rate for women was higher 2 per 100,000 per year than men, which was just 0.6. The median age at diagnosis was 61(7).

Our patient had early presentation of the disease. Primary erythromelalgia is an autosomal dominant disorder. It is caused by mutation of the voltage-gated sodium channel α-subunit gene SCN9A. Primary erythromelalgia is idiopathic or sporadicand secondary erythromelalgia is due to underlying neurologic, hematologic, or vascular problems.(8) The causes can be essential thrombocytosis, hypercholesterolemia, mushroom or mercury poisoning, and some autoimmune disorders. Among the secondary forms, its association with diabetes mellitus is infrequent and its significance is little known (9).

Our patient had erythromelalgia secondary to juvenile diabetes but the age of onset is 32yrs which is quite young. Patient used to give history of worsening of symptoms even when blood sugars were controlled.

Treatment with pharmacologic agents and surgery are ineffective except in the secondary group where treatment of the associated disorder generally results in a remission. Symptoms in the primary group can be minimized by appropriate environmental control with cooling and avoiding heat-producing situations that would raise skin temperature above a critical thermal threshold(10)

The diagnosis is based on the medical history and clinical findings – what about histological findings? The most useful oral medications for erythromelalgia are aspirin, propranolol, clonazepam, cyproheptadine, drugs inhibiting serotonin reuptake (venlafaxine and sertraline), tricyclic antidepressants (amitriptyline, imipramine), anticonvulsants (gabapentin), calcium antagonists (nifedipine, diltiazem), and prostaglandins (micoprostol). We had given our patient gabapentin and the patient was responding well (11).

Erythromelalgia is usually chronic, sometimes progressive, and disabling disease, which can greatly affect the quality of life. Some patients have stable disease and get better, or even experience full resolution of the disease, with time.(1)

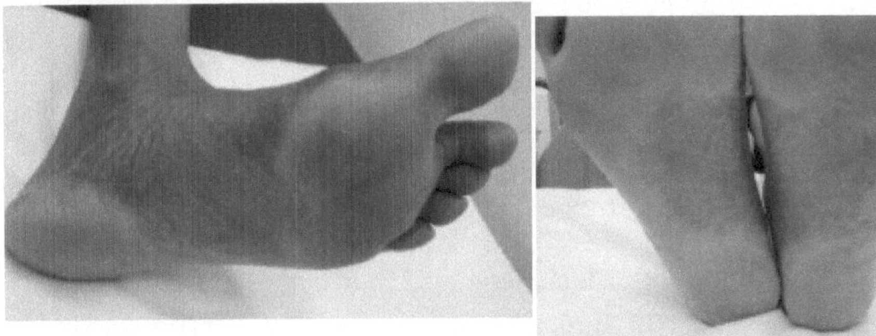

Fig 1: Symmetrical erythema, scaling, warmth and blanching on the instep and plantar surface of both feet   *Fig 2 After 1 month of therapy*

Despite multiple treatment options, erythromelalgia is a challenging disease to effectively manage. Early recognition and treatment may offer patients the best probability of achieving remission or significant improvement.(12) Living with erythromelalgia can result in a deterioration in quality of life resulting in the inability to function in a work place, lack of mobility, depression, and is socially alienating; much greater education of medical practitioners is needed. As with many rare diseases, many people with EM end up taking years to get a diagnosis and to receive appropriate treatment. EM remains a rare condition that most doctors are completely unaware of; consequently EM patients may take years to get proper pain control. Like many rare conditions the management of the condition is patient led as they are usually completely knowledgeable of their condition and what needs to be done

Conclusion:

Erythromelalgia if untreated has disabling consequences. This patient has unusual severe co-morbid conditions, which could be responsible for the development of this disease. We report this case for its rarity, unexplored aetiology and the challenges posed in its diagnosis and treatment.

References:

1.   Ljubojević S,Lipozencić J,Pustisek N. Erythromelalgia.Acta   Dermatovenerol Croat.2004;12(2):99-105.

2.   Rudikoff   D,   ,   Israeli A.Jaffe.Erythromelalgia:Response to serotonin reuptake inhibitors Journal of the American Acad Of Dermatol August 1997; 37(2) :281-283, .

3.   Lisa   M.Coppa,Kishwer   S.Nehal,James W.Young,Allan   C.Halpern.   Erythromelalgia precipitated by acral erythema in the setting of thrombocytopenia.Journal of the American Acad of Dermatol June 200; 48(6) :973-975,

4 Khalid F,Hassan S,Qureshi S,Qureshi W,Amer S.(2012)."Erythromelalgia: An   Uncommon Presentation   Precipitated   by   Aspirin Withdrawal".Case reports in Medicine 2012: 616125

5. James,William D. ; Berger,Timothy G. ; et al.(2006).Andrews' Diseases of the Skin: clinical Dermatology.Saunders   Elsevier.p.816.ISBN 0-7216-2921-0

6.   Berlin   AL,Pehr   K.Coexistence   of erythromelalgia and Raynaud's phenomenon J Am Acad Dermatol.2004 Mar;50(3):456-60.

7. Reed KB,Davis MD (January 2009)."Incidence of erythromelalgia: a population-based study in Olmsted   County,Minnesota".J   Eur   Acad Dermatol Venereol 23 (1):13–5.

8.   Michiels JJ,Drenth JP,Van Genderen PJ.Classification and diagnosis of erythromelalgia and erythermalgia.Int J Dermatol.Feb 1995;34(2):97-100

9.   Vendrell J,Nubiola A,Goday A,Bosch X,Esmatjes E,Gomis R,Vilardell E . Erythromelalgia associated with acute diabetic neuropathy: an unusual condition. Diabetes Res.1988 Mar;7(3):149-51.

10.   Thompson GH,Hahn G,Rang M Erythromelalgia. Clin Orthop Relat Res.1979 Oct;(144):249-54.

11. Cohen JS.Erythromelalgia: new theories and new therapies.J Am Acad Dermatol.2000 Nov;43(5 Pt 1):841-7

12. Buttaci CJ. Erythromelalgia: a case report and literature review.Pain Med.2006 Nov-Dec;7(6):534-8.

Wegener's Granulomatosis: A report of two Cases with different clinical and laboratory features

Ram H Malkani, Rahul Dixit, Maninder Singh Setia

Indian Journal of Basic and Applied Medical Research; June 2015: Vol.-4, Issue- 3, P. 109-112

Abstract

We present two cases of Wegener's granulomatosis (WG) with systemic involvement. Our first case, a 50 year old female, presented with painful vesicles on the left side of neck and chest. She was diagnosed as post-primary tuberculosis due to persistent cough and a nodular opacity in the left lower lobe of the lung. A wedge biopsy of the lung tissue did not show any mycobacteria, and an open biopsy showed granulomatous inflammation with necrosis. The serology for cytoplasmic antineutrophil cytoplasmic antibodies (c-ANCA) and perinuclear – antineutrophil cytoplasmic antibodies (p-ANCA) was negative and renal parameters were normal. Our second case, a 50 year old male, presented with fever, productive cough, and blood stained nasal discharge for the past 15 days with no cutaneous lesions. The renal biopsy showed cresentic glomerulonephritis and serum tested positive for c – ANCA. Both the cases were diagnosed as WG and managed using corticosteroids and/or cytotoxic medications. These cases represent the different clinical and laboratory features of limited and classical forms of WG respectively, and though the second case did not require extensive investigations, the first case posed a diagnostic challenge since one of the common differential diagnosis of nodular lung involvement with persistent cough in developing countries is tuberculosis.

Introduction

Wegener's granulomatosis (WG) is a multisystem disorder of unknown etiology characterised by necrotizing granulomatous inflammation and vasculitis involving both arteries and veins.(1) The disease is more common in males and seen in fourth and fifth decades of life; the estimated incidence of the disease in the population being 4 per million to 8.5 per million.(2,3) WG exists in two forms: 1) the classic form which affects the upper respiratory tract (URT), the lower respiratory tract (LRT), and the kidneys; 2) the limited form which affects only the URT and LRT.4 Apart from these organs, WG can also affect the skin, eyes, joints and the central nervous system.5 Detection of circulating cytoplasmic antineutrophil cytoplasmic antibodies (c-ANCAs) and histopathology of the affected organs are useful to diagnose WG at an early stage.(6) Indeed, the increase in estimates of WG has been attributed to increased clinical suspicions and availability of good laboratory tests.(2) We present two cases of WG presenting with different clinical and laboratory features to our clinic.

Case report

Our first case, a 50 year old female presented with painful vesicles on the left side of neck and chest (over the cervical dermatomes – two, three, and four) in November 2012. Thus, based on these findings, we diagnosed her to be a case of cervical herpes zoster (Figure 1a and b). The patient reported that she had cough for three months, seven years ago for which she was investigated. An initial X- ray of the chest showed the presence of a nodular opacity in the left lower lobe (Figure 2) and subsequently, the computerised tomography (CT) scan of the chest showed features suggestive of post-primary tuberculosis. The patient underwent a repeated CT scan at a different centre. The second scan showed pleural thickening and a mass in the lower lobe of the left lung. The patient was then diagnosed as case of non-small cell carcinoma of the lung by fine needle aspiration cytology. Subsequently, the patient was referred to specialised cancer centre. A repeat CT scan of the chest showed features suggestive of malignancy and a positron emission tomography

(PET) scan suggested an active disease in the lower lobe. A wedge biopsy of the lung tissue did not show any acid fast bacilli or other mycobacteria and an open biopsy of the lung tissue showed granulomatous inflammation with necrosis. The patient was diagnosed as a case of WG based on the above investigations. The serology for c-ANCA and perinuclear – antineutrophil cytoplasmic antibodies (p-ANCA) was negative. The serological investigations for renal parameters did not show any abnormalities. She was started on 40 mg of prednisolone daily; the dose was gradually tapered to 5 mg and she has been on this dose for the past five years. The patient was treated with valacyclovir in a dose of one gram three times daily for seven days for her current skin lesions. The patient did not follow-up after starting the therapy for herpes zoster. Our second case a 56 year old male, admitted in the nephrology department of our hospital and was referred to our department for dermatological evaluation. The patients presented to the hospital with complaints of fever, cough with expectoration, and blood stained nasal discharge for the past 15 days. We did not find any cutaneous lesions on examination of the patient. The patient, however, had a high serum creatinine (5.6 mg/dl), a patchy nodule in the lower base of the lung (as seen on X-Ray), and a cyst in the right kidney and cholelithiasis (as seen on the ultrasonography). The patient was initially managed by repeated dialysis with limited success (levels of serum creatinine did not reduce). glomerulonephritis and the patient's serum tested positive for c – ANCA. Thus, based on the above clinical features and investigations, the patient was diagnosed as a case of Wegener's granulomatosis.

The patient was started on a monthly pulse of methylprednisolone (1gram per day for three days) and cyclophosphamide (500 gram on day of pulse therapy) along with oral cyclophosphamide 50 mg on non pulse days. After three pulses (when the patient was referred to us) there was reduction in the nasal symptoms and the creatinine levels were within normal limits.

Discussion

The two cases of WG discussed above presented with different manifestations. The first case with the involvement of the upper and lower respiratory tracts presents a diagnostic dilemma, particularly in our clinical settings.(7) However, with the increasing awareness about the condition and introduction of serological markers like c - ANCA, the efficacy in diagnosing WG has greatly increased. However the sensitivity of c - ANCA is low (65-70%) in cases with limited WG and is often negative in about 10- 20% of the cases – this added to the diagnostic challenge in our case.(1, 6) Finally, a surgical procedure (open lung biopsy) was instrumental in helping us with the diagnosis of WG. Another feature which could have helped us with the diagnosis is therapeutic response to steroids and cytotoxics.(1) However, the differential diagnosis of tuberculosis (which will be very common in our settings) may prevent us from diagnosing WG based on a therapeutic response.

Furthermore, the cutaneous feature of herpes zoster in our patient may be due to immunosuppressive therapy rather than the disease itself. Our second case was representative of the classic form of WG. Though, the patient had upper and lower respiratory tract symptoms with high serum creatinine, the presence of c – ANCA and features of the renal biopsy were instrumental in final diagnosis of the condition. In both these cases introduction of cyclophosphamide and prednisolone resulted in rapid clearance of symptoms. To summarize we can say that Wegener Granulomatosis is a multisystemic disease with atypical course and manifestations, and should be considered as an important differential diagnosis of nodular lung lesions. Cutaneous features such as palpable purpurae (most common), papule plaque, ulceration, vesicles, urticaria like lesions, subcutaneous nodules and panniculitis are seen in up to 50 % of cases.8,9,10 Thus, patients who present with respiratory and renal symptoms and do not respond to conventional therapy should be investigated for WG. Though, serological tests such as c-ANCA may be useful in the confirmation diagnosis, its utility is limited in the 'limited' variety of WG and one may have to resort to more invasive procedures such as biopsies for confirmation of diagnosis.(6)

Acknowledgements: We would like to thank Dr. Rushi Deshpande for recommending the case.

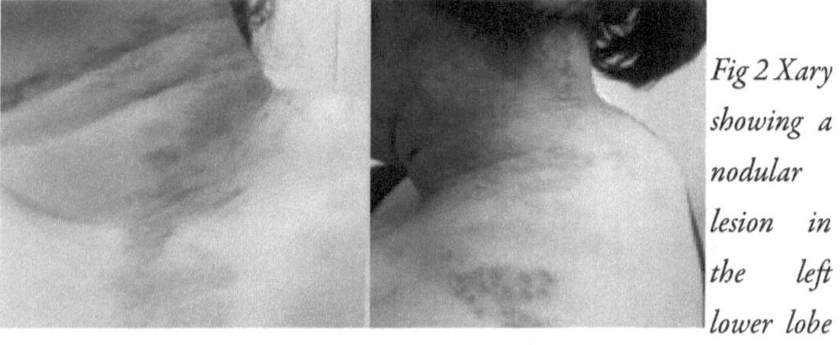

Fig 2 Xary showing a nodular lesion in the left lower lobe of the lung

Fig 1 a and b photograph of the vesicular lesion on the neck and chest

References

1. Dey A, Arunabha DC, Sudipta P, Susmita K, Mita S. A young lady presented with limited

pulmonary Wegener's granulomatosis. Lung India 2008; 25:168-71.

2. Aasarod K, Iversen BM, Hammerstrom J, Bostad L, Vatten L, Jorstad S. Wegener's granulomatosis: clinical course in 108 patients with renal involvement. Nephrol Dial Transplant. 2000 May; 15(5):611-8.

3. Watts RA, Carruthers DM, Scott DG. Epidemiology of systemic vasculitis: changing incidence or definition? Semin Arthritis Rheum1995; 25: 28-34.

4. Pradhan VD, Badakere SS, Ghosh K, Almeida A. ANCA: Serology in Wegener's granulomatosis. Indian J Med Sci 2005; 59:292-300.

5. Ghosh A, Bandyopadhyay D, Basu S, Majumdar A, Dutta S. ANCA-negative limited Wegener's granulomatosis. Indian J Dermatol Venereol Leprol 2004; 70:102-4.

6. Jashnani KD, Rupani AB, Deshpande JR, Karekar MD. Is positive c-ANCA mandatory for the diagnosis of Wegener's granulomatosis? Indian J Pathol Microbiol 2008; 51:307.

7. Singh YN, Malaviya AN, Sharma SK, Kumar A, Wali JP, Dash SC, Bhuyan UN. Wegener's

granulomatosis in northern India. J Assoc Physicians India. 1992 Sep; 40(9):594-6.

8. Hoffman GS, Kerr GS, Leavitt RY, Hallahan CW, Lebovics RS, Travis WD, et al. Wegener granulomatosis: an analysis of 158 patients. Ann Intern Med 1992;116:488-98

9. Daoud MS, Gibson LE, DeRemee RA, Specks U, el-Azhary RA, Su WP. Cutaneous Wegener's granulomatosis: clinical, histopathologic, and immunopathologic features of thirty patients. J Am Acad Dermatol 1994; 31:605-12.

10. Patten SF, Tomecki KJ. Wegener's granulomatosis: cutaneous and oral mucosal disease. J Am Acad Dermatol 1993; 28:710-8.

A Rare Overlap of Epidermolysis Bullosa Acquisita and Seronegative Rheumatoid Arthritis

Venisha B. Shah, Ram H. Malkani

Presented at DERMACON 2013

Epidermolysis bullosa acquisita (EBA) is an autoimmune subepidermal blistering disease of the skin and mucus membranes characterized clinically by blisters, scars, and milia at the trauma-prone areas.

We present you a case of 27 year old female, Nigerian resident who presented to dermatology OPD with complaints of recurrent itchy fluid filled lesions over scalp, upper and lower extremity since 3 years. History of itching prior to onset of lesion and healing of lesion with atrophy, scarring and hypopigmentation. History of loss of finger and toe nails over a period of 2-3 years. History of oral lesions with difficulty in swallowing. No history of rash prior to onset of symptom. History of joint pain with early morning stiffness since 4 years and was diagnosed as a case of Seronegative Rheumatoid Arthritis on Tab Methotrexate and oral steroid but non compliant with treatment.

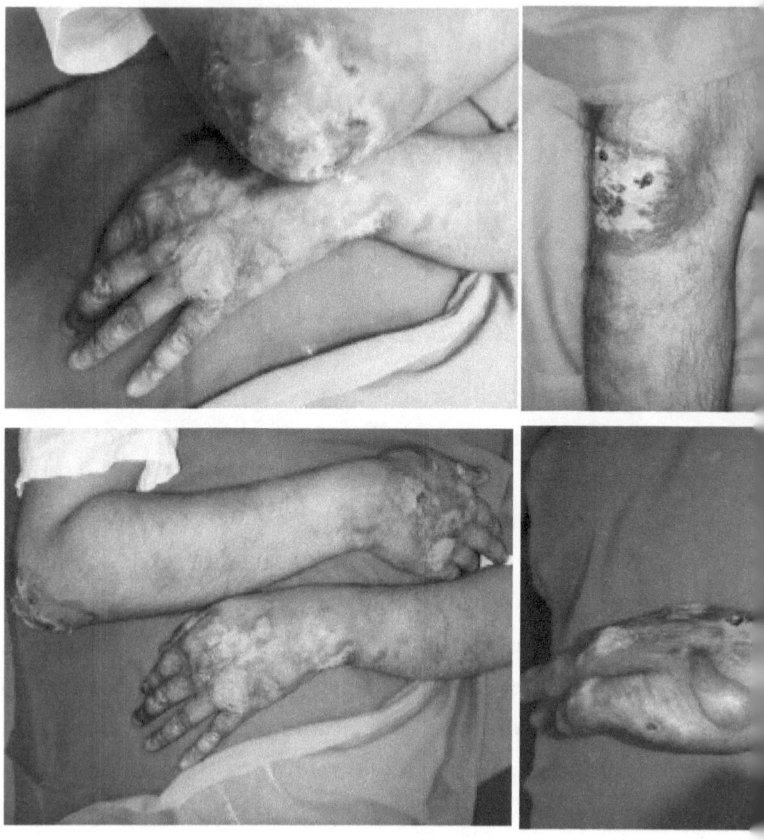

On examination there were fluid filled lesion over upper and lower extremity, atrophic scarring over dorsae of bilateral hands and contracture of right hand. On history and examination we made a provisional diagnosis of epidermolysis bullosa acquisita with seronegative rheumatoid arthritis.

On routine investigation Skin biopsy from an intact blister was taken which showed features suggestive of Epidermolystory.

Treatment was given in form of oral cyclosporine (50mg) thrice daily and tab colchicine (0.5mg) twice daily and tapering of oral steroids. Adjuvant therapy was given in form of topical treatment and physiotherapy for right hand.

We present this case for its rarity

Infections

Erythema Necroticans

Ram Malkani, Hemraj Chandalia, Arun Chitale

Bulletin of the Jaslok Hospital & Research Centre Vol XII no1 July 1987 p.24

Erythema Necroticans (ENL) is a severe kind of Type 2 reaction (Type III hypersensitivity in Coombs & Gell classification) seen in Lepraomatous Leprosy, where ENL lesions become vesicular or bullous and break down. Often there is oedema of face, hands and feet. The classical histological features of active ENL lesions are, in the upper dermis, increased vascularity with many dilated capillaries and in the lower dermis, intense infiltration with polymorphonuclear leucocytes (neutrophils) which have a predilection for surrounding blood vessels in invading their walls. There is swelling and odema of the lining (endothelium) of veins, arterioles and small arteries, (vasculitis).

In Erythema Necroticans, the invaded blood vessels undergo necrosis and obliteration of lumen (obliterative angiitis and endarteritis). Bacilli in ENL lesions are not numerous, as in the patient's leprosy lesions and are mostly fragmented and granular. Any or all of the following symptoms and signs may be associated with ENL, or may occur without ENL and all are manifestations of Type 2 reaction:

- Fever

- Malaise

- Nerve pain

- Periosteal pain (especially tibiae)

- Muscle pain

- Pain and swelling in joints (See leading article in the Lancet 1981, vol.l.Page 649 on 'Rheumatic manifestations of leprosy7)

- Rhinitis

- Epistaxis

- Acute iritis (Iridocyclitis)

- Painful dactylitis

- Swollen and tender lymph nodes (especially femorals)

- Acute Epididymo-orchitis and

- Proteinuria.

A patient may be in either Type 1 or 2 reaction when first seen. It may sound unusual, but there has been a publication from Los Angeles, reporting a series of 32 adults presenting for the first time with reaction and 22 (69%) presented with ENL.

In the present communication, we report a case of Erythema Necroticans presenting as the initial manifestation of leprosy in a diabetic patient recently seen by us. Erythema Nodosum Leprosum (ENL) is almost routinely seen in Lepromatous Leprosy patients, but occurrance of Erythema Necroticans is rather rare.

Case Report

63 year old male patient was admitted under a diabetologist with the history of diabetes mellitus for the last 15 years, for which initially he was on oral hypoglycemics, but for the last 8 years has been on insulin. The patient had not kept the diabetes under adequate control in the past. On admission his fasting blood sugar was 256 mg%. He had undergone an above knee amputation on the left leg 8 years back and a year back underwent, a below knee amputation on the right side. He was a nonalcoholic, but smoking almost 50 bidis (indigenous counterpart of cigarettes) per day. Surprisingly he had no history of hypertension or ischaemic heart disease. He had diminished sensation in both hands for the last 3 years. He was getting chills on and off for the last 2 years. His vision was diminished. His renal function showed impairment since the last 1 year. He complained of drowsiness, malaise and redness in the left eye on admission. On admission he also had nodules, large subcutaneous swellings on hands, forehead, face and abdomen. Some of them had ulcerated and some had healed leaving scars. He had been getting these lesions for the past few months on and off.

On examination the skin lesions were isolated, annular, erythematous nodules, swellings with central vesiculation or pustule formation. In some there was central necroses resulting in large ulcers forming a cavity within the nodules and swell ings. Elsewhere on the body were scars of earlier healed lesions.

The examination of the sensory system revealed loss of sensation below the wrists and thighs to pin prick. During hospitalisation he had intermittent fever for four days only. The redness in the left eye was diagnosed as iridocyclitis. Laboratory studies revealed, haemoglobin 14.8 gm%, WBC 19,58Cf, X-ray chest, ECG, Im~ munoglobulin levels, G6PD, Ultrasound of both kidneys and serum chemistry profile (except for blood sugar levels) were within normal limits. Mantoux was positive 10 x 10 mms. Swab culture from the wound (ulcers) grew Klebseilla and Staphylococci. Urine examination revealed RBCs and moderate proteins.

Skin biopsy (JH1667/86) obtained from one of the plaques revealed, thin epidermis and in the dermis were several large, centrally inflammatory lesions involving small sized blood vessels. The blood vessels had undergone necrosis and around them were compact concentric layers of neutrophils, lymphocytes and histiocytes. Fite Farrace stain showed few fragmented bacilli present in the upper dermis in the region of the infiltrate and the blood vessels. In view of the above findings a diagonoses of Erythema Necroticans in Lepromatous leprosy was made and the standard polytherapy for leprosy was instituted, which consisted of Tab. Dapsone 100 mg. one daily, Cap. Clofazamine 100 mgm one every alternate day (3 per week), Cap. Rifampicin

600 mg one daily on empty stomach for two weeks and then one, once a month on empty stomach along with oral cortisone, Tab. Prednisolone 60 mg/day, which was tapered as the reaction was subsiding.

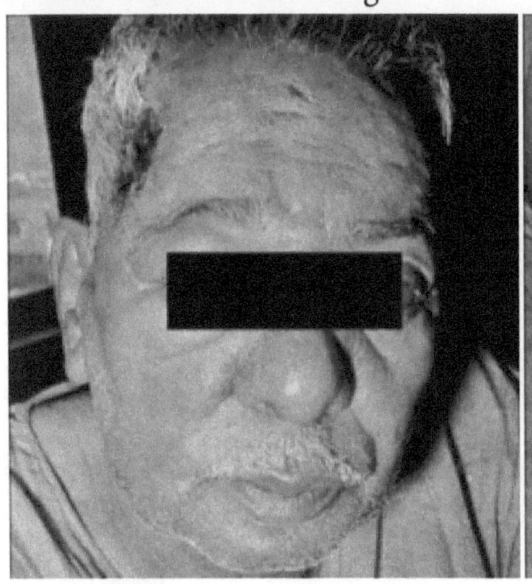

Fig1. Facial appearance of the patient

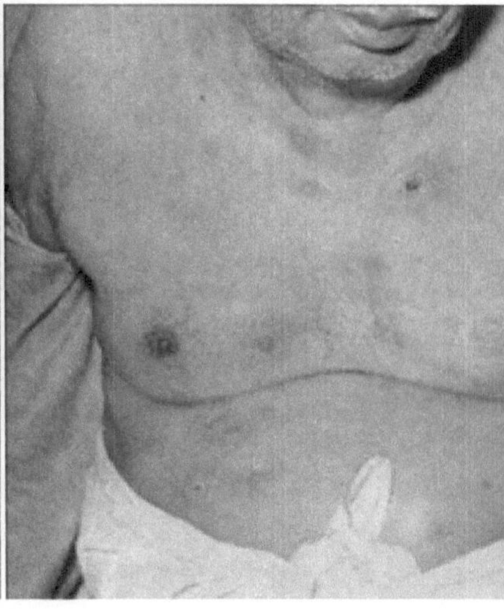

Fig 2. Erythema Necroticans lesion seen on th

Comments

A good deal is now known about the two main types of leprosy reactions - Reactional states and their immunological basis. The terminology presently accepted by the Leprologists for the two types of reactions is, Type 1 and Type II Lepra reactions.

Type 1 Lepra Reaction

This is a delayed hypersensitivity reaction which is an example of Coombs and Gell Type IV hypersensitivity reaction. Antigen from breaking down bacilli, reacts with T lymphocytes and this is associated with a rapid change in the cell mediated immunity (CMI). It is typically seen in Border line leprosy patients, because of their iminunological instability. If the reaction is associated with a rapid increase in specific CMI, as it is in patients under treatment, we speak of upgrading or reversal reaction. On the other hand, if the reaction is associated with a reduction in immunity, we speak of a downgrading reaction. Clinically there is erythema, swelling of some or all the leprosy skin lesions and new lesions may appear. There may be oedema of extremities, inevitably accompanied by neuritis. Systemic disturbances, such as malaise and fever are unusual. Histologically, in reversal reaction, there is oedema, reduced bacilli, and increased defensive cells and giant cells. In down grading reaction, there is increase in bacilli and replacement of defensive cells by macrophages.

Type II Lepra Reaction

It is an immune complex syndrome (an antigen - antibody reaction involving complement) which is a humoral body response. It is an example of Type III (Coombs and Gell) hypersensitivity reaction. It occurs almost exclusively in Lepromatous Leprosy. Clinically there is no change in the appearance of the Leprosy lesions, but there may be crops of erythematous nodules (Erythema Nodosum Leprosum) which come and go. Systemic disturbances are usual. It is very unusual to occur during the first 6 months of therapy. It tends to occur later during the course of the treatment, when leprosy lesions appear quiescent and all or most of the bacilli in the skin are granular. However, a patient may be in reaction when first seen, as was the case with our patient in this communication.

Discussion

Our patient had ulcerated inflammatory nodules, swellings which when biopsied had the classical features of Erythema Necroticans such as obliterative angiitis, endarteritis and few fragmented, granular bacilli. Urine examination of the patient had shown RBCs and protein. The findings were thought to be due to his long standing diabetes. Though immune complexes have been reported in the renal glomeruli during Type 2 reaction, our patient did not show immune complexes by flourescence microscopy in the EN lesions of the skin. The iridocyclitis in the patient was attributed to the Type 2 reaction.

Lucio phenomenon, a type of reaction confined to the diffuse nonnodular form of Lepromatous Leprosy chiefly encountered in the Mexicans was considered momentarily, because of the morphological resemblance of the skin lesions. The skirting difference being that the leprosys of Lucio phenomenon are always afebrile, have numerous bacilli in their skin lesions and the initial skin lesions is purpuric which undergoes necroses ulceration.

References

1. DESIKAN K.V. and JOB C.K.: Severe Lepra reactions, International Journal of leprosy, 36:32,1968.

2. REA T.H. and LEVAN N.E.: ENL as the initial manifestation of leprosy, Archives of Deimatology,lll:1575,1975.

3. DRUTZ DJ. and GUTMAN RA.: ENL and immune glomerulonephritis, American J of Tropical Medicine and Hygiene, 22:496,1973.

4. WATERS M.F.R.et al: Immune complexes in ENL,Intemational Journal of leprosy,39:417,1971.

5. WEMAMBU S.N.C et al: Flourescence microscopy in ENL,Lancet,3:933,1969.

6. MORAN C.J. et al : Type 2 reactions and immune complexes in leprosy ,Lancet,2:572,1972.

7. ROJAS-ESPINOSA O. et al: Serum sickness, Clinical and Exp.Immunology,12:215,1972.

8. RIDLEY MJ. and RIDLEY D.S. : Immunopathology of ENL, International Journal of leprosy, 47:161,1983.

9. LATAPI F. and ZAMORA A.C. : Lucio phenomenon, International Journal of leprosy,16:421,1948.

10. REA T.H. and LEAVAN N.E. : Lucio phenomeno - a report of 10 Mexican patients, Archives of Dermatology, 114:1023,1978.

11. Rea T.H.: Lucio phenomenon, leprosy review, 50:107,1979.

12. REA T.H. and RIDLEY D.S. : Histology of ENL and Lucio phenomenon - a comparison, International Journal of leprosy, 47:161,1979.

Chromomycosis

Ram Malkani, Ajay Kumar

Bulletin of the Jaslok Hospital & Research Centre Vol XIV No.4 April 1990 p.44.

Chromomycosis is a chronic cutaneous and subcutaneous infection of the skin and subcutaneous tissue caused by several fungi and characterised by production of slow growing lesions. Most common among species are *Phialophora verrucosa, P. pedrosoi, P. compactum, Wangiella dermatitidis and Cladesporum carionii.* The nomenclature of these fungi are not universally accepted and some have appeared in the literature as species of fomecaea or Rhinocladiella.

The causal fungi have been isolated from wood and soil and the infection usually results from trauma such as splinter of wood. The condition is usually found in rural communities. Adult male agricultural workers are most often affected but the condition has occurred in children also. On culture all species produce similar heaped up dark colonies with short serial hyphae, producing a grey, green or brown velvety surface resembling a mous pelt. The various causal agents are differentiated microscopically. The usual sites of involvement are exposed parts of the body particularly feet, legs, arms, face and neck.

A warty papule slowly enlarges to form a brownish warty plaque. The early lesion may occasionally be an ulcer.

Eventually after many months or years large hyperkeratotic masses are formed and these may be as much as 3 cm thick. Secondary ulceration is very frequent. The lesion is usually painless unless the presence of secondary infection causes pain or itching. Satellite lesions are produced by scratching and there may be lymphatic spread to adjacent areas. Haematogenous spread has occured but is rare and brain abscesses have been described. Secondary infection may eventually lead after several years to lymphatic stasis with production of elephantiasis.

On direct microscopy of KOH mounts or in biopsy specimens, the pathogen can be seen, irrespective of the species, as deeply pigmented thick walled sclerotic cells (Medlar bodies) and occur in pairs or clusters. Laboratory identification also depends on growth of the characterstic colonies on culture. Histopathology reveals the presence of dark brown thick healed spares in the dermis with granuloma .

Treatment is by complete surgical removal by excision or cryosurgery. Early localised lesions are treated by cautery or diathermy. Local infilteration with amphotericin B has been reported successful. It may also be given intravenously until a dose of 2 to 3 g is reached. 5-flourocytosine alone or with ketoconazole has given promising results.

CASE REPORT:

An eighteen year old male patient presented with complaints of nodules and ulcers around the ankle and foot bilaterally of eight months duration. Initially he had developed a nodular lesion near the medial malleolus of right side, which subsequently increased in size and broke to form an ulcer.

He developed a similar nodule in the vicinity of the old one and about 2 months later small nodules were formed on the dorsum of the left foot which in turn broke down to form ulcers with hyperpigmentation. All lesions were painless but he had itching in the ulcerated lesions. Before presentation he was given local and systemic antibiotics with supportive therapy but condition did not improve.

He did not have any systemic complaints nor any other skin lesions. Urine examination, blood counts and x-ray chest were normal. Hepatitis B antigen was positive. A biopsy was taken from the nodule. The histopathological picture was of markedly thickened epidermis with pseudoepitheliomatous hyperplasia. The dermis showed an exuberant granulation tissue with granulomatious reaction in the deeper dermis. The granulomas were composed of plasma cells, neutrophils, histiocytes with brown round thick walled bodies suggestive of chromoblastomycosis.

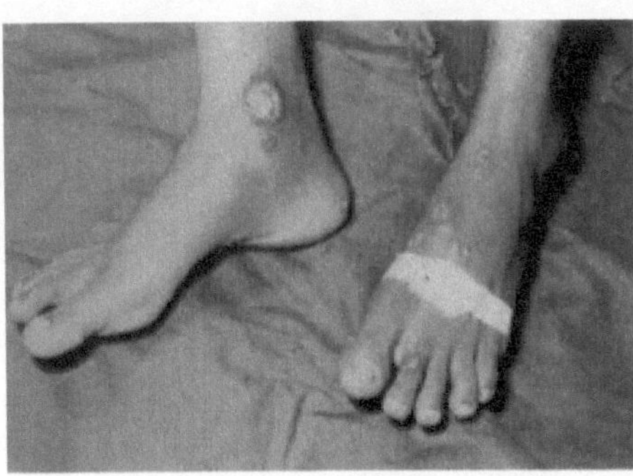

Fig. 1. Nodules leading to ulcer formation

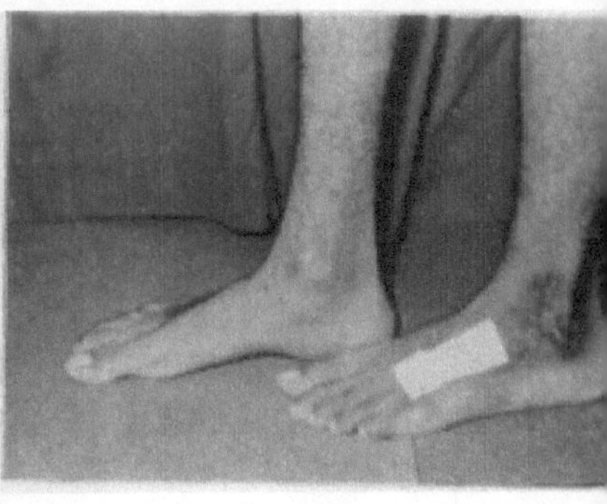

Fig. 2. Lesion resolving after treatment flucytosine

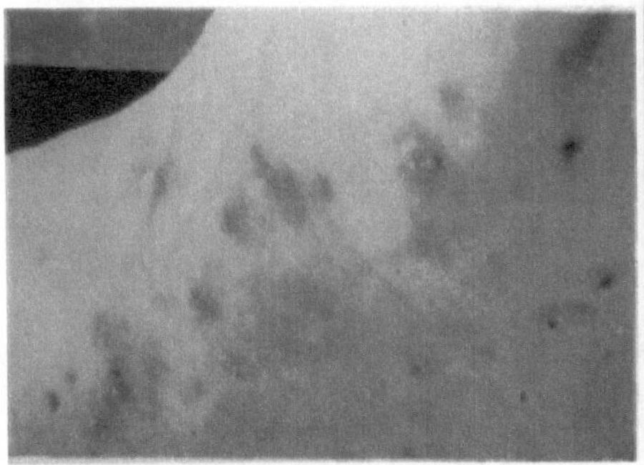

Fig. 3. Recurrence of lesion

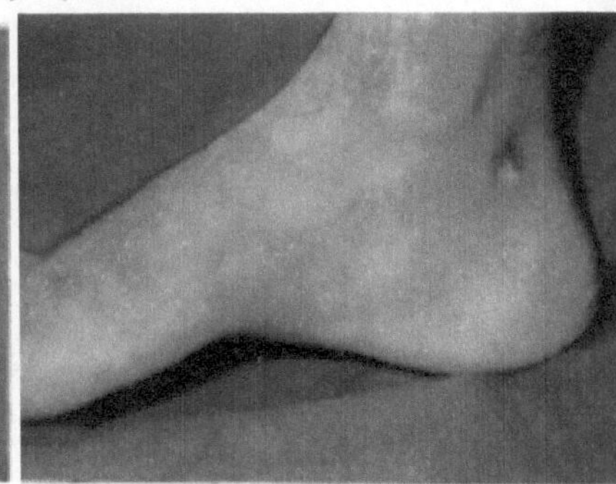

Fig. 4. Recurred lesion

He was given flucytosine 500 mg oral tablets 4 times a day on which dose the lesions improved. The lesions recurred again after 2 months time with appearance of nodules. Subsequently he was advised to take keticonezole orally 200 mg three times a day. The lesions subsided in about three weeks time thereafter.

REFERENCES

1. Carrion et al: Chromoblastomycosis and related infections. Int J Dermatol, 14: 27-32, 1975.

2. Vollum DI: Chromomycosis: A review. British J Dermatol, 96: 454-58, 1977.

3. Derbes VJ, Friedman L: Chromoblastomycosis, Dermatol Tropica, 3: 201-206, 1964.

4. Azulay RD, Serruya J:Haematogenous dissemination in Chromoblastomycosis. Arch Dermatol, 95: 57-60, 1967.

5. French AJ, Russel AR: Arch Dermatol Syph, 67:129-134, 1953.

Pseudo elephantiasis of the vulva of tubercular etiology-An unusual presentation

Ram H. Malkani, Ajay Kumar, G.N. Manusukhani

Bulletin of the Jaslok Hospital & Research Centre Vol XIV No. 4 April 1990 p.5.

SUMMARY

A seventeen year old unmarried girl developed secondary amenorrhoea, elephantiasis of the vulva accompanied by loss of appetite. Lymphangiogram and CT scan revealed destruction of left inguinal and internal iliac lymph nodes. On giving her antitubercular regimen the amenorrhoea was relieved, but the swelling persisted. It was excised surgically but recurred again.

INTRODUCTION

Elephantiasis is a condition of chronic lymphatic oedema with associated thickening and hypertrophy of the epithelial tissues of the vulva. The skin is rough, warty and verrucous. True elephantiasis is caused by the filarial worm Wucheraria bancrofti. It is also seen as an end result of any chronic infection which heals by fibrosis when it is called *Pseudo elephantiasis*. This is seen secondary to lymphogranuloma venereum, granuloma inguinal, tuberculosis, possibly syphillis, angioedema and recurrent erysipelas. The lymphatic drainage of the vulva is mainly to the superficial inguinal nodes, and from there to the deep inguinal and external iliac nodes. Lymphatics from deep tissues accompany the internal pudendal vessels to the internal iliac nodes.

CASE REPORT

A seventeen year old unmarried female presented with swelling of both labia which was of fifteen days duration. She had developed secondary amenorrhoea one year nine months prior to this. Her periods were regular before the amenorrhoea. She also had loss of appetite. She denied any history of sexual contact. Local examination revealed swelling of both the labia minora which was more on the left side. The swelling had a rough surface and there was no oozing or local inflamation. There was no plapable lymph nodes in the inguinal region. Her secondary sexual characters were normal. Investigations revealed a haemolgobin level of 12.7 gms% and WBC count of 10,300/cmm. Mantoux Test was positive showing an induration of 12 mm diameter. Serum biochemistry profile was normal. Radiographic examination of her chest and pituitary fossa and barium enema studies were normal, and so was the ultrasound examination of her pelvis. Follicular stimulating hormone, leutinising hormone and thyroid hormone levels were in the normal range.

A skin biopsy from the oedematous vulva revealed a slightly atropic epidermis, evidence of lymphectasia in the dermis and fibrosis (? secondary). A bilateral lower lyphangiogram was obtained, which revealed destruction of left inguinal and internal iliac lymph nodes. A CT scan of the pelvis revealed the same findings. She was administered oral Tetracyline 2 gm per day, a full course of diethylcarbamazine, oral corticosteroids, anti inflammatory and antihistaminic drugs, but the condition remained the same. As her symptom persisted, in view of her amenorrhoea, loss of appetite, positive mantoux and lymph node destruction, the possibility of tubercular etiology was considered and it was presumed that TB adenitis was responsible for her swelling. She was administered antitubercular regimen and given rifampicin 450 mg/day INH300 mg/day and streptomycin 0.75 gm/day. A month after this, her menstural periods returned and her appetite showed improvement. The size of the swelling remained same throughout the course of the therapy, which was stopped after a period of six months. This was followed by surgical exicision of the swelling. The swelling reemerged in the same region and persisted.

DISCUSSION

Genital elephantiasis occurs due to a variety of causes. It is caused by accumulation of fluid in the lymphatics leading to the thickening of the skin and sub cutaneous tissue. There is increase in both the stagnant lymphatic channels and in the supporting fat. True genital elephantiasis occurs secondary to chronic infection healing with fibrosis.

Our case presented with oedema of the vulva, amenorrhoea and anorexia. The cause of the swelling was demonstrated to be due to obstruction of lymphatic drainage. She had no history of sexual contact and no other skin lesion. She was investigated for the cause of her secondary amenorrhoea and her LH, FSH. Thyroid hormones and x-ray of pituitary fossa were found normal. A biopsy of the endometrium and a laparotomy to biopsy the pelvic glands were not carried out as it was not felt proper to carry out these procedures in an unmarried girl. The lymph node involvement, positive mantoux test and return of the menstruation on anti TB treatment was considered as a fair evidence of tuberculous etiology. The oedema of vulva did not subside inspite of treatment presumably as the lymph glands underwent fibrosis and the lymphatic obstruction continued to persist. It is possible for the same reason that swelling reappeared after surgical excision. Tuberculous infection of the genitals is uncommon and usually involves the fallopian tubes and endometrium in the females. Involvement of the vulva, penis and scrotum is still rare.

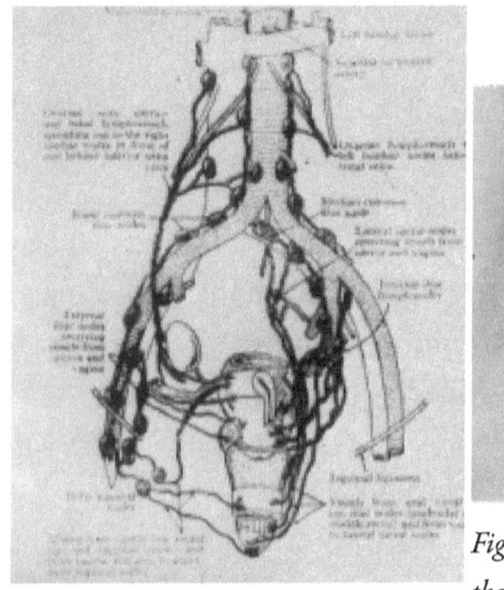

Fig. 1 : Lymphatic drainage of vulva and vagina

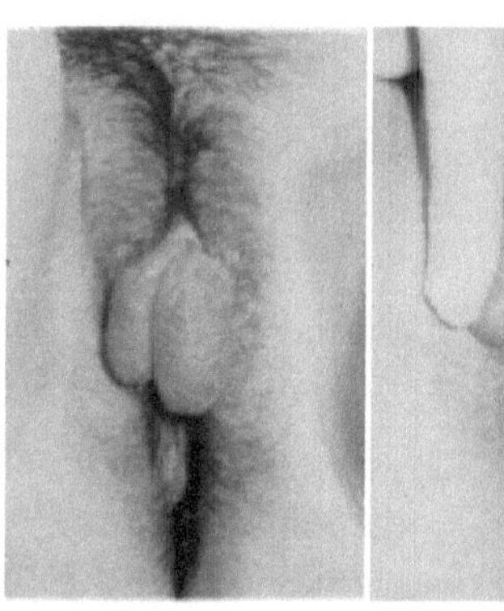

Fig. 2 : Swelling seen on the vulva

Fig. 3 : Me... the swelling

In a large series of 336 cases of tuberculoderma reported by Satyanarayana, there was no case of tuberculosis of the vulva. Rangaiah et al have described three cases of ulcers of the external genitalia in their series of tuberculous lesions in practice of Venerology. Most cases of genital tuberculosis have been observed in the age group of 20 to 40 years. Three types of tuberculosis of the vulva have been described. The ulcerative type is the commonest. Other two are the serpegenous scaly type and the hypertrophic type with oedema and elephantiasis.

There are two reports of elephantiasis of vulva of tuberculous etiology. Shah has reported a case where oedema of vulva occurred with associated superficial ulceration which healed on antitubercular regime. Naik et al have reported a case where oedema of vulva was associated with lupus vulgaris of the buttocks. Biopsy revealed a tubercular granuloma and the patient responded to antitubercular treatment.

This is apparently the first report of its kind where genital elephantiasis has occurred secondary to pelvic adenitis.

REFERENCES

1. Tindall V R: Jeffcvates principle of Gynecology, Butterworths, London, 1987; p 315.

2. Oromsby 0 S and Montgomery: Diseases of skin, Edn 8, Lea and Ferger, Philadelphia, 1954; p214.

3 Callamon F T and Wilson J F; Non Venereal Disease of Genitals, Charles C Thomas Publishers. Spring Illinois USA, 1956; p 72.

4. Satyanarayana B V: Tuberculoderma, Indian J Dermatol Venereal, leprol, 1963, 29: 25-41.

Disseminated Mycofoacterium Bovis Infection from BCG Vaccination of a patient with Combined Immunodeficiency

Nimita Talsania, Y.K. Amdekar, Ram Malkani

Bulletin of the Jaslok Hospital & Research Centre Vol XXVII No.4 April 2003 p.8.

Introduction

Disseminated mycobacterial infection after Bacillus Calmette- Guerin (BCG) vaccination is a very rare disorder, occurring mostly in patients with immunological deficiency. We report a case of disseminated BCG infection in a 4years 2 months old infant with severe combined immunodeficiency.

Case Summary

A 4 years and 2 months old male infant born in Bangalore, following a Lower section caesarean section (because of CPD, oligohydraminos), full term delivery, cried at birth. There were no neonatal complications.

Patient was initially well. Presented to us at 4 years and 2months of age with history of fever since the age of 2 years 2 months, intermittent, moderate grade (101-102°F) subsiding with syrup paracetamol. Maculopapular lesions on the thigh since last 2 months which became generalised. Skin lesions were noticed at the same time as fever. The skin lesions over the face, chest and abdomen became prominent in the last 1 month. There was excessive crying and irritability since 15-20 days. Developmental history of social smile present, recognised the mother, mild head lag was present. History of Immunisation: Received 2 doses of Hep-B, 2 doses of DPT, 3 doses of OPV. BCG given at birth, formed indolent nonhealing BCG ulcer since 1 month of age with bloody discharge.

The child had been medically investigated at Manipal Hospital, Bangalore 10 days before being presented to us. A skin biopsy was there suggestive of ? histiocytosis. Electron microscopy was not done. A liver biopsy was performed, but the sample was insufficient. Bone Marrow was normal. USG of the abdomen revealed moderate splenomegaly studded with multiple focal hypoechoic lesions. Other causes of fever were ruled out. HBs Ag, HIV, VDKL, Well Felix, Brucella IgM, Herpes IgM profile all were negative. The child was referred to us for further evaluation and treatment.

Examination

Local: There were 2 types of skin lesions affecting almost the whole body with greater density on the chest. There were fewer skin coloured papules with central crust, separate from each other, scattered on the face, trunk and scrotum. The second type of lesions, more in number, were indurated deep seated nodules. Some of them appeared bluish. There was a non-healing BCG ulcer with bloody discharge. Skin biopsy was performed earlier at Manipal and the site of the biopsy was found infected with abscess. Montoux test was negative.

At Jaslok Hospital the child was kept on breast feed and soft diet. IV antibiotics were given for 6 days. (Ceftazidime and Cloxacillin). Other investigations revealed anaemia (Hb-6.5), thrombocytopenia (platelet -23, 700), WBC-11, 400. Liver function was deranged.

Total proteins 3.7, Sr. albumin-1.7, SGOT-118, SGPT-33, GGTP-90, Total bilirubin-2.8, direct bilirubin-1.8. To assess the involvement of CNS, CSF analysis was done which was normal. CT Scan of the chest revealed ground glass opacities suggestive of Pneumocystis carinni pneumonia. The immune status was evaluated thoroughly which revealed severe immunoglobulin deficiency. IgG and IgA were absent. IgM levels were very low. T cell deficiency CDS, CD4 absent. CDS count just detectable. C3 and C4 normal. Biopsy was taken from 3 sites. Both the type of skin lesions, the skin coloured papules with crust and nodules were biopsed, for routine paraffin section. The skin coloured papules was sent for Electron microscopy. Skin biopsy was reported by a surgical pathologist and reviewed by a dermatopathologist. The report read by a dermatopathologist is as follows.

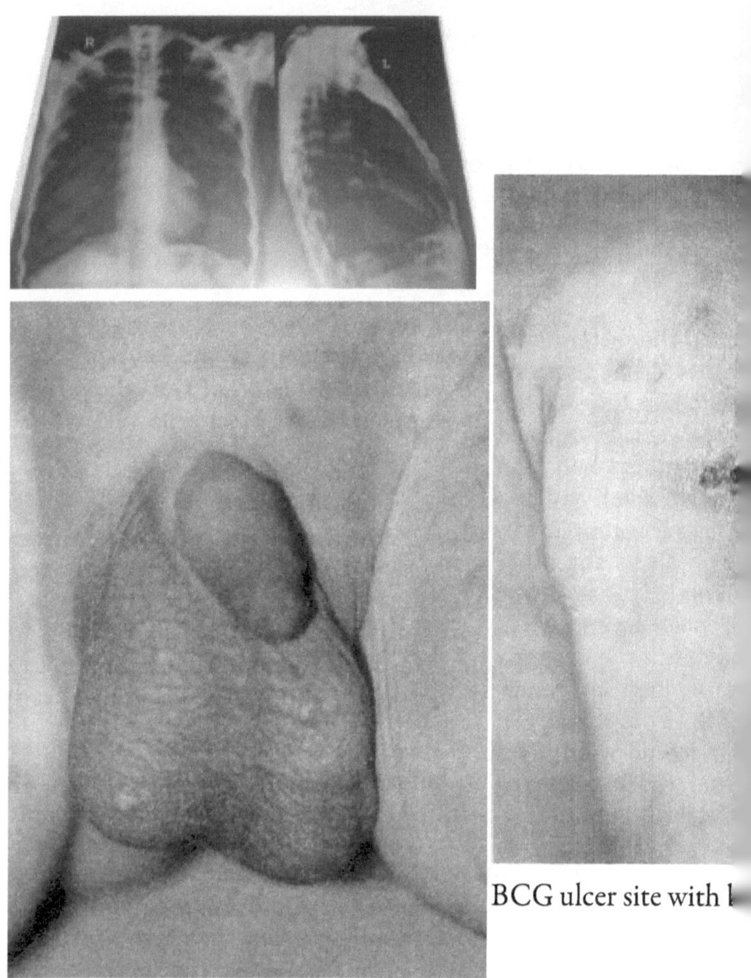

Papula Nodular lesion on the scrotum and thigh

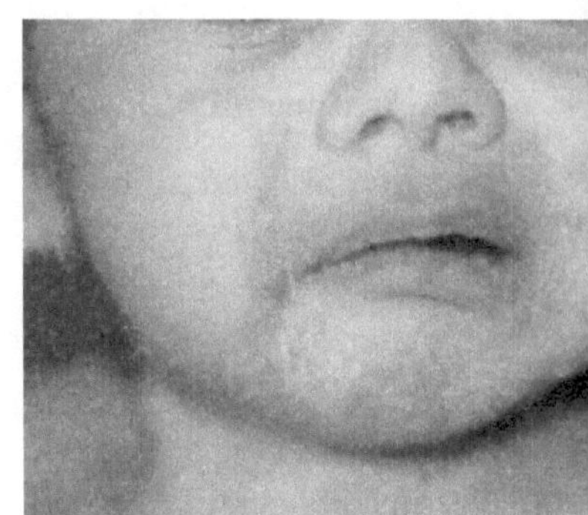

Papulonodular lesion on the face

Multiple papular lesion on the trunk and
abdomen.

Microscopy: Suppurative granulomatous inflammation
involving the deeper reticular dermis and sub cutaneous
tissue. The granuloma consists of numerous foamy
histiocytes admixed with lymphocytes and neutrophils.
Numerous large histiocytes (arrow) filled with bluish
granular and filamentous material also seen. The granulomas
are present in large nodular pattern without following the
neurovascular bundles and extend into the interstitum of
reticular dermis. The upper dermis and epidermis are
unaffected. Presence of large histiocytes packed with bacilli

favours the diagnosis of atypical mycobacteriosis in an immunocompromised host.

Z.N. Stain showed all histiocytes distended with bundles of Acid fast bacilli.

Electron Microscopy: Showed all histiocytes full of bacillary bodies in cross and longitudinal planes. Most are situated in autophagic vacuoles.

Histology

DNA-PCR send for mycobacteria from the blood and BCG vaccine site identified the organism as *Mycobacterium bovis*. In view of AFB bacilli seen from the skin biopsy, on PCR of BCG site and on blood PCR assay a diagnosis of TB was made. The child was advised anti tuberculosis treatment. Keeping abnormal liver function in mind the child was started on the following drugs.

INH- 5 mg/kg/day.

Ethb- 20mg/kg/day.

Ofloxacin- 15mg/kg/day.

Inj. Streptomycin- 25mg/kg/day.

A blood transfusion of the whole blood was given before discharge.

Discussion

Severe combined immunodeficiency (SCID) is a serious human immunodeficiency disorder. It is a group of congenital disorder in which both the T and B cells are defective. Most common type is linked to X chromosome making this form, affect only males.

For the first few months of the life the child with SCID, is protected by maternal antibodies received during pregnancy and breast feeding. As early as 2-3 months, child begins to suffer from recurrent severe infections. Even our patient presented with fever at 2years 2 months of age when maternal antibodies started waning.

BCG vaccine contains live mycobacteria derived from a strain of mycobacteria bovis attentuated through years of serial passage in culture by Calmette and Guerin at the Pasteur Institute.(3)

Effective containment of the attenuated BCG bacilli requires intact T-lymphocytes and macrophages functions. In the absence of effective host immune function injected bacilli can proliferate unchecked and spread throughout the body. Even our case presented with, unresolved infection at the injection site and its spread to the other organs. Regional lymph node spread can be the early indicator of host immunodeficiency. With dissemination most severely affected organs are liver, spleen, bone marrow, lungs, skin and CNS. In our case liver, spleen and skin were involved with Myco Bovis. Bone marrow and CNS were normal. Lungs were infected with *Pneumocystis carinni* pneumonia an indicator of immunodeficiency.

Infection with M. bovis if disseminated is generally considered opportunistic and is a marker of immunodeficiency.(5) In immune deficient patients with systemic mycobacterial infection virtually any of the mycobacteria may induce skin lesions in upto 10% of patients.(5)

Disseminated BCG disease has historically been a disease of infants, but cases now occur in adults and elderly coinfected with HIV(6).

BCG vaccination leads to complication which includes local abscesses, urticaria, erythema multiforme, generalised maculopapular rash or purpuric rashes, chronic ulcer, lichen scrofulosorum, papular tuberculides, lichen nitidus, lupus vulgaris, keloid and basal cell carcinoma. (7)

Cutaneous tuberculosis can manifest as follows.

Mycobacteria marinum can occasionally present as disseminated ulcer or small abscesses in an immunocompromised host. *Mycobacteria ulcearns* can present as itching nodules on the arms or legs which then break down to form an ulcer. *Mycobacterium avium* intracellulare which frequently cause disseminated disease rarely presents as heterogeneous skin manifestation as nodules, ulcer, pustules and abscess. *Mycobacterium hemophilum* also has tendency to involve the skin.

Long Vulgaris can rarely occur as a result of BCG vaccination. Buttocks, thighs and legs are more common sites of involvement. The initial lesion vulgaris is a soft erythematous nodule slightly elevated above the surface. A few surrounding nodule may appear later and coalesce to form a soft plaque.(9)

Lichen Scrofuloderm: Tiny, perifollicular lichenoid papules in groups. The papules are flat well defined, firm, and often asymptomatic.

Disseminated TB of the skin: A sudden eruption of small, brownish scaly lesions appear extensively but irregularly over the body. Ulcer develops when caseation occurs. A deeper form affects the subcutis, though resembling erythema induratum. The index case is an example of disseminated TB.

Unfortunately, the child succumbed to the disease a month after presenting with the lesions when the article was being written.

References

1. The SCID Homepage .htm Lymhocyte courtesy of Art Anderson. Primary Immune deficiency webring.

2. Severe combined immunodeficiency. Autors. Rebecca. J.Prey.

3. Epidemiologic Notes and Reports of disseminated Myco.bovis infection from BCG vaccination of a patient with HIV. Weekly April 26, 1985/34(16);227-8.

4. Disseminated BCG infection 3 recent Canadian cases. Canada Communicable disease report. Volume 24-9, May 1998. BCG Live Systemic Revised 7/20/995.

5. Bacterial infection in HIV.Infections may be localised or widespread easily identified or elusive,

and have a variety of manifestations Clay J. Cockerell, MD. From the May 1995 JLAPAE.

6. Disseminated BCG disease after vaccination. Talbot EA, Purkins MD, Silva, SF, Frothingham.

7. Textbook of Dermatology. 4th edition by Arthur Rook/D.S. Wilkinson, F.J.G. Ebling/ R.H. Champion, J.L. Burton. Blackwell Scientific Publications.

8. Harrison's Principle of Internal Medicine. 14th edition. Fauci, Braunwald, Isselbacher, Wilson, Martin, Kaspen, Hauser, Longo. International edition.

9. Indian Association of Dermatologist, Venerologist and Leprologist. Textbook and Atlas of Dermatology Vol-1 2nd edition. Editorial in chief R.G. Valia. Assistant Editor Ameet R. Valia, Project Director K. Siddappa. Published by Bhalani Publishing House.

Cutaneous presentation of atypical mycobacterial infection – An interesting case

Sneh L Thadani, Om Shrivastava, Ram H Malkani

Published in the Journal of Saifee Hospital, Mumbai

Acknowledgements: We would like to acknowledge Dr. Maninder Singh Setia for editorial help with this article.

ABSTRACT

Environmental mycobacteria are the causative factors of an increasing number of infections worldwide. We report an interesting case of a 29 year old woman with a localized recurrent soft tissue swelling due to *Mycobacterium abscesses*. The patient presented with ulcers on the lower abdomen that had developed over a surgical scar since the past two years; these ulcers healed with a puckered scar. Microbiological investigations revealed the presence of atypical mycobacterium in the lesions. On further sub speciation, M. abscesses was identified. The patient was treated with Isoniazide (300 mg), Rifabutin (300 mg), Clarithromycin (500 mg), Levofloxacin (500 mg), for a duration of 18 months. Post treatment, a gradual but complete recovery was noted in the patient. The case is being reported for its uncommon clinical presentation and the

associated etiological agent that has been recently
subspeciated.

INTRODUCTION

Atypical or non-tuberculosis mycobacterium consist of a
heterogeneous group of acid fast bacilli found in the water,
soil, plants, and faeces of healthy animals. [1] The increased
prevalence of atypical mycobacterial infections as recently
observed may be a due to a higher numbers of surgical/
invasive procedures, immunocompromised state, and/or
antibiotic resistance. [2] These patients often present with
wide spread infection involving the skin and subcutaneous
tissue. *Mycobacterium abscesses* is an atypical mycobacterium
classified as a rapid grower. It may cause infections at
injection and tattooing sites, andfollowing implants,
catheterization, and other forms of surgical instrumentation.
[3,4] However, it is not known to be transmitted from
person to person.[1] We present a rare case of ulcers due to
this organism developing at the site of a previous operation.

CASE REPORT:

A 29 year old female presented to the dermatology
department with itching in both upper and lower limbs for
the past four months. She also complained of recurrent
ulcers over the lower abdomen for two years that had
developed over an operation scar (operated for caesarean
section). These had started as painful lesions which later
ruptured to form ulcers and finally healed with hyper
pigmented puckered scars (Figures 1 and 2). The patient

also complained of high grade fever associated with the occurrence of lesions, a weight loss of about 13 kilograms, and three miscarriages.

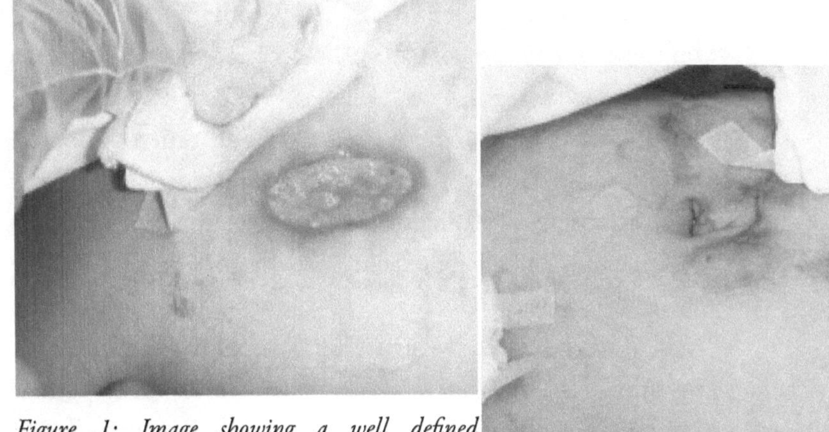

Figure 1: Image showing a well defined granulomatous ulcer (dimensions 4 X 3 cm) with minimal slough, and an erythematous and indurated border

Figure 2: Image showing a healed puckered

The patient had consulted many physicians for these complaints; she was treated by various antibiotics for the same. However, there was little improvement in the lesions. Subsequently she consulted an infectious disease specialist. At this stage a detailed microbiological examination was performed and multiple repeated specimens from the ulcer were sent for culture (Lowenstein – Jensen medium). Atypical mycobacterium was identified in the culture growth; a sub speciation led to the identification of mycobacterium abscesses. A computerized tomography scan of the abdomen revealed pyaemic pockets in the anterior abdominal wall; however, these did not communicate with the peritoneal cavity. The patient also had a low hemoglobin

(9.3 g%) and an erythrocyte sedimentation rate of 20 mm at the end of one hour. The skin biopsy from the lesions showed fibrosing granulation tissues with tissue neutrophilia - it was not suggestive of any active inflammation. Based on these, a diagnosis of atypical mycobacterial ulcers due to *Mycobacterium abscesses* was made.

In view of the above clinical and microbiological findings, the patient was started on isoniazide (300 mg per day), rifabutin (150 mg twice a day), clarithromycin (500 mg per day) and levofloxacin (500 mg per day). All these medications were given for 18 months. In addition, the patient was treated with prednisolone for a period of 2 months, to control the high grade fever. The patient responded well to these medications, the lesions healed, and no new lesions had occurred till the last follow-up of the patient [April 2011].

DISSCUSSION:

This interesting case has been presented for the following reasons: 1) recurrent ulcers over surgical scars should arouse a suspicion of atypical mycobacterium infections; 2) sub speciation will be important to identify the organisms particularly if they have been recently identified as was seen in our case; and 3) treatment for these infections is usually long term often dictated by clinical improvement.

Atypical mycobacteria, belonging to the phylum actinobacteria, have been described since 1950's. These are classified into two different types the rapid growers and slow growers.[5] The latter, comprising of about 60 species, are distinguished from slow growers by their capacity to produce a visible culture in a few days on an ordinary medium. M. abscesses is a rapid grower which was earlier thought as a type of M.chelone. However, it has recently been described as an individual organism. [5,6] It is a gram positive non-motile acid fast rod, grows in starch based medium, and the colonies appear as light yellow streaks.The pus samples collected in our patient grew colonies on LJ medium as smooth and rough, white to greyish and nonphotochromogens. M. abscesses provokes a large spectrum of soft tissue infections and infections of the locomotor apparatus after surgeries, at sites of injection of drugs, and disseminated broncho pulmonary infections in immunocompromised patients such as graft recipients.[7] It may affect all age groups, and occur equally in male and female patients. They are severe and especially difficult to treat, because of the resistance to many antibiotics. [1,2,4]

As seen in our patient, there were chronic recurring abscesses which were resistant to antibiotics like amoxicillin and clavulanic acid, and other broad spectrum antibiotics. In general no specific criteria exist for the treatment of infections caused by Non Tuberculosis mycobacteria. The treatment is usually medical in nature; however, adjunctive surgical interventions may be needed to control deep infections. The duration of therapy depends on patient response. The antimicrobials are administered singly or in combination. Some of the suggestions for treatment are: 1) Monotheraphy with clarithromycin 500mg bid; 2) Minocycline 100mg bid; or 3) Doxycycline 100mg bid was reported successful. In our patient based on pus cultures isoniazide (300 mg per day), rifabutin (150 mg twice a day), clarithromycin (500 mg per day) and levofloxacin (500 mg per day) were given. Drug resistance varies and has been reported with all classes of antibiotics. A multidrug approach which includes clarithromycin, rifampicin and or ethambutol has also been suggested and is often used to minimize drug resistance or in severe cases. [1,2,3]

In sum we would like to suggest that a differential diagnosis of atypical mycobacterium should be considered in a presentation of post incisional abscess, not responding to several antibiotics; a delay in the diagnosis should not be made. In a sub continent like ours, where the prevalence of tuberculosis is so high, such patients should be treated with both anti kochs drugs and specific atypical mycobacetria antibiotics for a prolonged period of time.

Refrences:

1). Abbas O, Marrouch N, Kattar MM, Zeynoun S, Kibbi AG, Rached RA, Araj GF, Ghosn S. Cutaneous non-tuberculous Mycobacterial infections: a clinical and histopathological study of 17 cases from Lebanon.2011 Jan;25(1):33-42. doi: 10.1111/j.1468-3083.2010.03684.

2) Streit M, Böhlen LM, Hunziker T, Zimmerli S, Tscharner GG, Nievergelt H, Bodmer T, Braathen LR. Disseminated Mycobacterium marinum infection with extensive cutaneous eruption and bacteremia in an immunocompromised patient.2006 Jan-Feb;16(1):79-83.

3) Dr Varghese , Atypical Mycobacterial injection abcess. MJAFI 2003;59:246-247

4) Sousa TS, Matherne RJ, Wilkerson MG. Case report: cutaneous nontuberculous mycobacterial abscesses associated with insulin injections. J Drugs Dermatol. 2010 Nov;9(11):1439-42.

5) Van Ingen J, de Zwaan R, Dekhuijzen R, et al. Region of difference1 in nontuberculous Mycobacterium species adds a phylogenetic andtaxonomical character. J Bacteriol 2009;191:5865-7. [PubMed]

6) Esteban J, Ortiz-Pérez A (December 2009). "Current t reatment of atypical mycobacteriosis". Expert Opin Pharmacother 2009 Dec ; 10(17):2787-99

7) Carmen Cantisani,1 Antonio G. Richetta,1 Andrea Bitonti,1 Pietro Curatolo,1 Gianfranco Ferretti,2 Carlo Mattozzi,1 Melis Luca,1 Emidio Silvestri,1 Stefano Calvieri. Recurrent cutaneous abscesses in two Italian family members,doi:10.4081/idr.2010e11/ Pubmed:2010-08-04 12:10:43/views:370

8) Atypical Mycobacterial Infection Among HIV Seronegative Patients in PondicherryP. Sivasankari1, Annie B. Khyriem, K. Venkatesh and Subhash Chandra ParijaDepartment of

Microbiology, Jawaharlal Institute of Postgraduate Medical Education and Research (JIPMER),Pondicherry, India and School of Engineering and Technology, Bharathidasan University1, Tiruchirapalli,Indian J chest dis allied sci.2006 apr – jun;48(2):107-9

9) Emily Berger MD, Priya Batra MD, Jonathan Ralston MD, Miguel R Sanchez MD, Andrew G Franks Jr MD , Atypical mycobacteria infection in an immunocompromised patient. Dermatology Online Journal 16 (11): 21

10) Street ML, Umbert-Millet IJ, Roberts GD, Su WP. Nontuberculous mycobacterial infections of the skin. Report of fourteen cases and review of the literature, J Am Acad Dermatol. 1991 Feb;24(2 Pt 1):208-15.

Cutaneous Malakoplakia - A Rare Entity!

Ishita Patani, Ram Malkani

Presentated at CUTICON 2010, an annual conference of the Maharashtra branch of the IADVL

HISTORY:

54 year old, married female presented with h/o recurrent, painful ulcers over the lower abdomen since 10 months. Has been treated in the past for the same with antibiotics and steroids. H/o healing of the ulcers with scarring.

ON ENQUIRY:

- No h/o constitutional symptoms
- No h/o similar lesions elsewhere in the body
- No h/o similar complaints in family members
- No h/o any major medical or surgical illness
- Not on any chronic medications

ON EXAMINATION:

Single, well defined, indurated, erythematous, approximately 5cm x 3cm in its largest diameters, pus filled ulcer with central eschar formation on the lower abdomen. Local

tenderness present. Few well defined cribriform scars on the
lower abdomen Hair, Nails – No abnormality detected.

INVESTIGAT

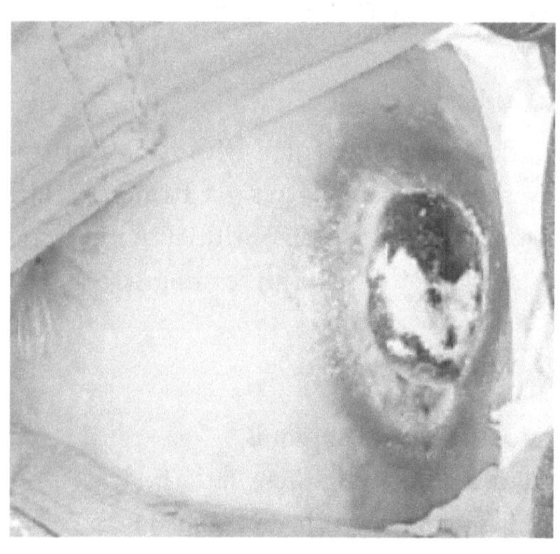

- Haemogra
Within   no.
limits
- Blood Sug
Normal
- ESR - 69 m
- LFT and
– Normal
- Urine rou
& microscop
Normal
-    ANA
Negative
- RA Fact
non reactive
- Chest X r
No   abnorm
detected
- HIV I &
ELISA
Negative
-    HBsAg
Negative

PROVISIONAL DIAGNOSIS:

Pyoderma Gangrenosum, Carbuncle, Vasculitis, Ecthyma

Skin Biop
Histopatl

Biopsy show
dense and
tuberculoid
granulomat
infiltrate w
of suppurat
Granuloma
up of lym
plasma
histiocytes
epitheloid
occasional
and foreig
giant cells.
epidermis
moderate s
psoriasiforn
The dermi
abundant f
and pro
granulation
the deep
several h
show
basophilic
intracytopl
inclusion l

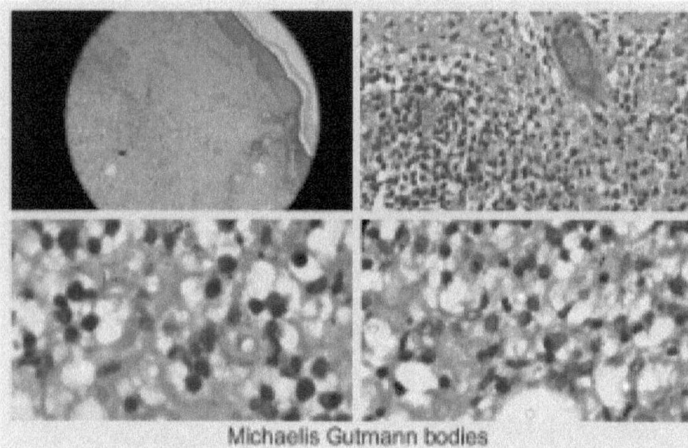

Michaelis Gutmann bodies

size 2-5 microns (Michaelis Gutmann bodies) suggestive of MALAKOPLAKIA.

FINAL DIAGNOSIS: CUTANEOUS MALAKOPLAKIA

TREATMENT:

Oral antibiotics and Ascorbic acid.

REVIEW OF LITERATURE:

Cutaneous malakoplakia is a rare entity with less than 50 cases reported in the literature.

HISTORY:

First described by Michaelis and Gutmann in 1902. In 1903, it was named 'malakoplakia' by Von Hansemann. The term malakoplakia originates from the Greek 'malakos' (soft) and plakion (plaque). Malakoplakia of the skin was first described by LeClerc and Bernier in 1972. Malakoplakia is an uncommon inflammatory condition usually affecting the genitourinary tract, gastrointestinal tract, but may rarely involve the skin.

Usually associated with immunosuppression most of the cases presented in the setting of organ transplantation, others include patients with connective tissue disorders (15%), neoplasm (10%), diabetes mellitus (10%), and chronic debilitating/immunodeficiency disorders – HIV, hepatitis C, sarcoidosis (18%).

CUTANEOUS SITES: Perineum (40%), abdominal wall/thorax (20%), head and neck (20%), extremities (10%), and axilla (10%).

PATHOGENESIS:

Secondary to an acquired bactericidal defect in macrophages. Defect appears to involve the function of the monocytes in endocytosis and intracellular bacterial digestion which results in accumulation of bacterial degradation products and a granulomatous reaction. Decreased intracellular cyclic guanosine monophosphate (cGMP) level may interfere with adequate microtubular function and lysosomal activity. The Michaelis-Gutmann bodies represent an accumulation of non-exocytosed phagolysosomes that have undergone calcification and contain a dense calcium hydroxyapatite core with variable amounts of iron and are considered pathognomonic for malakoplakia.

STAINS : Periodic acid-Schiff (PAS), VonKossa stain for calcium, and Perls Prussian blue iron stain.

IMMUNOHISTOCHEMICALLY: cells are positive with CD68, lysozyme and á-chymotrypsin.

HISTOLOGICAL: 3 stages :

1st - inflammatory
    2nd - "classic" - abundant Michaelis-Gutmann bodies
    3rd - progressive fibrous tissue

ORGANISMS:

Most commonly isolated are gram negative organisms *E. coli* Others: *Pseudomonas, Proteus, Klebsiella, Staphylococcus, Rhodococcus, Mycobacterium* etc.

CLINICAL PRESENTATION:

Papules or plaques - yellow to pink or skin coloured, abscesses, erythematous papules, subcutaneous nodules, ulcerations, or masses, nonhealing surgical wounds and sinus tract formation.

CLINICAL COURSE:

Benign clinical course with a mean duration of skin lesions of 4-6 months. Draining sinuses, persistence of disfiguring skin lesions, and involvement of visceral organs constitute significant morbidity.

TREATMENT:

Antibiotics that concentrate in macrophages e.g., ciprofloxacin and trimethoprimsulfamethoxazole, as well as penicillin, and clofazimine Antibiotic therapy directed against gram-negative bacteria, especially E. coli in combination with surgery provides the best chance of cure.

Excision of skin lesions and drainage of abscesses

Ascorbic acid used to increase the intracellular cGMP improve macrophage function.

Acknowledgments Dr Uday Khopkar

REFERENCES

1. Ahmad Z Shawaf, Lamis A Boushi, Thaer Hassan Douri. Perianal Cutaneous malakoplakia in an immunocompetent patient. Dermatology Online Journal 16 (1): 10

2. Kohl SK, Hans CP. Cutaneous malakoplakia. Arch Pathol Lab Med. 2008

3. Shaktawat SS, Sissons MC. Malakoplakia of the appendix, an uncommon entity at an unusual site: a case report. J Med Case Reports. 2008 May 29;2:181.

4. Teeters JC. Rectal and Cutaneous malakoplakia in an orthoptic cardiac transplant recipient. J Heart Lung Transplant – 01-APR-2007; 26(4): 411-3 (Abstract)

5. Sandy Flann, Jane Norton, Andrew Charles Pembroke. Cutaneous malakoplakia in an abdominal skin fold. J Am Acad Dermatol 2010 May;62(5):896-7

Cutaneous Myiasis

Reshma T. Vishnani, Venisha B. Shah, Ram H. Malkani

Poster at CUTICON 2011, Poster at DERMACON 2012

A 61 year old male Nigerian resident presented to us with complains of red raised itchy lesions over his back and right elbow since 8 days. The lesions were preceded by an insect bite and history of similar lesion in neighbors was present. No history of oozing or pain around the lesion. No history of any systemic complaints. On history and examination, provisional diagnosis of insect bite reaction, papular urticaria, perforating granuloma annulare and perforating folliculitis were considered.

A skin biopsy was done and patient was given topical mupirocin and oral antihistamines. Routine histopathology revealed moderately dense nodular mixed infiltrate of lymphocytes, eosinophils, neutrophils in mid dermis surrounding a large cavity lined by chitinous material. The cavity revealed parts of a larva of a fly surrounded by numerous neutrophils and collagen degeneration. Overlying epidermis showed spongiotic psoriasiform hyperplasia, the above findings were consistent with cutaneous myiasis. Thus a final diagnosis of Cutaneous Myiasis was made, most probably due to Diptera fly genus *Cordylobia anthropophaga*. Occlusion therapy in the form of liquid paraffin gauze dressings helped in the extrusion of the larvae along with a single dose of oral ivermectin (200μg/kg).

The focus of this presentation is to create awareness and vigilance towards this interesting condition which is rarely seen.

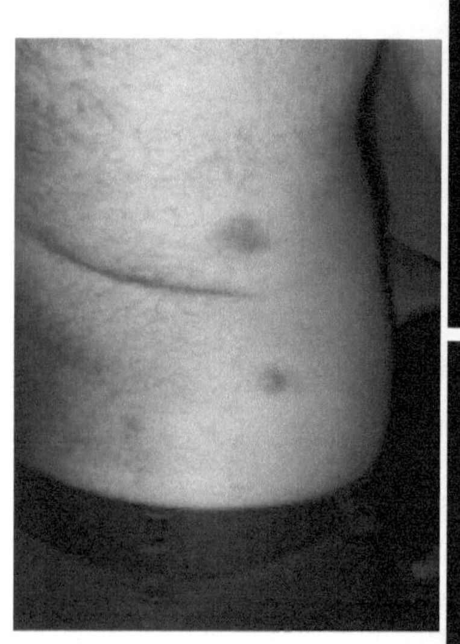

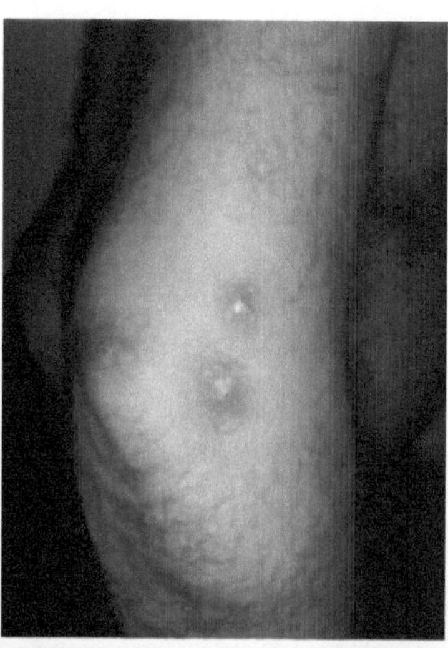

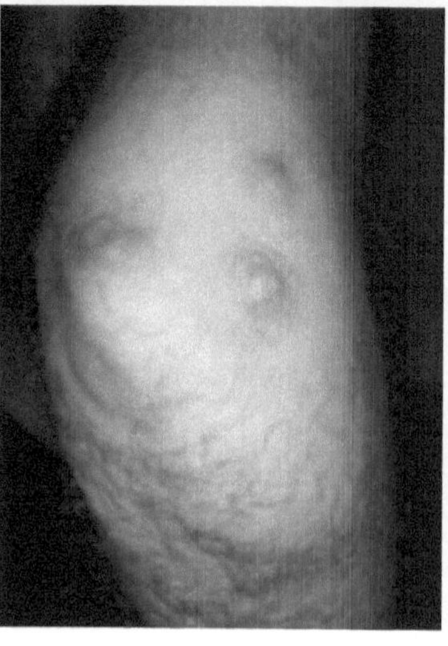

A Rare Case of Actinomycetoma

Priyanka Ghuge, Ram Malkani

National Conference of the IADVL, Maha, CUTICON 2012

National conference of the IADVL DERMACON 2013

We present you a case of a 56yr old male, who presented to the dermatology OPD with complaints of swelling and nodules over the left foot since 6 yrs with h/o discharge of white granules, recurrent nodules since 6 years following injury with broken glass. No h/o pain, fever. On investigating 3yrs back USG revealed resolving hematomas with small pockets of collections likely pyogenic. MRI revealed ill defined inflammatory lesions in the medial aspect of the foot with focal nodular enhancement seen in the subcutaneous plane. He was treated with multiple courses of antibiotics with partial improvement. Based on the previous history we kept a provisional diagnosis of actinomycetoma and eumycetoma.

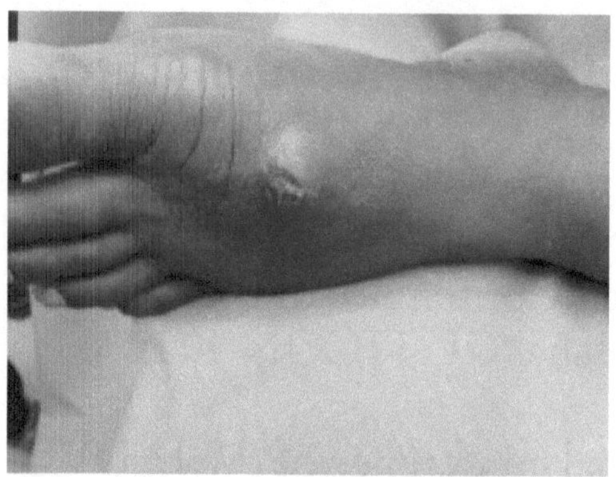

Investigations done: 1) CBC, ESR, LFTs, RFTs-normal. 2) Multiple pus samples did not reveal any growth. Several attempts made to culture the granules also did not yield growth. 3) Multiple lesional skin biopsies taken; majority of them inconclusive; however a couple of them were consistent with a biopsy from periphery of Mycetoma.

Hence based on a strong clinical suspicion of Actinomycetoma in view of whitish granules being discharged, Welsh regime (Inj. Amikacin 15mg/kg bd,T.Bactrim1.5mg/kg bd for 21 days. f/b T.Bactrim bd for 15 days) was started. 3 cycles completed. Patient started responding after completion of 1cycle and is under observation and regular follow up.

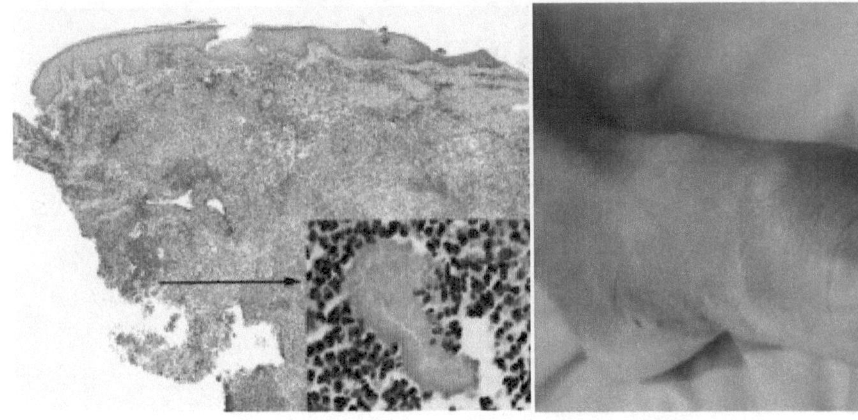

We present this case to highlight difficulties in reaching a definitive histopathological and/or mycological diagnosis of mycetoma despite a diligent search based on clinical suspicion and the merits of welsh regime in managing cases of Mycetoma.

Malignancy

Follicular Mucinosis

V L Aswani, R H Malkani

Ind J Dermatol VenereolLeprol1995; 61
:159-62

Introduction

The first series of patients with alopecia rnucinosa was presented by Pinkus in 1957.[1] He described six cases of slowly enlarging inflammatory plaques with alopecia and root sheath mucinosis. A few years later Jablonska et al[a] suggested the name follicular mucinosis, because alopecia is not always an apparent or prominent feature.

Clinically follicular mucinosis (FM) may start as grouped follicular papules or plaques that are hypopigmented, slightly erythematous, scaly and eczematous or there may be a solitary nodule. The plaques and nodules are generally firm, but may be soft, Sometimes mucin can be squeezed out of affected follicles. If a hair bearing area is involved non-scarring alopecia may result. The most commonly affected areas are the head and neck, but with multiple lesions the trunk and extremities may also be involved. Rarely, follicular papules may be generalised without obvious grouping. There is usually little or no pruritus. Rare cases of local dysesthesia have been reported.[3]

A coexisting lymphoma is associated with follicular mucinosis in about 15% of cases.[4]

Case Report

A 62-year-old male presented with multiple, discrete skin coloured to reddish papules on the face, neck and lower arms that were associated with mild itching for 1 year. There was no hisotry of photosensitivity. He had diabetes which was under control with diet and exercise. There was no history of drug intake prior to the onset of the disease.

His vital parameters were within normal limits. Cutaneous examination revealed discrete, skin coloured to slightly erythematous, follicular and nonfollicular papules on the face, neck and lower arms. They ranged in size from 2-5 mm and were firm in consistency. Some of the hair follicles were accentuated but did not contain keratin plugs; some were without hair. Systemic examination revealed no abnormality.

A complete blood count was within normal limits. The fasting and postprandial blood sugar levels were 100 mg and 130 mg respectively. Liver and renal function tests were normal.

A skin biopsy showed dilated hair follicles with mucinous changes and the formation of cystic cavities in the outer root sheath surrounded by a predominantly lymphocytic infiltrate and a few epithelioid cells. One section revealed a large cystic cavity formed due to mucinous degeneration of the outer root sheath containing degenerated outer root sheath cells, lymphocytes and eosinophils. A mucicarmine stain did not show mucin.

Patient was given dapsone, 100 mg orally daily.(5) After one week of treatment he had no new lesions, after two weeks the lesions had reduced in size and by the end of the month they had resolved.

Discussion

Our patient presented with discrete, firm, follicular and nonfollicular papules, some with accentuated follicular prominences, on the sun exposed parts of the body, suggesting a differential diagnosis of papular polymorphic light eruption and papular discoid lupus erythematosus. It was only on skin biopsy that the diagnosis of follicular mucinosis was made.

No mucin could be demonstrated on staining with the mucicarmine stain as it can be removed during fixation on account of its solubility in water. Staining of a frozen section is required in such cases.

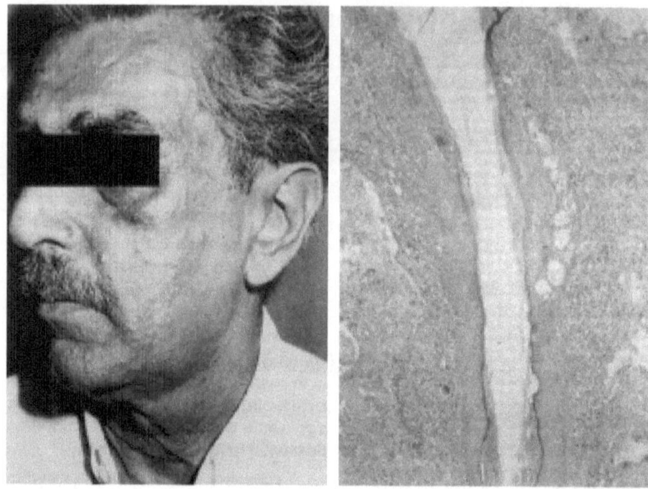

Fig 1 Skin coloured to erythematous follicular and non-follicular papules of the face and neck

Fig 2 Mucinous degeneration with formation of cystic cavities in the outer root sheath is seen (H&E x20)

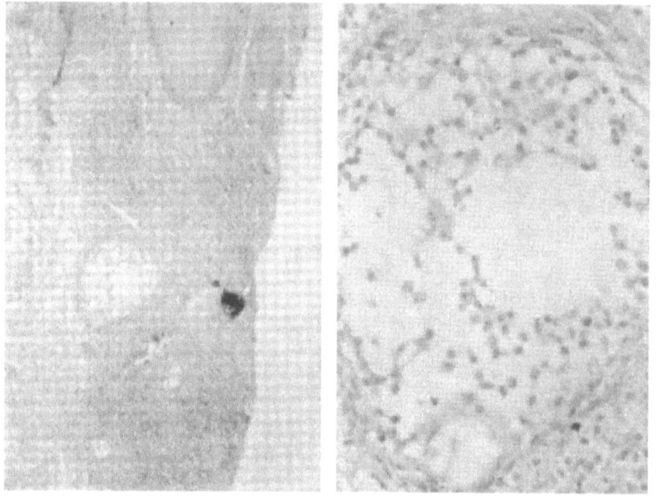

Fig 3 Transverse section of hair follicule showing cyctic space surrounded by mononuclear

Fig 4 Cystic cavity showing degenerate root sheath cells lymphocytes and eosinophils (H&E x450)

infiltrate

The disease has been known to assume one of three possible clinical courses

(a) Spontaneous resolution after 2 months to 2 years, without any recurrence,

(b) A chronic course with the persistence of individual lesions or the appearance of new lesions for over 2 years, but with no sign of the development of reticulosis, or

(c) An association with reticulosis.

In a study by Nickoloff ,[6] the following histologic criteria were found in benign juvenile idiopathic FM, in contrast to FM associated with mycosis fungoides:

(1) The lymphocytic infiltrate was generally confined to the follicular, perifollicular or perivascular zones with no extension into the epidermis.

(2) Within follicular epithelium there was a dense collection of lymphocytes with occasionally atypical appearing nuclei but never as Pautrier microabscesses.

(3) There was the absence of a significant associated plasma cells or eosinophil containing inflammatory dermal infiltrate.

Our patient responded well to treatment with dapsone, but no mode of therapy is consistently effective. Other modalities include topical, intralesional, or systemic steroids; superficial X-ray therapy, and PUVA therapy. In patients with FM and a lymphoma, therapy should be directed at the malignancy.

References

1. Pinkus H. Alopecia mucinosa: Inflammatory plaques with alopecia characterized by root sheath mucinosis. Arch Dermatol 1957; 76: 419-26.

2. Jablonska S, et al. Mucinosis follicularis. Hautarzt 1959; 10: 27-33. 3. ArnoldHLJr. Dysesthesiainalopecia mucinosa : A possible diagnostic sign. Arch Dermatol 1962; 85: 409-10.

4. Emmerson RW. Follicular mucinosis: A study of 47 patients. Br J Dermatol 1969; 81: 395-413.

5. Kubka RK, Stewart TW,. Follicular mucinosis responding to dapsone. Br J Dermatol 1974; 91: 217-20

6. Nickloff BJ, et al Benign idiopathic vs mtcosis fungoides associated folicular mucinosis. Pediatr Dermatol 1985; 2: 201-6

Recalcitrant pruritus as primary manifestation of synchronous Hodgkins lymphoma and Langerhans cell histiocytosis

Afsha A Topal, Ram H Malkani, Ganapathi Bhat, Reshma T Vishnani

Acta Medica (Hradec Kralove).
2012;55(2):104-6

Abstract

We present a 73 year old female with intractable pruritus and nonspecific cutaneous rash for a period of 9 months. She had recieved symptomatic therapy with no improvement. A complete examination revealed axillary and abdominal lymphadenopathy. A biopsy confirmed the diagnosis of Hodgkins lymphoma with Langerhans cell histiocytosis. She received 5 cycles of chemotherapy with resolution of pruritus and reduction in axillary and abdominal lymphadenopathy. The patient presented 6 months later with relapse and succumbed to the illness.

Simultaneous occurrence of Langerhans cell histiocytosis and Hodgkins lymphoma may lead to misdiagnosis. The awareness of such an association is important to make an accurate diagnosis and guide appropriate therapy.

CASE REPORT

A 73 year old lady presented with generalised pruritic rash since a duration of 9 months. She had recieved various topical and systemic symptom oriented medications with no significant benefit. She had experienced weight loss of around 15 kgs in the last 6 months and low grade fever for 1 month. Cutaneous examination revealed multiple erythematous excoriated papules, few showing scaling, over extremities (extensor/flexor), chest, abdomen and back(Fig 1 and 2). Scalp and flexures were spared. General examination revealed firm, discrete and nontender left axillary lymphadenopathy. Initial investigations revealed anaemia (Hb: 10.4), a normal complete blood count and hypoproteinemia(Serum Total Protein- 6.7g/dl, Serum Albumin- 3.4g/dl). A skin biopsy from an erythematous papule showed spongiotic epidermis, a moderate superficial and deep perivascular infiltrate composed of lymphocytes, monocytes and several eosinophils, with no evidence of Langerhans cell histiocytosis or Hodgkins lymphoma(Fig 3). Ultrasound of abdomen showed multiple hypoechoic retroperitoneal lymphnodes and multiple hypoechoic splenic deposits suggestive of a possibility of lymphoma. Positron emission tomography(PET) scan revealed evidence of high grade active disease in bilateral axillary, mediastinal, perihepatic, periportal, retroperitoneal, and bilateral iliac group of lymphnodes, involvement of the spleen, liver, left ischial and sacral bones(Fig 4). Bone marrow biopsy (posterior iliac crest) was normal. Axillary lymph node biopsy was reported as Langerhans cell histiocytosis with expression of S100 and CD 1a. But, due to the strong clinical suspicion, the biopsy specimen was resectioned and reviewed by the same histopathologist. It showed CD30 positive Reed-Sternberg cells which were negative for CD 15, LCA, CD 20 and CD 3(Fig 5). On the basis of these findings the patient was diagnosed as Classical Hodgkins lymphoma, Stage IV according to the Ann Arbor classification and treated with pulsed injectable methylprednisolone followed by chemotherapy. She was given 1 cycle of CEPP (cyclophosphamide, etoposide, procarbazine, and prednisone) followed by 5 cycles of COPP (cyclophosphamide, vincristine, procarbazine, and prednisone), after which she achieved complete remission. There was resolution of pruritus and reduction in axillary and abdominal lymphadenopathy on abdominal ultrasound. A repeat PET scan did not reveal any disease activity. The patient presented 6 months later with history of itching and lethargy since 3 weeks. USG Abdomen showed multiple hypoechoic lesion in liver and spleen, multiple lymphnodes seen at porta and in suprapancreatic region. Repeat PET scan showed evidence of high grade active disease in left axillary lymphnode, mediastinal, retroperitoneal lymphnodes and involvement of the spleen and liver. The patient was treated in relapse with 3 cycles of etoposide, procarbazine and prednisone and started on Tab. Chlorambucil 2mg daily. Repeat USG Abdomen showed multiple hypoechoic lesions in liver. Eventually, the patient developed septicaemia and succumbed to the disease.

Discussion

Hodgkin's disease (HD) is rare in the elderly. In population based studies, the proportion of HL patients over age 60 years has ranged from 15% to 30%(1). Several studies have shown that Hodgkin's disease in older adults has a poorer prognosis than in younger adults(2). Walker et al reanalysed data from the American College of Surgeons Patterns of Care Study (Kennedy et al, 1985) and found that advanced age remained an independent predictor of poor prognosis, even after correction for histological subtype, stage of disease, B symptoms and treatment(3). The most established prognostic tool in HL is the International Prognostic Score (IPS), which uses 7 adverse clinical prognostic factors, including age older than 45 years, to predict outcome(4). Epstein–Barr virus has been suspected as an aetiological agent in the pathogenesis of Hodgkin's disease for some years, however the relationship between EBV-associated (EBV-positive) Hodgkin's disease and prognosis is controversial. Studies have demonstrated an association between EBV positivity and a poor prognosis of Hodgkin's disease in older patients(5). Elderly individuals are recognized to have lower immunocompetence than younger people and may therefore have more difficulty in controlling the growth of an EBV-associated tumour than younger patients.

Generalized pruritus is noted in approximately 30% cases of Hodgkins lymphoma(6) and maybe the only presenting symptom(7). Smith et al and White et al found that specific skin involvement in Hodgkins lymphoma is rare, occurring in 0.5% and 3.4 %respectively (8,9).

Nonspecific cutaneous symptoms maybe seen in upto 50% of patients(10) and include eczema(11), hyperpigmentation, prurigo, icthyosis, vasculitis, bullous eruption, erythema nodosum and generalized hyperhidrosis(12). Gobbi et al proposed inclusion of severe pruritus among Ann Arbor criteria for definition of the B-clinical category due to the intrinsically poor prognosis related to severe pruritus(6). But it was retrospective analysis from 1971-1979 years and pruritus was not added to B symptoms.

Langerhans cell histiocytosis has been described in association with a variety of other tumor types, preceding, after or synchronous with the other tumor. The most common associations are with malignant lymphomas and leukaemias(13). Most commonly, the diagnoses are concurrent, with the lymphoma being of Hodgkin type. This association is rare, and has been estimated to be 0.3% for Hodgkin lymphoma (14). Shin et al discussed the relationship between these two conditions and proposed various possibilities(15):

Hodgkins disease induces Langerhans cell histiocytosis

Radiotherapy and/or chemotherapy for Hodgkins disease leads to the development of Langerhans cell histiocytosis

Langerhans cell histiocytosis may represent a specific cell mediated immune response to Hodgkins disease

A common etiological agent induces both Hodgkins disease and Langerhans cell histiocytosis

In concurrent occurrence of these two diseases, Langerhans cells are smaller than regular ones in histopathologic examination and this makes the differential diagnosis more difficult(16). PET imaging is not of much help in differentiating these two conditions, since both conditions show increase uptake of glucose(17). Hence, histopathology and immunohistochemistry are essential to distinguish these two conditions.

In our case, the presence of the characteristic pruritus, which is strongly suggestive of Hodgkins disease and the knowledge of the synchronous occurrence of these two conditions helped us reach the correct diagnosis. An accurate diagnosis in such cases guides the physician in the choice of therapy (conservative in Langerhans cell histiocytosis versus aggressive in Hodgkins lymphoma).

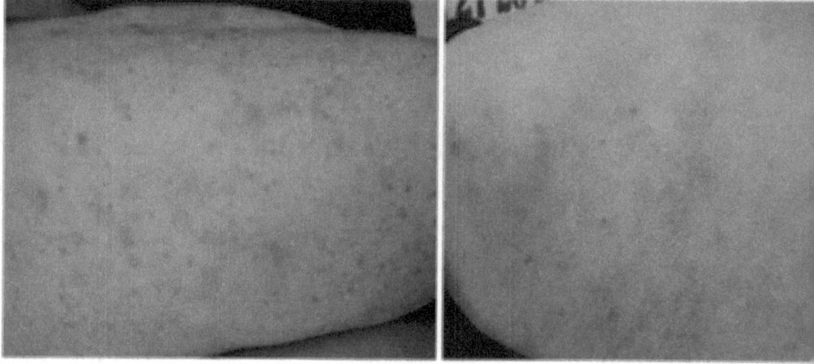

Fig 1: Multiple erythematous papules, few excoriated over the thigh

Fig 2: Few excoriated papules, underlying erythema over the upper

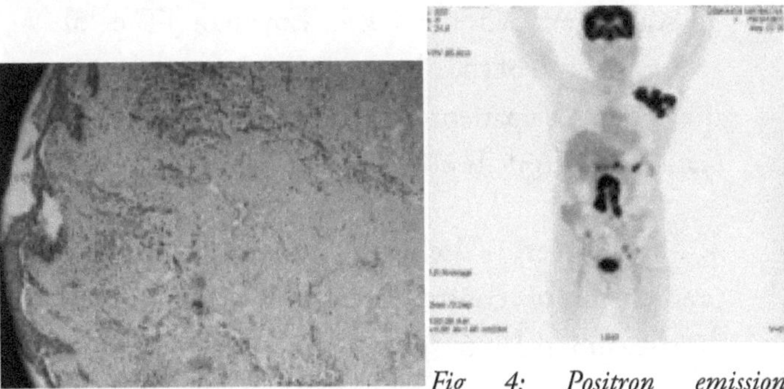

Fig 3: A skin biopsy from an eythematous papule showed spongiotic epidermis, a moderate superficial and deep perivascular infiltrate composed of lymphocytes, monocytes and several eosinophils

Fig 4: Positron emission tomography (PET scan) revealed evidence of high grade active disease in bilateral axillary , mediastinal, perihepatic, periportal, retroperitoneal, and bilateral iliac group of lymphnodes

Fig 5. Left axillary showed Reed-Sternb of classical Hodgkins

References

1. Evens AM, Sweetenham JW, Horning SJ. Hodgkin lymphoma in older patients: an uncommon disease in need of study. Oncology 2008; 22(12):1369-1379.

2. Gail L. Stark,1 Katrina M. Wood,2 Fergus Jack,1 Brian Angus,2 Stephen J. Proctor1and Penelope R. Taylor1 on behalf of the Northern Region Lymphoma Group Hodgkin's disease in the elderly: a population-based study British Journal of Haematology, 2002, 119, 432–440

3. Walker A, Schonfeld ER, Lowman JT et al 1990. Survival of the older patient compared with the younger patient with Hodgkins disease. Cancer 65, 1635-1640

4. HasencleverD, DiehlV. A numerical index to predict tumor control in advanced Hodgkin's disease. Blood 1996 (suppl 1, abstr); 88: 673a

5. Thorley-Lawson DA, Gross A. Persistence of the Epstein-Barr virus and the origins of associated lymphomas. N Engl J Med 2004;350:1328-1337.

6. Gobbi PG, Attardo Parinello G, Lattanzio G Rizzo SC, Ascari E. Severe pruritus should be a B symptom in hodgkins disease. Cancer 1983:51:1934-6

7. O Donell BF, Alton B, Carnney D, Loughlin S. Generalized pruritus when to investigate further. J Am Acad Dermatol 1993;28:117

8. Smith JL Jr , Butler JJ. Skin involvement in hodgkins disease cancer 1980;45:354-61

9. White RM, Patterson JW. Cutaneous involvement in hodgkins disease. Cancer 1985;55:1136-1145.

10. Szur L, Harrison CV, Levene GM, Samman PD . Primary cutaneous hodgkins disease Lancet 1970;1:1016-20

11. Callen JP, Bernadi DM, Clark RA, Weber DA. Adult onset recalcitrant eczema: marker of noncutaneous lymphoma or leukaemia J Am Acad Dermatol 2000;43:207-10

12.Rubenstein M, Duvic M. Cutaneous manifestations of hodgkins disease. Int J Dermatol 2006;45:251-6

13. Egeler RM, Neglia JP, Arico M et al. The relation of langerhans cell histiocytosis to acute leukaemia, lymhomas and other solid tumors. Hematol Oncol Clin North Am 1998;12:369-78

14. Barnes BF, Colby TV, Dorfman RF. Langerhans cell granulomatosis associated with malignant lymphomas. Am J Surg Pathol. 1983;7:529-533.

15. Myung S. Shin, Scott E. Buchalter, Kang-Jey Ho. Langerhans' cell histiocytosis associated with Hodgkin's disease: A case report.. J NatI Med Assoc.1994;86:65-69

16. Adu-Poku K, Thomas DW, Khan MK, Holgate CS, Smith MEF. Langerhans cell

histiocytosis in sequential discordant lymphoma. J Clin Pathol 2005;58(1):104-6.

17. Naumann R, Beuthein BaumannB, Fischer R, Kittner T, Bredow J, Kropp J et al. Simultaneous occurrence of Hodgkins lymphoma and eosinophilic granuloma, a potential pitfall in positron emission tomography imaging. Clin lymphoma 2002 ;3(2):121-4

Skin - a mirror of internal disease

Reshma T. Vishnani, Ram Malkani

Presented at CUTICON 2011

History:

73/F presented with c/o generalized itching with rash for 8-9 months, initially on the extremities then spreading to the rest of the body.

H/o fatigue, weight loss (15kgs) since 6months, low-grade fever since 1month.

Patient was a k/c/o bilateral plantar psoriasis for 32 years, well maintained on topical treatment. H/o taking AKT for 9 months on suspicion of pulmonary TB 8 years ago and has iron deficiency anemia.

Examination: Multiple erythematous scaly papules with excoriations over upper and lower limbs (extensor/flexor), chest, abdo, back with a few crusted lesions. Palms/soles/scalp/mucosa spared.

Provisional diagnosis: Dermatitis herpetiformis or pruritus due to iron deficiency anemia was made.

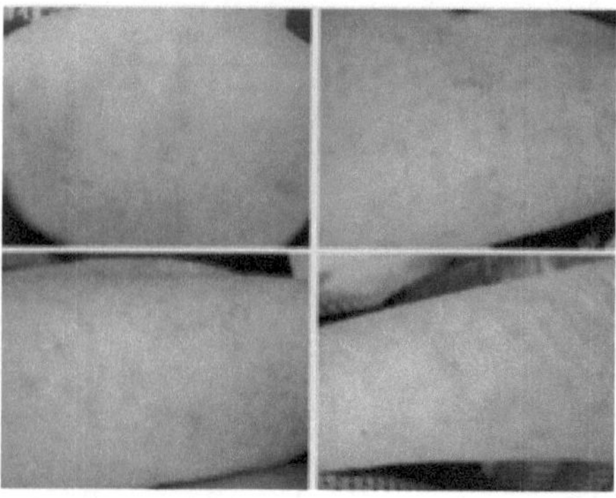

Investigations:

a) Low Hb, a low normal WBC (5300), normal differentials and platelets.

b) Skin biopsy: showed a moderately severe superficial and deep perivascular infiltrate of lymphocytes, eosinophils, several eosinophils lying scattered in the interstitium of reticular dermis and deep vascular plexus were also seen.

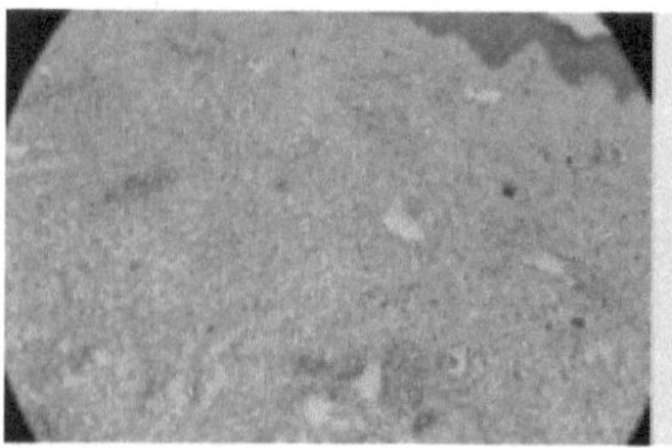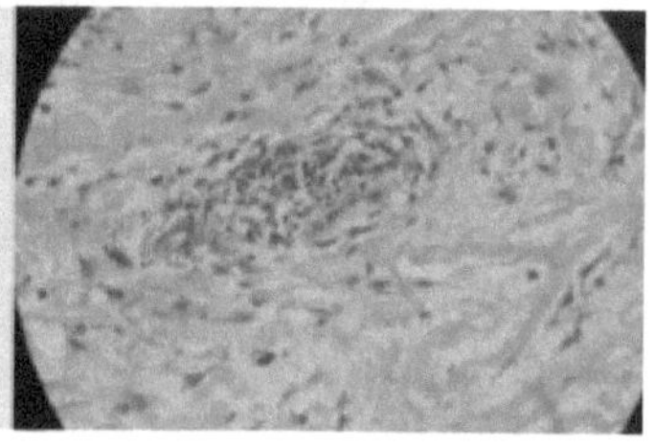

Further investigations done, since patient's response to oral antihistamines was not satisfactory and biopsy report was not conclusive.

- General- pallor + Systemic- Abdo- Mild hepatomegaly - left axillary lymphadenopathy Rest-WNL

- USG Abdo: showed multiple hypoechoic retroperitonal lymph nodes and multiple hypoechoic deposits in spleen suggestive of a possibility of lymphoma

- Repeat routine investigations revealed a fall in Hb and WBC and increase in eosinophils

- LDH: 530U/ml H, CA-125: 44.4U/ml H, CA 19.9: 5.19 U/ml, CEA: 1.05 ng/ml

- PET scan: showed evidence of high grade active disease in bilateral axillary group of lymph nodes, mediastinal, perihepatic lymphnodes, spleen, lymphnodes at splenic hilum, periportal, retroperitoneal, bilateral iliac group of lymphnodes, left ischium and sacrum. These findings were suggestive of Lymphoma

- Whole Body CT-PET showed multiple enlarged homogenously enhancing lymphonodal masses in left axilla and pectoral region, mediastinum, periportal, perisplenic, peripancreatic, retroperitoneal, bilateral iliac are highly suggestive of lymphoma. Ill-defined osteolytic lesion in sacrum and left ischial bones could represent skeletal lymphomatous deposits.

Multiple hypodense splenic lesion and focal hypodense lesion with peripheral enhancing in segment 2 and 4A are suggestive of lymphoma deposits

- Skeletal survey and bone marrow examination: normal.

Axillary lymph node biopsy by an oncosurgeon was done and reported as Langerhans cell Histiocytosis (LCH). (S-100 and CD1a focal +ve).

Treatment:

Patient was thus referred to the Hematology-oncology clinic and was treated with Inj Methylprednisolone 1gm for 3 consecutive days.

Skin lesions improved, patient subjectively better and left axillary lymph nodes were decreased.

? Recurrence of itching and lethargy after 5 months.

? Review left axillary lymph node biopsy was s/o classical Hodgkins disease, Reed-Sternberg cells express CD30 and were negative for CD 15, LCA, CD 20 and CD 3. Previous biopsy was reviewed showed no evidence of Hodgkin's disease

Treatment:

She was given 1 cycle of methylprednisolone followed by CEPP followed by 5 cycles of COPP. Unfortunately patient expired in the following few months.

Discussion:

Systemic disease is detected in approximately 10-50% of all patients seeking medical attention for pruritus

Among patients with malignancy, lymphoproliferative disorders, particularly Hodgkin's disease (H.D) are the most important and well-known causes of unexplained pruritus.

Pruritus, although not considered as a B symptom by definition, indicated poor prognosis.

Cause: Pruritogenic mediators released due to the autoimmune response against malignant cells-leukopeptidase and bradykinin

Poor response in our patient- because ABVD considered gold standard could not be given due to age of patient.

Cimetidine 1gm (200mg at meal times and 400mg at bed time) can be used to treat pruritus in Hodgkin's disease, till chemotherapy is given

Langerhans cell histiocytosis: Age range: 10-15 years of age, very rare in adults (1 in 560,000). M:F= 2:1. Bone involvement in the form of painful swellings is the most common presentation. Skin manifestations are in the form of scaly erythematous rashes or papules in intertriginous areas and scalp. Other sites: - Bone marrow, lymph nodes, endocrine glands and lungs.

Mediators and Transmission of itch:

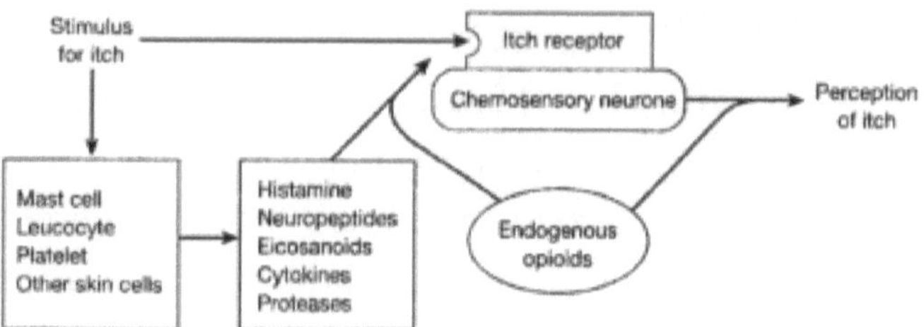

Conclusion:

We present this case, for its rarity and also to create awareness and potential suspicion towards the varied causes of skin lesions, some of which may be the earliest manifestations of a grave underlying systemic condition.

Reference:

1. Rubenstein M, Madeline D. cutaneous manifestations of Hodgkin's disease. Int J Dermatol 2006,45: 251-256

2. Omidvari SH, Khojasteh HN, Mohammadianpanah M, Monabati A, Mosalaei A, Ahmadloo N, Long-term pruritus as the initial and sole clinical manifestation of occult Hodgkin's disease. Indian J Med Sci 2004 Jun;58(6):250-2.

3. Ulla Kapilin1, Kristian Thestrup-Pedersen1, Torben Steiniche2 and Hans Lomholt, Skin Markers for Hodgkin's Disease, Acta Derm Venereol 2005; 85: 345–381

4. J P Aymard, P Lederlin, F Witz, J N Colomb, R Herbeuval, and B Weber, Cimetidine for pruritus in Hodgkin's disease. Br Med J. 1980 January 19; 280(6208): 151–152.

Neutrophilic Eccrine Hidradenitis in a patient of Chronic Lymphoid Leukemia

Priyanka Ghuge, Rusina Karia, Ram Malkani

To be published

INTRODUCTION:

Neutrophilic eccrine hidradenitis has been first described by Harrist et al. in 1982[1] and Flynn et al. in 1984[2]. NEH is associated with an underlying malignancy in 90% of cases[3] most common being AML on chemotherapy. The most frequently described cases are those where patients were receiving cytarabinecontaining induction chemotherapy for AML. Most cases are associated with a state of peripheral neutropenia. Very few case reports are available with the classic presentation.

A 45 year old male patient presented with multiple, reddish, small, slightly painful eruptions involving the upper and lower limbs and lower back since 3-4 days. The eruption began on the lower limbs and progressed to involve the other areas in a span of 2-3 days. Lesions were asymptomatic except for slight pain on pressure. Patient was a known case of Acute Myelogenous Leukemia, diagnosed 1 year back. There was history of 2 cycles of Chemotherapy received with Injection Cytarabine and Injection Daunorubicin. Patient was admitted at present in view of AML blast crisis and has received the 3rd chemotherapy cycle with the same drugs 15 days back. There was history of similar episodes following the previous chemotherapy cycles, which were milder in nature and were followed by complete resolution of the lesions by the end of 3 weeks, leaving behind only dark coloured spots.

On cutaneous examination, there was evidence of multiple well defined erythematious macules and papules, some coalescing to form plaques, measuring 0.5cm to 2cm in size, present over the extensor aspect of the lower limbs Fig 1 (a) Presence of erythematous, ill-defined nodules, of 1cm in size over the dorsal aspect of fingers and lower back was present Fig 1(b). Deep dermal tenderness was mildly positive.

A differential diagnosis of drug eruption, erythema nodosum, vaculitis and neutrophilic eccrine hidradenitis was considered

Histopathological examination revealed a spongiotic epidermis with mild hyperkeratosis. There was dense periappendageal neutrophilic infilterate present in the dermis, particularly involving the eccrine coils. Dermal edema present Fig. 2(a) 2(b), 2(c) There was no evidence of vasculitis. Patient was febrile and had peripheral neutropenia.

Based on these observations a diagnosis of Neutrophilic Eccrine Hidradenitis was confirmed.

Patient was treated with oral Prednisolone 0.5mg/kg/day for 7 days. There was partial resolution of the lesions after which he was lost to follow up.

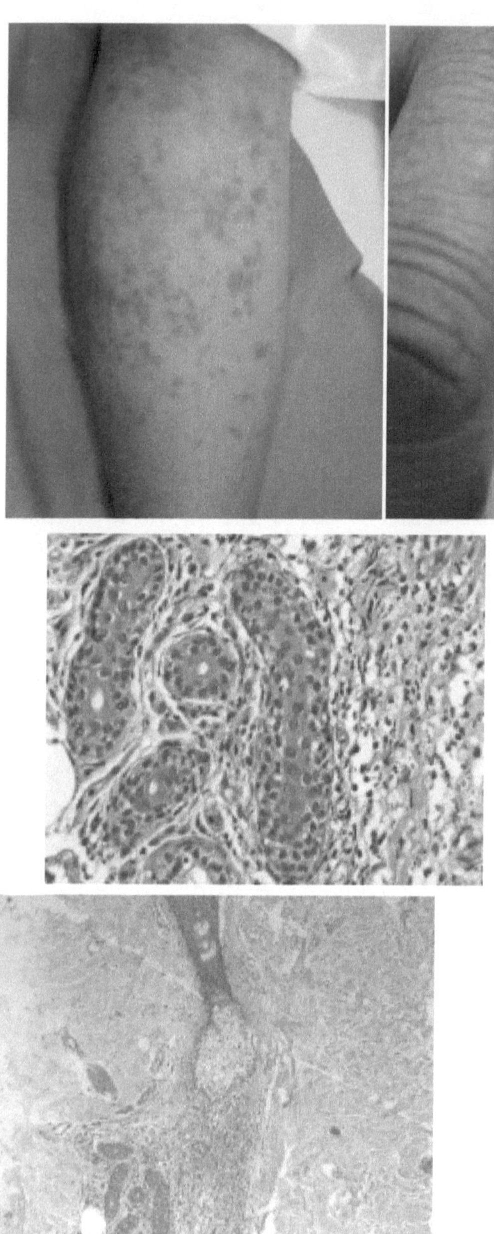

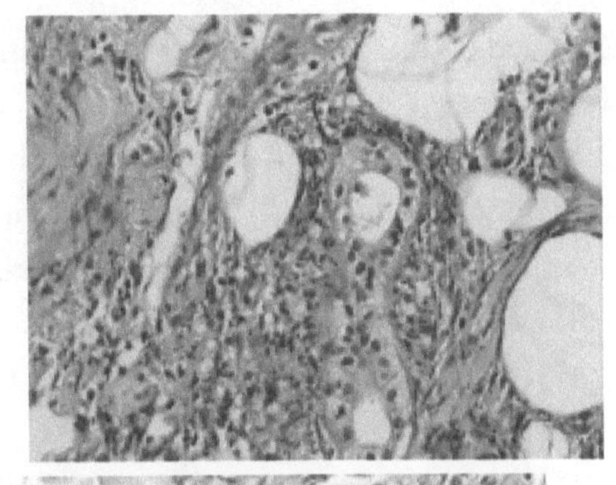

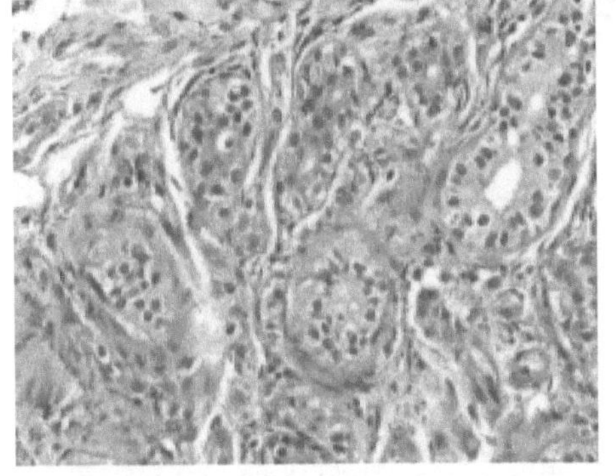

Discussion:

Neutrophilic eccrine hidradenitis (NEH) is a dermatoses affecting the eccrine glands in particular. It has been known to occur most commonly in patients undergoing chemotherapy for malignancies. It is a rare condition, but characterised by acute, self-limited, inflammatory neutrophilic dermatosis and has beenmost commonly described in association with patients of acute myelogenous leukemia (AML) receiving chemotherapy.[1]

Neutrophilic eccrine hidradenitis has been first described by Harrist et al. in 1982[1] and Flynn et al. in

1984. NEH is associated with an underlying malignancy in 90% of cases[2], most common being AML on chemotherapy. Other hematologic malignancies with a known association include acute myeloid leukemia, chronic lymphocytic leukemia, Hodgkin's and non-Hodgkin's lymphoma, as well in solid tumors such as osteogenic sarcoma, testicular carcinoma, metastatic breast cancer and Wilms tumor[3]. The most frequently described cases are those where patients were receiving cytarabine containing induction chemotherapy for AML. Some other drugs like bleomycin, mitoxantrone, anthracyclines, decitabine, zidovudine[5] and acetaminophen, which have also been described as being associated with NEH.

There are some case reports of infectious causes for NEH. Infectious agents like HIV[4], Gram-positive cocci, Streptoccoccus spp., Serratia marescens, Nocardia spp., Enterobacter cloacae and Staphyloccocus aureus have beenreported in patients who presented classical histological features of NEH.

NEH usually presents 2 days to 3 weeks following the initiation of chemotherapy, although a period of as long as 2 years following therapy is also known[4]. It can either present in a localized distribution involving the limb or trunk, or be generalized. General presentation is that of erythematous papules and plaques but the morphology may be very variable, which may be multiple or solitary, painful or asymptomatic.

Patients are usually febrile and neutropenic at the time of presentation.[6]

The diagnosis is histological with the biopsy demonstrating a dense neutrophilic infiltrate in the eccrine unit, dermal edema, and necrosis of the eccrine coils and glands. The mechanism by which the eccrine sweat unit is affected remains unknown. One hypothesis underlines direct cytotoxic effect of the drugs. Toxic byproducts are secreted through sweat, and thus, by neutrophilic chemotaxis induced by cellular damage, neutrophilic infilteration of the eccrine coils and glands occurs. Consequently, the toxic concentration of the drugs within the eccrine gland may lead to necrosis of the epithelial cells[7]. Even so, no studies that evaluated the drug concentration in sweat glands were found.

Another hypothesis describes NEH as a part of the neutrophilic dermatoses spectrum[8] as a paraneoplastic condition. As mentioned, NEH has also been described in a healthy population[9]. Therefore, a possibility of underlying sweat gland abnormalities was formulated.

NEH is a self-limiting condition. Associations other than malignancy or chemotherapy have been made in the literature. The treatment is symptomatic and mainly consists topical or systemic corticosteroids for a short duration.[7]

However, corticosteroids should be used with caution in patients with peripheral neutropenia. Pain can be managed with usual analgesic medication if tender lesions are present.

As for the prevention of possible recurrences of NEH with the same drug use, one case report encourages use of Dapsone, which inhibits neutrophil chemotaxis, in a dose of 100 mg daily beginning 48 h before the treatment[10].

We have reported here a febrile neutropenic patient undergoing chemotherapy for acute myelogenous leukemia who presented with classic neutrophilic eccrine hidradenitis. We emphasize the necessity of a prompt diagnosis in order to prevent the use of multiple antibiotics and inadvertent use of other drugs. In our case, cytarabine was the drug likely responsible for NEH.

References

1) Shear NH1, Knowles SR, Shapiro L, Poldre P. J Am Acad Dermatol. Dapsone in prevention of recurrent neutrophilic eccrine hidradenitis. 1996 Nov;35(5 Pt 2):819-22.

2) Bailey DL1, Barron D, Lucky AW. Pediatr Dermatol. Neutrophilic eccrine hidradenitis: a case report and review of the literature. 1989 Mar;6(1):33-8.

3) Fitzpatrick JE1, Bennion SD, Reed OM, Wilson T, Reddy VV, Golitz L. J Cutan Pathol. Neutrophilic eccrine hidradenitis associated with induction chemotherapy. 1987 Oct;14(5):272-8.

4) Bachmeyer C1, Reygagne P, Aractingi S. Dermatology. Recurrent neutrophilic eccrine hidradenitis in an HIV-1-infected patient. 2000;200(4):328-30.

5) Bachmeyer C1, Aractingi S. Clin Dermatol. Neutrophilic eccrine hidradenitis. 2000 May-Jun;18(3):319-30.

6) Wong GC1, Lee LH, Chong YY. Ann Acad Med Singapore. A case report of neutrophilic eccrine hidradenitis in a patient receiving chemotherapy for acute myeloid leukaemia. 1998 Nov;27(6):860-3.

7) Thorisdottir K1, Tomecki KJ, Bergfeld WF, Andresen SW. J Am Acad Dermatol. Neutrophilic eccrine hidradenitis. 1993 May;28(5 Pt 1):775-7.

8) Wallach D. Rev Med Interne. Neutrophilic dermatoses. 2005 Jan;26(1):41-53.

9) Belot V1, Perrinaud A, Corven C, de Muret A, Lorette G, Machet L. Presse Med. Adult idiopathic neutrophilic eccrine hidradenitis treated with colchicine 2006 Oct;35(10 Pt 1):1475-8.

10) Shear NH, Knowles SR, Shapiro L, Poldre P. J Am Acad Dermatol. Dapsone in prevention of recurrent neutrophilic eccrine hidradenitis. 1996 Nov;35(5 Pt 2):819-22.

Drug Reactions

Management of pemphigus with gold compounds

Ram Malkani, Ajay Kumar

Bulletin of the Jaslok Hospital & Research centre Vol XIV No. 4 April 1990 p.28.

At one time all blistering diseases of the skin were considered to be pemphigus, but with improved diagnostic techniques in modern histopathology and more recently immunohistochemical methodology, pemphigus has become a distinct entity clearly separable from a large variety of other bullous disorders. Pemphigus is an auto immune disease which involves skin and mucous membrane, in which there is scantholysis and blister formation within the epidermis. Immunoglobulins and complement are found bound to the intercellular substance in the perilesional epidermis.

Introduction of corticosteriods have greatly reduced the mortality of this condition. Many therapeutic agents have been used with varying success to manage patients with pemphigus. Currently systematically administered corticosteriods are used most commonly. A retrospective review of the side effects caused by systematically given corticosteroids in pemphigus patients showed a substantial morbidity and mortality. The major difficulty is managing these patients in achieving a balance between risks associated with high dose steriod therapy and poorly controlled disease.

A variety of immunosuppressive agents have been used in an attempt to reduce steroid requirement. These are methotrexate, azothioprine and cyclophosphamide.

The value of systemic gold therapy in the management of patients with pemphigus was first reported in 1973 by Penneys et al. Most patients received cryotherapy for less than one year at the time of that report, the results of the same group of patients were presented after three years of treatment in 1976. The preparation used is sodium aurothiomalate given intramuscularly. Sodium aurothiomalate and other gold salts are used mainly for their anti-inflamatory effect in active progressive rheumatoid arthritis in which condition their experience is maximum. It is given deeply intramuscularly. Initially 10 mg is given to test the patient's tolerance. Seven days later 25 mg intramuscularly is given. If satisfactory, this is followed by doses of 50 mg at weekly intervals until signs of remission occurs and there is a drop in ICS antibody titres or toxicity develops, or a total of 1 g of gold has been given without effectively lowering the corticosteriod dose. Maintenance therapy consists of 50 mg of gold sodium thiomalate intramuscularly every 2 to 4 weeks.

Reports indicate a wide range of incidence of adverse effects with the drug. Authors consider that with careful treatment about one third of patients will experience adverse effects. The most common side effects involve the skin and mucous membranes, with pruritus and stomatitis being the most prominent. Other adverse effects are on the haemopoietic, renal, pulmonary and gastro intestinal systems. In treatment of these adverse effects chelating agents such as dimercaprol may be employed.

Gold is contraindicated in exfoliative dermatitis, systemic lupus erythematosus and severe renal or hepatic disorders. Patients with a history of haematological disorders or who have previously shown toxicity to heavy metals should not be given gold salts, so also to any severely debilitated patient.

It is recommended that patients with diabetes mellitus and those with congestive heart failure should be adequately controlled before gold is given. Conditions such as proteinuria, pruritus and rash arising during treatment should be allowed to resolve before gold treatment is continued. Patients with a history of urticaria, eczema or collitis should be treated with caution. It is generally recommended that gold salts should not be given to patients who are pregnant or those who are breastfeeding. Concurrant administration of gold salts with other therapy capable of inducing blood disorders should be undertaken with caution if at all. Patients should be warned to report the appearance of sore throat, purpura, rash or malaise.

Urine should be tested for albumin before each injection and blood should be examined for signs of depressed haemopoiesis. Annual chest x-ray should be carried out.

CASE REPORT:

A 35 year old female patient presented with recurrent attacks of blistering lesions all over the body for 5 years. The blisters occurred in the oral cavity, scalp, chest and back and sometimes over the proximal limbs. There was no fixed interval between attacks.

Before presentation she was clinically and histopathologicaly diagnosed as pemphigus vulgaris and was given courses of systemic corticosteriods with the administration of high doses of steriods upto 160 mg per day, till the disease would come under control, after which the dose would be tapered and a maintenance dose advised. She continued to get recurrences with no specific factor precipitating the condition. On term administration of steroids she had adverse effects in the form of Cushingold features, amenorrhoea and obesity.

It was comtemplated to give her systemic gold therapy considering her adverse effects to corticosteroids, her recurrences and the encouraging reports of chryrotherapy in the literature.

Before initiating therapy she was investigated and her urine exam, blood counts, x-ray chest, and biochemical parameters liver and renal function were found to be in the normal range. A urine test confirmed that she was not pregnant.

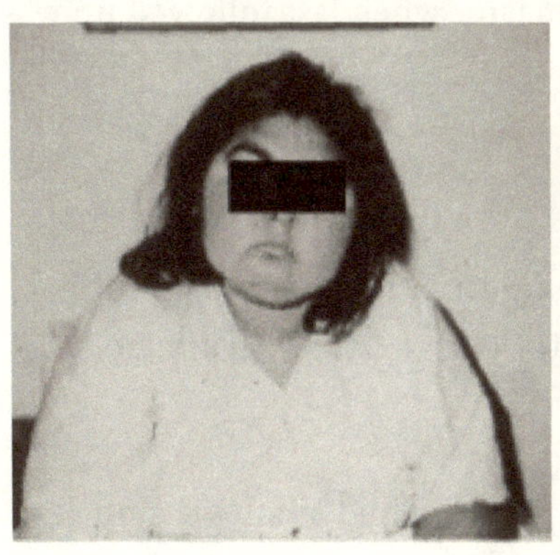

Fig. 1: Features of Cushingold appearance upon long term steroid administration

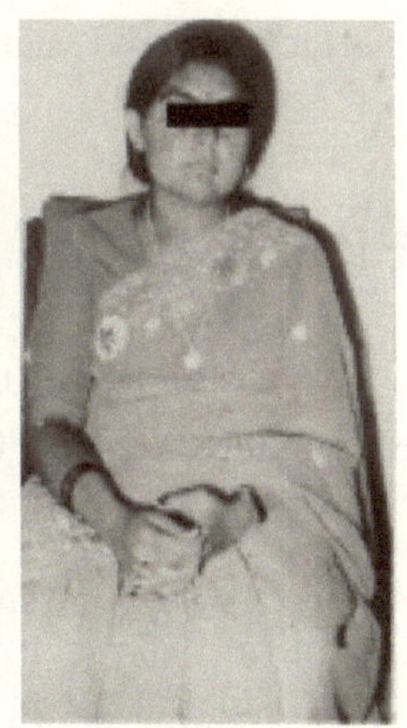

Fig. 2: Improvement in patients condition after gold therapy.

Treatment was initiated with a test dose of Sodium aurothiomaleate 10 mg intramuscularly and observed for seven days. It was well tolerated with no adverse effects. She was then given 25 mg intramuscularly and observed for another week when no adverse effect was observed. Subseqently she was given 50 mg of sodium aurothiomaleate at weekly intervals. Her oral steriods were gradually tapered off.

She did not experience symptoms of any adverse effects during the course of treatment. Her urine was examined and close watch was kept on the complete blood count before each injection. Both these were found to be normal.

After eight injections she developed signs of remission and her amenorrhoea improved. Subsequently she was advised maintenance dose of 50 mg once in two weeks for 4 such injections, she became free of symptoms and the adverse effects of steriods therapy improved. The gold therapy was then withdrawn and she did not develop any further attack till two years later when last followed up was done.

REFERENCES

1. Ryan J G : Pemphigus: A 20 year survey of experience with 70 cases. Arch Dermatol 104:14-20, 1971.

2. Krain L S : Pemphigus: Epidemiologic and survival characteristics of 59 patients, 1955-1973. Arch Dermatol 110 : 862 - 865, 1974.

3. Level W F, Goldberg H S : Treatment of pemphigus vulgaris with methotrexate. Arch Dermatol 110 : 862 - 865, 1974.

4. Roenigk H H, Deodhar S : Pemphigus : treatment with azothioprine : clinical and immmunological correlation. Arch Dermatol 107 :353 - 357, 1973.

5. Mckelvy E M Hasegawa J : Cyclophosphamide and pemphigus vulgaris. Arch Dermatol 103 :198 - 200, 1971.

6. Pennys N S, Eaghtel W S, Indrin S et al : Gold sodium thiomaleate treatment of pemphigus. Arch Dermatol 108 : 56 - 60, 1973.

7. Penny N S, Eaghtein W S, Frost P: Management of pemphigus with gold

compounds. Arch Dermatol 112 : 185 - 187, 1976

Drug hypersensitivity syndrome to leflunomide

Rahul Bade, Priyanka Ghuge, R.H. Malkani

Presented at CUTICON 2012

Abstract

We are presenting a drug hypersensitivity syndrome due to tab leflunomide used for an indication of psoriasis ina 51yr old female who presented with a generalized red mildly itchy scaly rash , associated wit intermittent fever and chills, oral ulcer and deranged liver function test.

Case Report:

A 51 Year oldfemale patient, known case of psoriasis, was admitted to the hospital with history of generalized red midly itchy rash associasted with intermittent high grade fever and chills with oral ulcer since 6days. 2 months prior to admission to hospital she was onTab leflunomide 20mg once a day, in the course of the treatment patient developed generalized erythematous maculopapular rash and few purpuric lesions (since 4 days).with deranged liver function test (raised AST, ALT, Bilirubin) with mild splenomegaly and hepatomegaly and bilateral moderate pleural effusion with underlying collapse lung , bilateral axillary , inguinal periportal and peripancreatic lymphnode . Lab investigation hb 11,wbc 7530(N-53, E-24.6,L-18,M-2,B-0), platelet 146, g6pd neg, anti dsDNA NEG, ASO neg, CRP 77. INR(1.7), S.Lipase(891) A provisional diagnosis of drug induced drug rash was made .After initial improvement with steroids and supportive care she developed erythroderma with a fatal outcome.

Discussion:

Lefunomide is a isoxazole immunomodulatory agent approved by the USFDA since 1998 for the treatment of psoriasis and rheumatoid arthritis. It is an inhibitor of pyrimidine synthesis and has antiproliferative and anti-inflammatory properties(1).

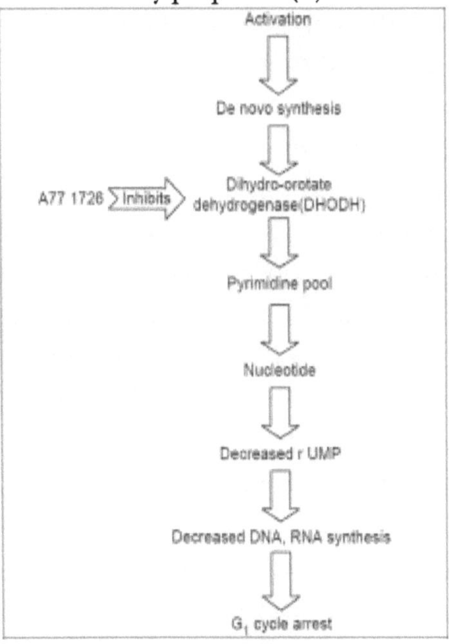

Figure 1: Schematic diagram showing the mechanism of action of leflunomide

Leflunomide is converted to its active metabolite A771726 with a half life of more than 2 weeks(1) . A771726 undergoes enterohepatic recirculationin healthy subjects and 90% of the drug is excreted by 28days, but in some, may be present for much longer (2). As detectable A771726 may be present in the body for months and years, the ability to eliminate it rapidly and effectively with cholestyramine is important which was done in our patient to (8g three times daily) can reduce the half life to 1 to 2 days(3). Leflunomide is available in 10 mg, 20 mg, 100mg, the standard recommendation is to start therapy with loading dose of 100mg daily for 3 days, then switch to 20 mg daily, despite recommendation, most clinicians no longer prescribe the loading dose, as its believed to increase drugs GIT toxicity (3) as it was done with our case to. Contraindications of the drug are hypersensitivity to drug or to inactive ingredient (eg lactose), pregnancy, preexisting liver, renal, bone marrow or immune status dysfunctions, moderate to severe bacterial, fungal or viral infections(4). Most serious side effect is liver damage ranging from jaundice to hepatitis, which can be fulminant, severe liver necrosis and liver cirrhosis were severe, fatalities are know(4, 5). Aslo very importaant is a relative high incidence of myelosuppression with leukopenia and or hypoplastic anemia, thrombocytopenia, infections(TB, PCP, pneumonia) leading to sepsis and death of the patient. Cutaneous reactions upto steven johnson and toxic epidermal necrolysis maculopapilar rash with nail discolouration are noted. Others are alopecia, git discomfort, intertial lung disease.(4-6)

In our case we observed fever, skin rash and internal organ involvement. Skin lesions were purpuric rash which progressed to erythroderma. The patient also had lymphadenopathy, diarrhea, eosionophilia, hyperbilirubinemia. Leflunomide was stopped the patient was treated with systemic steriods and supportive IV fluids and topical creams. Patient received oral cholestyramine 4mg tid chloestyramine causes leflunomide clearance by interfering with biliary secretion. The patient showed a characteristic pattern of events like delayed onset of lasting skin rash and internal organ involvement, our diagnoses was delayed hyper sensitivity syndrome. We had kept a differential diagnosis of viral hepatitis, viral rash, after initial improvement the patient succumbed.

Conclusion:

This case is been reported to create awareness regarding the above mentioned drug, which has caused serious fatalities.

And also the importance of IV or oral cholestyramine to hasten the clearance of the drug

References:

1) Mehta V, Kisalay S,Balachandran C . Leflunomide.Indian J Dermatol Venereol Leprol 2009;75:422-4.

2) Mladenovic V., Domljan Z., Rozman B., et al: Safety and effectiveness of leflunomide in the treatment of patients with active rheumatoid

arthritis: Results of a randomized, placebo-controlled, phase II study.Arthritis Rheum1995; 38:1595-1603.

3) Rozman B.: Clinical experience with leflunomide in rheumatoid arthritis.J Rheumatol1998; 25(Suppl 53):27-32.

4) http://en.wikipedia.org/wiki/leflunomide

5) Leflunomide hepatotoxicity. European Agency for the Evaluation of Medicinal Products (EMEA), March 2001.

6) Leflunomide: Serious hepatic, blood, skin and respiratory reactions.Australian Adverse Drug Reactions Bulletin2001; 20:(Feb)

7) Uppal M, Roy R,Srinivas CR. Leflunomide induced drug rash . 2004;49:154-5

8) Agrawal S, Agarwalla A. Dapsone hypersensitivity syndrome: a clinicoepidemiological review. J Dermatol. 2005 Nov; 32(11):883-9.

9) O Sener,L Doganci,M Safali,B Besirbellioglu,F Bulucu,A Pahsa Severe Dapsone Hypersensitivity Syndrome J Investig Allergol Clin Immunol 2006; Vol. 16(4): 268-270

10) Richardus JH, Smith TC. Increased incidence in leprosy of hypersensitivity reactions to dapsone after introduction of multidrug therapy. Lepr Rev. 1989;60:267-73.

Dapsone induced Hemolysis in Glucose-6-Phosphate Dehydrogenase (G6PD) deficient individual

Namita D. Talsamia, B.C. Mehta, Ram Malkani

Bulletin of the Jaslok Hospital & Research Centre, Vol XXVII No.2 October 2002.

Introduction

G6PD is the commonest congenital enzyme defect. It affects millions of people throughout the world. We report a case of dapsone induced hemolysis in G6PD deficient individual.

Case Summary

A 67 years old male, a known diabetic (for 10 years) and hypertensive had consulted a dermatologist for his skin problem. Patient was diagnosed as a case of Lichen planus and was started on local steroid and oral dapsone.

Few days later patient came with complaint of giddiness, chest pain and breathlessness since a day. Patient was rushed to a cardiologist. EGG was taken and was within normal range. He was admitted in Nanavati Hospital ICU. Patient also had 3 episodes of vomiting and complained of change in the colour of urine to to reddish yellow since last 3-4 days. There was no history of other urinary complaint of fever.

On admission patient appeared icteric, there was edema on the feet. In systemic examination liver was palpable 2 finger spaces below the right costal margin. Rest of the systems appeared normal.

Patient was thoroughly investigated. His random blood glucose on admission was 402 mg%, routine blood investigation were as follows: Hb-5.2 gm%, PCV-15.8, WBC-45,600, neutrophil-76%, SGPT- 89, SGOT-223, Alkaline phosphate-209. Urine routine for renal study showed bile salts present, bile pigment present, sugar+, acetone +ve, proteins +++, urobilinogen normal amount. Other investigations done were Sr. crea'tinine 2.2 mg%, LDH-2144, Reticulocyte count 10.6%, USG normal, G6PD status normal, Coombs test negative. Sr. ammonia 82mg/dl, Sr. ketones negative, Gamma gultamyl transfearse 94 u/1. Other causes of anaemia were ruled out, malarial parasite negative, urine for homosiderin and porphobilinogen were negative. ANA -ve.

Patient was diagnosed as a case of autoimmune hemolytic anaemia was given blood transfusion. Diabetes was controlled through insulin injections. Keeping that in mind he was started on steroids. Gradually steroids were tapered, insulin reduced. Patient recovered in 6 days and steroids were stopped. And was started on oral hypoglycemic drugs. Later it was discovered that he had taken dapsone, probably he was a case of G6PD deficiency.

Discussion

G6PD deficiency is a common condition that presents with a hemolytic anaemia and affects millions of people throughout the world, particularly in Africa around the Mediterranean, the Middle East and South East Asia(1).

In G6PD defect lies in the hexosemonophosphate shunt (HMP shunt). The enzyme G6PD holds a vital position in the HMP shunt oxidizing glucose-6-phosphate to 6-phosphogluconate with the reduction of NADPH. The reaction is particularly important in red cells where it is the only source of NADPH which is used via glutathione to protect the red cells from oxidative damage(1).

G6PD gene is located on the X chromosome. Thus the deficiency state is a sex linked trait. There is considerable genetic heterogenecity among affected individuals and over 400 variants of G6PD deficient have been described. Mutations are mostly single amino acid substitutions. The most common types with normal activity are called type B+ . Among the clinical significant G6PD variants the most common called A-type is due to 2 base substitutions . Mild form is characterized by hemolytic episodes triggered by infection or drug exposure. More severe enzyme deficiency such as the Mediterranean variety, results in hemolysis when susceptible individuals develop anaemia with hemolysis in absence of a secondary cause. Hemolysis is self limiting as the young red cells newly produced by the bone marrow have nearly normal enzyme.

Clinical problem arises only when the affected individual is subjected to some type of environmental stress. Most often, hemolytic episodes are triggered by viral or bacterial infections. The mechanism is unknown. In addition, drugs or oxidant that pose an oxidant threat to the RBC cause hemolysis in individual deficient in G6PD.

Anti malarials - Primaquine, Dapsone, Sulfonamides, Analgesic-Acetamilid. The patient may experience an acute hemolytic crisis-within hours of exposure to the oxidant stress. The anaemia when it occurs, may be rapid in onset, becoming obvious between 2 and 10 days after exposure to the precipitating agents . In severe cases, hemoglobinuria and peripheral vascular collapse can develop. Acute hemolytic episodes are characterized by sudden onset of severe pallor, icterus and red colored urine . Patient also developed hemolytic crisis with pallor, icterus and red coloured urine. When hemolysis occur hemoglobin liberated into the plasma is bound mainly by the alpha-2 globulin, haptogolbuin, to form a complex too large to.be lost in the urine. It is taken up by the liver and degraded. Some Hb is partially degraded and bound to albumin to form methaemoalbumin. If all haptoglobin has been consumed, free Hb may be lost in the urine. Since only the older population of RBC is rapidly destroyed, the .hemolytic crisis is usually limited even if the exposure to the oxidant continues. Diagnosis is usually done by enzyme assay. Test should not be done till some week after a crisis as the young RBC may have sufficient enzyme to make the result appear normal. Screening test may fail to detect the decrease levels of G6PD which occur in female heterozy.

Auto immune hemolytic anaemia is caused by anti-body to RBC's. Warm autoimmune hemolytic anaemia is caused by IgG auto antibody. Maybe idiopathic or associated with underlying malignancy, collagen vascular disease or drug use. The clinical presentation is weakness, jaundice, moderate splenomegaly. Severe hemolysis may be associated with fever, chest pain, syncope, hemoglobinemia . Coomb's test the ability of anti-IgG or anti- C3 antisera to agglutinate the patient's RBC is determined. The presence or absence of IgG or C3 may give important information about the origin of immune hemolytic anaemia. Rarely, neither IgG or C3 may be found on RBC of patient (Coomb's negative hemolytic anaemia). Direct Coomb's test is positive in 98% of the patients. Non immune hemolytic anaemia is caused by infections like malaria, Clostridium perfingens septicemia, Drugs like dapsone and salazopyrin.

Diabetes ketoacidosis appears to require insulin deficiency coupled with a relative or absolute increase in glucagons concentration. It is often caused by cessation of insulin intake, but it may result from physical stress like infection, trauma, surgery or emotional stress despite continued insulin therapy. Clinically ketoacidosis begins with anorexia, nausea and vomiting, coupled with an increased rate of urine formation. Abdominal pain may be present. The initial examination usually shows Kussmaul respiration (hyperventilation together with signs of volume depletion). Rarely, the latter is sufficient to cause vascular collapse and renal shut down. Leukocytosis, frequently is very marked, is a feature of diabetic acidosis pre se and may not indicate infection. Laboratory evaluation reveals metabolic acidosis with an elevated anion gap with serum ketones present(2,6).

Dapsone (4,4'-diaminodiphenylsulfone) inhibits bacterial folic acid synthesis. It is well absorbed orally and distributed well throughout the body. Dapsone is cleared by acetylation in the lever, with genetic variation. The hemotoxicity of dapsone which includes hemolysis in G6PD deficient individual. Agranulocytosis, is thought to be due to the metabolism of dapsone to its hydroxylamine metabolite by specific cytochrome P450 enzymes. The extent to which the dapsone is converted to its toxic metabolic depends on the activity of these cytochrome P450 enzymes in the individual which determines the individual susceptility to the adverse effect. Other side effect includes gastrointestinal intolerance, headache, pruritis, peripheral neuropathies, nephritic syndrome, fever and rash. Dapsone can cause severe hemolytic anaemia in HIV patients who are G6PD deficient and can create a functional anaemia in others through induction of methomoglobinemia. The protective effect of Vitamin E on the hemolysis associated with dapsone treatment is under trial.

Another serious idiosyncratic adverse effect is the dapsone hypersensitivity syndrome. Drug hypersensitivity syndrome is a severe idiosyncratic reaction to a drug defined by the clinical triad of fever, rash and internal organ involvement (most commonly the liver and the hematologic system). It occurs in a relatively small proportion of patients but is associated with considerable morbidity and mortality. Although this reaction to dapsone is rare considering the widespread use of the drug (particularly in patients receiving multidrug therapy for leprosy), it ranks high among drugs that cause this syndrome. Dapsone-induced hypersensitivity syndrome usually appears four or more weeks after initiation of therapy. Symptoms include a mononucleosis - like rash with fever and lymphadenopathy. Involvement of other organs varies and includes the liver (hepatomegaly, icterus, hepatitis and hepatic encephalopathy), lymphadenopathy, eosinophilia and others. The course of the disease is also variable, but it may last four weeks or more and fatalities have been reported. Examthematous skin eruptions usually resolve within two weeks of stopping dapsone, although patients in whom Stevens-Johnson syndrome or toxic epidermal necrolysis develops have increased morbidity and mortality.

Our patient was a case of G6PD deficiency (not known) was given dapsone for lichen planus which was a triggering factor for hemolysis. He went into acute hemolytic crisis presenting to us with pallor, icterus, breathlessness. Red cell breakdown lead-to decrease in hemoglobin level to 5.2. There was increase in Sr. bilirubin (indirect-7.65) pointing towards hemolysis, increased serum LDH level, hemoglobinuria presenting as red coloured urine and increased retieulocytes to 10.6% showing compensated erythropocisis.

The hemolysis was a stress factor for precipitating diabetic keto acidosis in a known diabetic, so he presented with kussumal breathing (hyperventilation breathlessness), which was confirmed by a high blood sugar level of 402 mg% and urine sugar positive, urine ketones positive and proteinuria. The markedly increased WBC count (45,600) is per se because of metabolic acidosis and not infection.

Auto immune hemolytic anaemia was a misdiagnosis since Coomb's test was negative. The normal G6PD status at that time is explained by increased reticulocytes (erythropoeisis) compensating for hemolysis. The younger

RBC (reticulocytes) had a normal enzyme level giving a false negative result.

References

1. Kumar and Clark Clinical medicine. 4th edition. Edited by Parveen Kumar and Michael Clark Page 381.

2. Harrison's Principle of Internal Medicine. 14th edition. Fauci, Braunwald, Isselbacher, Wilson, Martin, Kaspen, Hauser, Longo. International edition. Page 338, 663-664, 424, 382-388.

3. Oxford handbook of clinical medicine. Murray Longmore. Ian Wilkinson 5th edition. Estee torok. Update service at http://www.oup.co-u/ OHCM. Pa^e 640.

4. Screening for G6PD prior to dapsone therapy. Todd P, Samartung IR, Pembrok A. Department of dermatology, King's College Hospital, London, UK. PUMED.

5. PMID:1739229 Arch dermatol 1992 Feb:128(2) 210-3. The protective effect of vitamin E on the hemolysis associated with dapsone treatment in patients with dermatitis herpetiformis. Prus- sick R, Ali MA, Rosenthal D. Guyatt G.

6. Manual of medical therapeutics: 25th edition. Department of Medicine Washington. University School of Medicine. St. Louis, Missouri. Gregory A. Edwald, Clark R. Mekenzie. Editors.

7. Davidson's Principle and Practice of Medicine. Edited by Christopher R. W. Edward laria A.D. Bouchier, Christopherhaslett. Editor in;ehief.

8. API textbook of medicine. Editor-in-chief G.S. Sainani, Associates editors: Philip Abraham, F.D. Dastur, V.R. Joshi, R.D. Lele, Late P.J. Mehta, Sukumar Mukerjee, P.S. Shankar,

9. Dapsone. Ronni Wolf, Hagit Matz1, Edith Orion1, Binhur Tuzun^, Yalcin Tuzum3 Dermatology Online Journal 8(1):2. The Dermatology Unit, Kaplan Medical Center, Rechovot, Israel, 2. The Department of Dermatology, Trakya University, Medical Faculty, Edrine, Turkey, 3. The University of Istanbul, Cerrahpasa Medical Faculty, Istanbul Turkey.

10.   http://dermatology.cdlib.org/ DOJvol8numl/ reviews/dapsorie/wolf.html

Dapsone syndrome : A case study

Dipti Desai, Ram Malkani, Vijay Aswani

Bulletin of the Jaslok Hospital & Research Centre, Vol XXVI No. 4 April 2002.

A 47-year-old woman developed fever, dermatitis, lymphadenopathy and hepatitis a few days after taking dapsone. She was investigated and diagnosed as 'dapsone syndrome'

Introduction

Dapsone is amongst the most widely used sulfones prescribed by various dermatologists and physicians the world over in millions of patients suffering from a variety of skin disorders . The major toxic side effects of dapsone include hemolysis, agranulocytosis, dermatitis, hepatitis and psychosis. Besides a distinct hypersensitivity reaction to dapsone usually occurring within 6-8 weeks of therapy presenting with exfoliative dermatitis and resembling infectious mononucleosis has been well documented. The "DDS syndrome" clinically resembling infectious mononucleosis was first described in 1949 by Lowe and Smith.(1) The incidence of dapsone hypersensitivity reported was 0,3% to 0.6% at rehabilitation centre in Thailand in 1982, which increased to 3.6% after introducing MDT at the same centre.(2) Allday and Barnes emphasized that dermatitis is always present although hepatitis, glandular enlargement and mononucleosis may be absent.(3)

The signs and symptoms of dapsone syndrome include cutaneous manifestations in the form of erythroderma, maculopapular eruptions, erythema multiforme, toxic epidermal necrolysis, Stevens Johnson syndrome, lymphadenopathy, anaemia, methaemoglobinemia, hepatic dysfunction, sometimes conjunctivitis, arthralgias and white tonsillar membrane. A generalised exanthematous eruption with predominance of pustules has been reported with dapsone. This syndrome is usually self limiting, but potentially a serious reaction. Few fatalities have been reported.

A syndrome similar to serum sickness is known to occur several days after therapy with sulfonamides too. However the latent period is more in sulfones. A case of DOS syndrome with widespread pustular eruption has been reported in a case of cutanous polyarteritis nodosa after 5 weeks of dapsone therapy.(4)

Case Report

A 47-year-old woman presented to us with pruritic scaly rash. Three months back she was seen by a dermatologist and was diagnosed as dermatitis herpetiformis and was treated with tab dapsone and tab prednisolone. Patient felt better initially but after a week she came with new complaints of fever, chills, malaise and an extensive pruritic scaly rash with swelling in the neck. The patient was brought to us at this stage. Dapsone was stopped.

The patient had all her vital parameters within normal limits. Pallor was significant and icterus was present. There was no edema of the feet. She had a generalised cutaneous exfoliation with extensive scaling and underlying erythema. Oral cavity and genitals were normal. The cervical and axillary lymph nodes were palpable. Her Hb. was only 5.4g%. Differential leucocyte cognt was N60 L13 M4 E23, ESR :86 mm/first hr. Reticulocyte count 9%, metamyelocyte 6%, myeloblast 7%, promyetQblast 5%. Liver parameters were moderately raised, SGCK 187 u/L, SGPT 326.8 u/L, LDH 703 unit/L, Total protein 6.58 gm%, albumin 2.2 gm%. Peripheral smear showed spherocytes. Heinz bodies were detected and so also methemoglobin. Autaagglutinin and cold agglutinin titres were 2048 u and 256 u respectively, Both direct and indirect Coomb's tests were positive. USG showed splenomegaly. Blood sugar, renal parameters, ANA test, x-ray chest were" all normal or negative. Skin biopsy was non-specific.

With all these features, a diagnosis of dapsone syndrome was made and she was put on tab. Prednisolone 40 mg/alt days in tapering doses for 1 month. The patient responded very well within a few days.

Discussion: Dapsone syndrome or 'DDS syndrome' is an idiosyncratic reaction to dapsone known to occur after prolonged exposure to dapsone which is usually within 6-8 weeks or more. Although the exact cause of dapsone syndrome is unknown, it is considered to be a hypersensitivity reaction. Richardus and Smith have mentioned the following criteria to diagnose a case of dapsone hypersensitivity.(2)

1.The symptoms appear within 8 weeks after commencement of dapsone and disappear after the discontinuation of the drug 2.The symptoms cannot be ascribed to any other drug given simultaneously with dapsone 3. The symptoms are not attributable to lepra reaction 4. No other disease liable to cause similar symptoms is diagnosed 5. Two of the following signs and symptoms are present: fever, skin eruption, lymphadenopathy, liver pathology (hepatomegaly, jaundice, and/or abnormal liver function tests).(2)

Dapsone is metabolized primarily via two pathways: N-acetylation and N-hydroxylation (oxidation).

N-acetylation had been shown not to determine total clearance of dapsone. Dapsone N-hydroxylation is mediated primarily by human liver microsomal enzymes P4503A4,2C6 and 2C11. This pathway is thought to be the initial step in the formation of toxic intermediate metabolites such as nitrosamines and possibly other compounds that can induce hemolytic anemia and methemoglobinemia. A toxic metabolite of dapsone, hydroxylamine depletes glutathione within G6PD deficient cells and then causes peroxidation reactions leading to rapid hemolysis which could be responsible for the methemoglobinemia.(4) It is presumed that these molecules are also important in the pathogenesis of Dapsone Hypersensitivity syndrome (DHS). A reduction in quantity of activity of N-hydroxylation enzyme system results in decreased total clearance of dapsone. Population studies show extensive interindividual variation in this ability; both genetic and environmental factors are probably involved.

Increased age and preexisting liver disease (i.e. cirrhosis) offer relative protection against adverse events because of decreased enzyme activity and therefore, decreased production of toxic metabolites. It is likely, but not proven, that these are also protective factors in the development of DHS.(5)

In the present case, all the criteria for dapsone syndrome were met. Treatment basically involves discontinuation of dapsone and instituting steroid therapy which should be gradually tapered. The variety of manifestations involved in hypersensitivity to dapsone and its increasing incidence make it necessary for dermatologists and internists to be familiar with the same.

References

1. Sharma VK, Kaur S. Dapsone syndrome in India. Indian Lepr 1985; 57:807-813.

2. Sule G. Dapsone syndrome. Ind J Dermatol Venereol Leprol 1992; 58:376-378.

3. Keneth Thomecki, Charles Catalano. Dapsone hypersensitivity. ArchDermatol 1981; 117 : 38 - 39.

4. Ronald Prussick, Neil Shear. Dapsone hypersensitivity syndrome. J AmAcad Dermatol Aug 1996 ; 346 - 349.

5. Antibaaerial agents. Martindale The Extra Pharmacopia Ed: JamesReynolds 31st Edition. 220-222.

Toxic Epidermal Necrolysis

Neeraj K. Tulara, Ram Malkani

The Jaslok Hospital and Research Centre Annual Bulletin, 2005, p 169

Described in 1956 by Alan Lyell, toxic epidermal necrolysis (TEN) is a rapidly evolving mucocutaneous reaction characterized by widespread erythema, necrosis, and bullous detachment of the epidermis resembling scalding.

TEN represents the most severe variant of a disease spectrum that consists of bullous erythema multiforme (EM) and Stevens-Johnson syndrome (SJS). Each of the disorders shares common features including widespread distribution of skin lesions, predominantly on the trunk and face with involvement of one or more mucus membranes.

A classification system based largely on the extent of epidermal detachment and morphology of the skin lesions helps in differentiating the disease entities.

- Bullous EM - Epidermal detachment less than 10% of body surface area involved with typical localized target lesions or "raised atypical targets

- SJS - Epidermal detachment less than 10% of body surface area involved with widespread erythematous or purpuric macules or flat atypical targets

- Overlap SJS-TEN - Epidermal detachment between 10-30% of body surface area with widespread erythematous or purpuric macules or flat atypical targets

- EN "with spots" - Epidermal detachment greater than 30% of the body surface area with

- widespread purpuric macules or flat atypical targets

- TEN "without spots" - Epidermal detachment greater than 30% of the body surface area in

- large epidermal sheets and without purpuric macules or target like lesions.

Histopathologic examination is necessary in differentiating these disorders from other severe bullous skin diseases such as staphylococcal scalded skin syndrome or paraneoplastic pemphigus. Initial emergency department management is therefore supportive

Pathophysiology

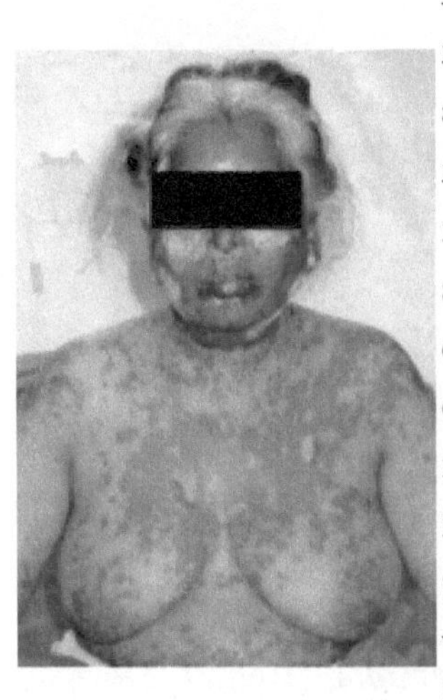

Multiple pathophysiologic mechanisms have been proposed, although an immunecomplex mediated phenomenon is likely responsible. One accepted theory suggests that accumulation of drug metabolites in the epidermis of genetically predisposed individuals induces an immunologic process analogous to that, which occurs in graft-versus-host disease. GD8+ T lymphocytes and macrophages activate an inflammatory cascade, leading to widespread apoptosis of epidermal cells.

Frequency

- Internationally: Worldwide, 0.4-1.2 cases per million population occur each year.

Mortality/Morbidity

TEN has a mortality rate of 30-40%. Epithelial loss results in vulnerability to bacterial and fungal infections and predisposes to septicemia, the leading cause of morbidity and mortality. Mucosal membranes are affected to a varying extent and can cause GI hemorrhage, respiratory failure, ocular abnormalities, and genitourinary lesions. Significant fluid loss from extensive skin lesions as well as an inability to tolerate oral intake can lead to hypovolemia, acute tubular necrosis, and shock.

A severity-of-illness score that estimates the risk of death in TEN has been developed and validated (SCORTEN).

- Age >40 years

- Heart rate > 120 beats per minute

- Cancer or hemopathy

- Involved body surface area >10%

- Blood urea nitrogen >10 mmol/L (10 mEq/L)

- Serum bicarbonate <20 mmol/L (20 mEq/L)

- Blood glucose 14 mmol/L (252 mg/dL)

- Mortality rates based upon the number of positive criteria are as follows: o0 to 1 factor = 3% o2 factors = 12% o3 factors = 35% o4 factors = 58% o5 or more factors = 90%

Age

SJS and TEN usually occur in adults but may be seen in children. Age older than 40 years is an independent risk factor for mortality.

History

Most cases of TEN are drug induced, typically occurring within the first 8 weeks of therapy: Fewer than 5% of patients report no history of medication use. Both SJS and TEN are generally preceded by a day to several-day prodrome of high fever, cough, sore throat, and malaise. As the disease progresses, mucosal membrane involvement (seen in all cases of SJS and in 90% of cases of TEN) becomes evident. The most frequently affected mucosal membrane is the oropharynx followed by the eyes, and genitalia. Oral cavity involvement typically presents as sore or burning sensations. Intake may be limited because of pain associated with the oropharyngeal lesions. Genital involvement may result in painful urination. Other mucosal surfaces such as the esophagus, intestinal tract, or respiratory epithelium may be affected.

The Cutaneous eruption develops rapidly, evolving from a papular exanthem or widespread erythematous and purpuric macules to confluent blisters and epidermal detachment. The lesions predominate on the torso and face, sparing the scalp. Pain is often the predominating symptom.

Physical Examination

Physical examination findings may include the following:

- Pyrexia may be present.

- Cutaneous manifestations may present as a generalized papular exanthem, purpuric macules, atypical target like lesions, bullae, or erosions.

Skin lesions rapidly coalesce producing large blisters. These lesions may wrinkle, slide laterally, and separate with slight pressure (Nikolsky sign). The underlying denuded skin is erythematous and tender.

• Involvement of the oral mucosa results in edema and erythema, followed by blistering. Ruptured blisters may form extensive hemorrhagic erosions with grayish white pseudomembranes or shallow apthous like ulcers.

• Ocular involvement varies in severity and can result in mild inflammation, conjunctival erosion, purulent exudates, or pseudomembrane formation.

• Involvement of respiratory epithelium may result in bronchial hyper secretion, hypoxemia, interstitial infiltrates, pulmonary edema, bacterial pneumonia, and bronchiolitis obliterans.

Causes

Medications are the major precipitating cause of TEN. Many drugs are cited in the literature as the causative agent. However, no laboratory test is able to confirm a specific drug etiology. A causal link is suggested when TEN occurs during the first 4 weeks of medication therapy, usually between 1-3 weeks. The most widely implicated medications are as follows:

- Sulfonamide antibiotics
- Anticonvulsants (Phenobarbital, phenytoin, carbamazepine, valproic acid)
- Oxicam non steroidal antiinflammatory drugs (NSAIDs)
- Allopurinol
- Antiretroviral medications
- Corticosteroids

Additionally, infectious agents (i.e., Mycoplasma pneumoniae, immunizations, and bone marrow or solid organ transplantation are potential etiologies

Lab Studies

- No definitive or specific emergent laboratory tests are indicated. Basic laboratory tests may be helpful in planning symptomatic or supportive therapy.

- Diffuse skin involvement may cause significant fluid loss and electrolyte abnormalities. Renal failure can result from hypovolemic shock or sepsis.

- Surveillance cultures of blood, skin, and urine should be obtained.

Imaging Studies

- No specific imaging studies are indicated.

- Chest radiography should be performed in the setting of respiratory distress because tracheobronchial inflammation may predispose to diffuse interstitial pulmonary disease or pneumonia

Other Tests

- Skin biopsy, harvested at the earliest possible stage, is important in establishing an accurate diagnosis and directing specific therapeutic modalities. Therefore, early involvement of a dermatologist and dermatopathologist is recommended

Prehospital Care

- Prehospital care is similar to that of burns.

In severe TEN, the barrier function of the skin is compromised. Thus, contamination and evaporation must be minimized. The patient should be treated as a patient with extensive burns is treated, that is, with the application of sterile coverings.

- Emergency Department Care

- Fluid and pulmonary status must be carefully monitored.

- Early recognition, prompt withdrawal of the causative agent, and referral to a burn center is key to successful outcome. Emergency department care should be directed at minimizing fluid and electrolyte loss and preventing secondary infection.

• Aggressive fluid and electrolyte management, pain control, and meticulous skin care are important. Patients with extensive skin involvement require reverse isolation and a sterile environment.

• Areas of skin erosion should be covered with non-adherent protective dressings such as petroleum gauze.

• Respiratory distress may result from mucosal sloughing and edema and may necessitate endotracheal intubation and ventilation.

• Silver sulfadiazine should be avoided because it is a sulfonamide derivative and may precipitate TEN.

• Antibiotic prophylaxis is not indicated unless sepsis or staphylococcal scalded skin syndrome is strongly suspected.

• Use of systemic steroids is controversial. There is no convincing evidence that steroid therapy is helpful.

- Although controversial, use of IVIG may demonstrate favorable outcome.

- Immediately discontinue any potentially offending medications (if identified).

Consultations

In general, patients with TEN benefit from a team approach to diagnosis and management, including a dermatologist, dermatopathologist, a burn surgeon, and an intensivist.

- Because the diagnosis of TEN indicates significant BSA involvement, patients should be admitted to a burn unit.

- Dermatologists may assist with diagnosis, biopsy, and inpatient treatment.

- Inpatient ophthalmology consultation is useful for assisting in the treatment of ocular manifestations and longterm sequelae.

Further Inpatient Care

Continuance of supportive care is initiated in the ED. The mainstay of treatment is supportive care until the epithelium regenerates. Supportive measures include isolation, fluid and electrolyte balance, nutritional support, pain management, and protective dressings. Anesthetic mouthwash may alleviate the discomfort associated with oral erosions. Meticulous wound care is necessary to prevent secondary infection. Cutaneous lesions heal in approximately 2 weeks; mucosal membrane lesions take longer.

Transfer

Transfer to intensive care unit or burn unit may be necessary for those patients who manifest with homodynamic instability or involvement of greater than 20-25% BSA.

Complications

Numerous complications can arise as a result of the widespread cutaneous and mucosal membrane inflammation and necrosis.

Skin: Epithelial loss predisposes to septicemia (Pseudomonas aeruginosa, S aureus, gram-negative species, and Candida albicans)

Mucosal membranes: Ulceration of various mucosal membranes results in pain,' scarring, and stricture formation. Affected surfaces include oral, ocular, and urogenital mucosa.

Pulmonary: Inflammation of respiratory epithelium results in bronchial hyper secretion, hypoxemia, interstitial infiltrates, pulmonary edema, bacterial pneumonia, and bronchiolitis obliterans.

Gastrointestinal: GI hemorrhage results from intestinal inflammation.

Renal: Hypovolemia results from poor oral intake and/or septic shock results in renal hypo perfusion, acute tubular necrosis, and renal insufficiency.

Prognosis

The overall prognosis of TEN is poor, with a mortality rate as high as 40%. Major sequelae are generally limited to the affected organ systems, that is, the skin and mucosal membranes. Mucosal lesions characteristically heal with scarring.

Cutaneous: Scarring may occur in areas of infection or over pressure points. Post- inflammatory hyper pigmentation and nail growth abnormalities are frequent sequelae.

Ocular: Complications generally result from abnormal keratinization of the tarsal conjunctiva. A Sjogren like syndrome with decreased lacrimal secretion causes dry eye and predisposes to corneal abrasions and corneal scarring with neo-vascularization. In addition, patients have been reported to have palpebral synechiae, entropion, or symblepharon (adhesion of the eyelids).

Oral: Oral and lip lesions usually heal without complications, but stricture in the throat and esophagus are reported.

Genitalia: Vulvovaginal synechiae and phimosis have been reported in the literature

Bibliography:

• Ayangco L, Rogers RS: Oral manifestations of erythema multiforme. Dermatol Clin 2003 Jan; 21(1): 195-205[Medline].

- Bachot N, Roujeau JC: Differential diagnosis of severe cutaneous drug eruptions. Am J Clin Dermatol 2003; 4(8): 561-72[MedIine].

- Magina S, Lisboa C, Leal V, et al: Dermatological and ophthalmological sequels in toxic epidermal necrolysis. Dermatology 2003; 207(1): 33-6[MedlineJ.

- Neff P, Meuli-Simmen C, Kempf W, et al: Lyell syndrome revisited: analysis of 18 cases of severe bullous skin disease in a burns unit. Br J Plast Surg 2005 Jan; 58(1): 73-80|MedlineJ.

- Prendiville J: Stevens-Johnson syndrome and toxic epidermal necrolysis. Adv Dermatol 2002; 18: 151-73[Medline].

- Roujeau JC, Guillaume JC, Fabre JP, et al: Toxic epidermal necrolysis (Lyell syndrome). Incidence and drug etiology in France, 1981-1985. Arch Dermatol 1990 Jan; 126(1): 37-4.

Lymphomatoid drug eruption due to levofloxacin

Reshma T. Vishnani, Ram Malkani

Won the Best poster award at the National Conference of the Indian Association of Dermatologists, Venereologists and Leprologists held in Jan 2013

History & Examination

25 y/o/f presented with c/o widespread itchy rash for 1 week. H/o cold, cough with expectoration & fever 10 days prior to presentation, for which she had received antihistamines and paracetamol for a week. Started Tab. Levofloxacin (500mg) OD five days prior to onset of rash. Within 24 hours of 1st dose of Levofloxacin she c/o generalised itching, f/b the development of an extensive rash, initially over the trunk, later involving the extremities. Past h/o Pulmonary Koch's 8yrs ago, received AKT for 9 mths. H/o developing a skin rash during AKT following introduction of Levofloxacin as second line treatment, which resolved on withdrawal of the drug.

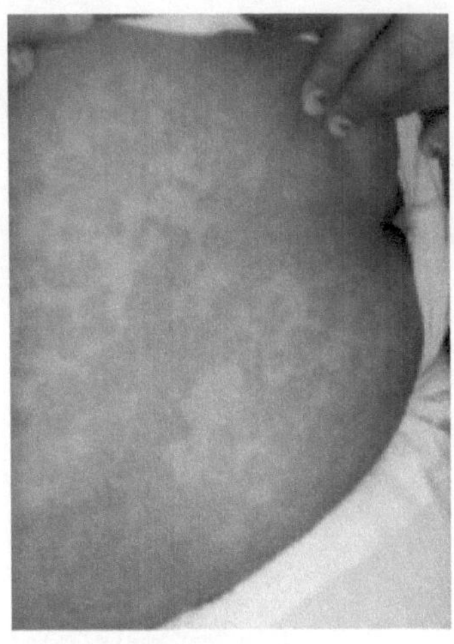

Well defined erythematous maculopapules and coalescing plaques over extremities and trunk (truncal)

Histopathology & Immunohistochemistry

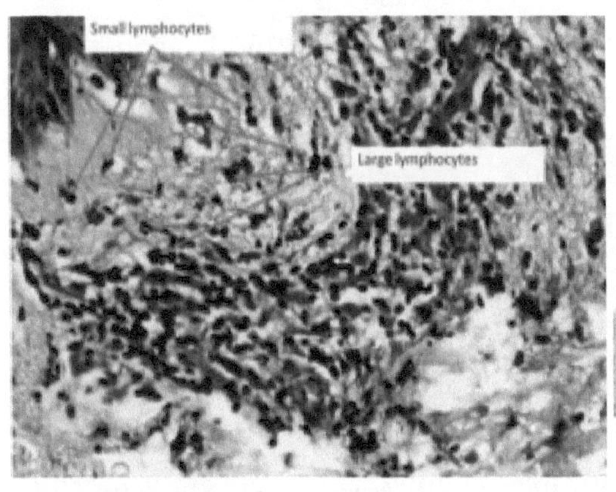

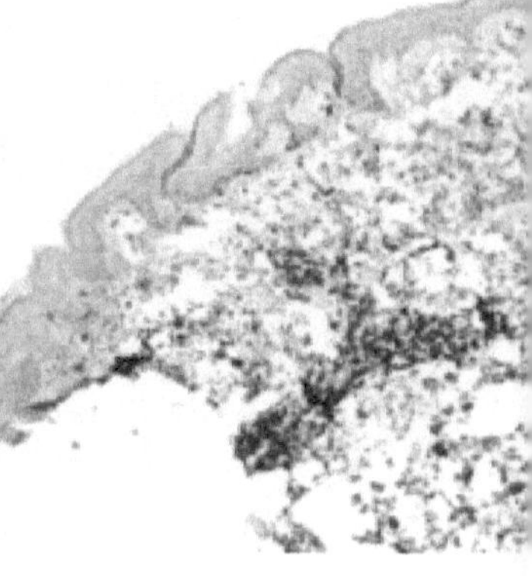

Moderately dense superficial and deep perivascular and periappendageal infiltrate of small and large lymphocytes. Few eosinophils and neutrophils scattered in the infiltrate.

Revealed the infiltrate to be T cell ri virtually staining all the cells Very mi CD 20 positive B cells

Final Diagnosis & Treatment

Based on the above history, histopathology and immunohistochemistry a final diagnosis of drug induced pseudolymphoma (Lymphomatoid Drug Eruption) secondary to levofloxacin was made.

Levofloxacin was withdrawn and patient was started on oral steroids, given in tapering doses over a period of 2 weeks along with anti-histamines.

Discussion

Cutaneous Pseudolymphoma (CPL) is a process that simulates lymphoma, primarily histologically but sometimes clinically, has a benign biologic behaviourand does not satisfy criteria for malignant lymphoma. CPLs are classified as T-cell (band like and nodular pattern) and B-cell (nodular pattern).Lymphomatoid drug eruption is a bandlike cutaneous T-cell pseudolymphoma.

Causes of CPL: idiopathic, drugs, infections, foreign agents and photosensitivity. Drug induced pseudolymphoma are classifed as anti-convulsants induced and those induced by drugs other than anti-convulsants. In CPL caused by drugs other than anti-convulsants. Appearance of eruption ranges from 1-11 months, clinically patients may have varied eruption from localised papules or single or multiple nodules and plaques, generalised papulonodularlesion or exfoliative erythroderma. The early onset of symptoms in our patient can be attributed to the prior exposure to Levofloxacin as second line AKT drug, eight years ago.

Pathogenesis: Current evidence indicates that the drugs depress immunologic function, Impair immunosurveillance which leads to abnormal proliferation of lymphocytes, increased suppressor T-cell activity and hypogammaglobulinemia. Extensive search of literature did not reveal any report of lymphomatoid hypersensitivity reaction following levofloxacin in an immunocompetent patient. Pseudolymphoma being a benign condition should be differentiated from malignant lymphoma in order to avoidunnecessary treatment with chemotherapy

Reference:

1. Ploysangam T, Breneman DL, Mutasim DF. Cutaneous pseudolymphomas. *J Am Acad Dermatol.* Jun 1998;38:877-95; quiz 896-7

2. Bordello RT, Santa Cruz DJ. Cutaneous pseudolymphomas. *Dermatol Clin.* Oct 1985;3(4):719-34.

3. Esparza EM, Takeshita J, George E. Lymphomatoid hypersensitivity reaction to levofloxacin during autologous stem cell transplantation. *J CutanPathol.* 2011 Jan;38(1):33-7

4. Albrecht J, Fine LA, Piette W. Drug-associated lymphoma and pseudolymphoma: recognition and management. *Dermatol Clin.* Apr 2007;25(2):233-44

Myocarditis: A rare complication in DRESS syndrome

Rahul Dixit, Ram Malkani

Presented as a poster at the National conference of the IADVL DERMACON 2013

Introduction:

DRESS (Drug reaction with eosinophilia and systemic symptoms) is defined bytriad of fever, skin rash and internal organ involvement. It is usually associated with antiepileptics, antiretrovirals ,dapsone, sulfonamides and allopurinol

Aims and objectives:

To highlight the importance of myocarditis due to DRESS syndrome which may sometimes prove fatal

Case history:

60 year old lady presented with fever andrashes all over bodyfor 2 days. History of allopurinol intake for 1 month.

- O/E: Generalized erythematous exfoliation all over body.

- No mucosal involvement.

- Lab Investigations: Leukocytosis, marked eosinophilia, raised ESR and liver enzymes.

- Chest X- ray : mild cardiomegaly

- USG abdomen : mild splenomegaly.

- Four days later she had chest pain and breathlessness.

- Creatinine kinase : marginally raised

- ECG :T wave inversion.

- Therefore, a diagnosis of myocarditisdue to DRESS syndrome was made.

Discussion:

DRESS syndrome is a severe idiosyncratic drug reaction.

Diagnostic criteria:

- Drug-induced skin eruption

- Eosinophillia, Absolute Eosinophil count >1500/dl, or atypical lymphocytes

- Atleast 1 of the following : Enlarged lymph nodes at least 2 cm, hepatitis, interstitial nephropathy, interstitial lung disease or myocardial involvement.

Withdrawal of the offending drug and oral steroids are the mainstay of treatment. Recurrences have been reported

Conclusion:

Thus, we suggest although a rare complication, myocarditis should always be considered when a patient of DRESS syndrome develops chest pain.

REFERENCES

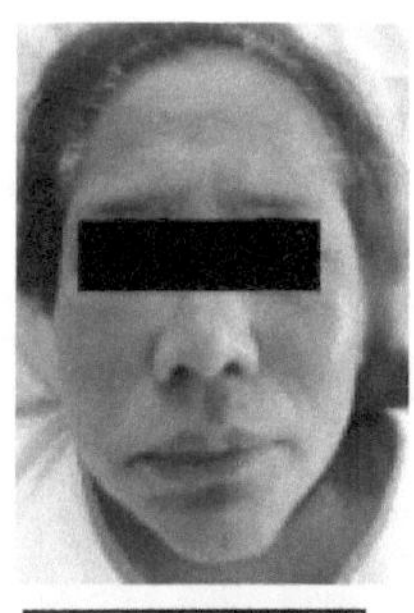

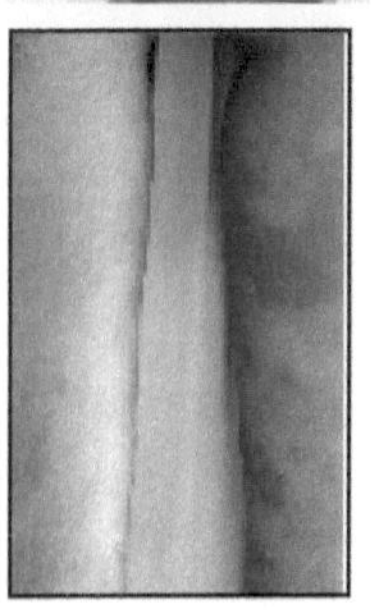

1. Bocquet H, Bagot M, Roujeau JC. Drug-induced pseudolymphoma and drug hypersensitivity syndrome (Drug Rash with Eosinophilia and Systemic Symptoms: DRESS) Semin Cutan Med Surg 1996;15:250-7.

2. Valencak J, Ortiz-Urda S, Heere-Ress E, Kunstfeld R, Base W. Carbamazepine-induced DRESS syndrome with recurrent fever and exanthema. Int J Dermatol 2004;43:51-4.

A rare complication of Rituximab therapy in Pemphigus vulgaris

Devakar D , Banodkar P, Malkani R

Presented as a poster at the National conference of the IADVL DERMACON 2013

ABSTRACT

Bronchiolitis obliterans organizing pneumonia (BOOP) is an inflammation of bronchioles we present the case of a patient on rituximab therapy for pemphigus vulgaris, which is known but a rare complication of monoclonal antibody therapy.

CASE REPORT:

A 45 year old male patient was admitted to the medicine ward with h/o breathlessness for 1 year. Breathlessness aggravated since 15days and h/o fever for 15 days. Breathlessness was grade 2 for 6 months which progressed to grade 3-4 since 15 days. It was not associated with diurnal/ postural variation. He c/o blurring of vision since 15 days simultaneously with onset of fever. No H/o TB/TBC/HT/ DM/ATOPY/ALLERGY.

He is a known case of pemphigus vulgaris for a year when he had developed lesions over the chest, back, scalp and oral mucosal membrane. Pemphigus vulgaris was confirmed by skin biopsy. The cutaneous lesions cleared with gradual tapering of doses of methyl prednisolone over a period of 2 to 3 months but mucosal lesions marginally improved over a period of 6 months. He was started on Inj. Rituximab 500mg weekly IV for 4 weeks in Jan 2011 and 5th dose was given on 13th April 2011 and 6th dose was scheduled for 13th July 2011. His oral lesions subsided but he c/o of raw sensation over the palate on and off for the last 6 months. Blurring of vision had increasingly progressed over the past 15 days.

On admission, dermatology reference was given. O/E no active cutaneous lesion of pemphigus was seen. However on oral examination an erythematous plaque was seen on the hard palate Patient was started on inj .monocef 1gm BID, tab. Ciplar BID, tab. Amino fit OD, tab. Zempred 40mg OD.

INVESTIGATIONS:

- HB – 13.4 g/dl
- ESR – 90mm HG (raised)
- Sr. creatinine – 0.7
- Total protein – 5.6 mg/dl (reduced)
- Total albumin – 3 mg/dl(reduced)
- SGOT – 53 (raised) SGPT – 95 (raised)

14/06/10   15/03/11

Anti desmoglien 156.8(up to 14 U/ml) 3.81

Anti desmoglien 3124 (up to 14 U/ml) 8.10

- Urine routine – occasional RBC's /HPF

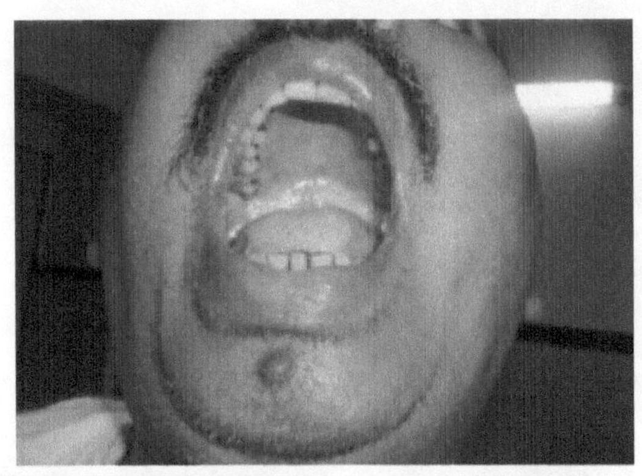

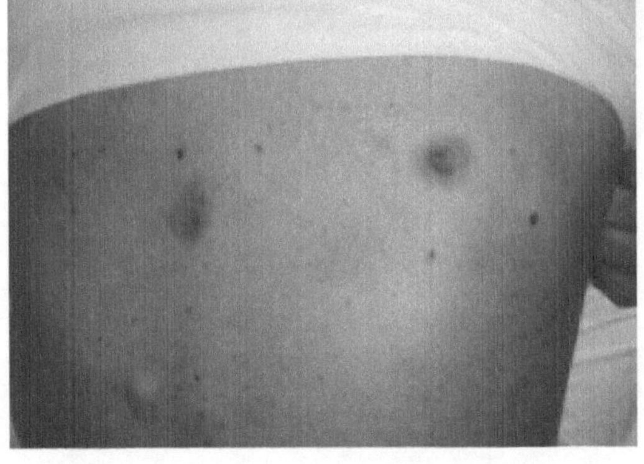

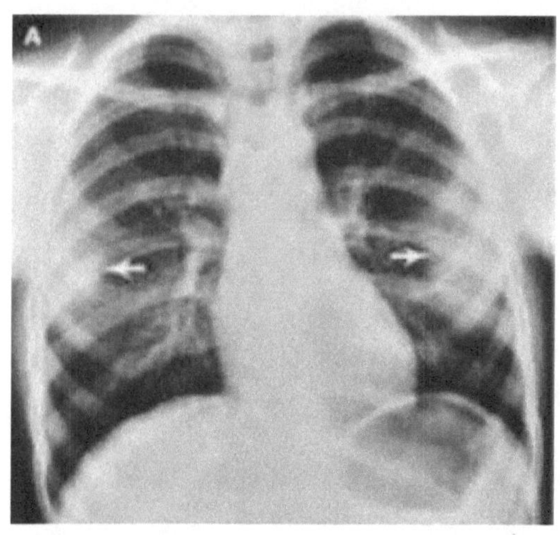

CHEST X-RAY PA VIEW: minimal bilateral pleural effusion with collapse / lower lobe consolidation.

HRCT: basal consolidation seen with suggestion of sub pleural bronchiolar oblitarans organizing pneumonia (BOOPS)

Patient was referred to ophthalmologist in Jaslok hospital no impression of CMV RETINITIS was given hence the CMV IgM and CMV DNA PCR assay was advised which concluded the diagnosis of CMV RETINITIS.

DISCUSSION:

Bronchiolitis obliterans organizing pneumonia (BOOP) is an inflammation of the bronchioles (bronchiolitis)[1] and surrounding tissue in the lungs. It is an non infectious pneumonia.[2] BOOP is often caused by a preexisting chronic inflammatory disease like rheumatoid arthritis. BOOP can also be a side effect of certain medicinal drugs, e.g. amiodarone. BOOP was discovered by Dr. Gary Epler in 1985 [3].

It is also known as cryptogenic organizing pneumonia (COP),[4][5] and some sources recommend using the latter term, to reduce confusion with bronchiolitis obliterans.[6]

The clinical features and radiological imaging resemble infectious pneumonia. However, diagnosis is suspected after there is no response to multiple antibiotics, and blood and sputum cultures are negative for organisms.

Organizing refers to unresolved pneumonia (in which the alveolar exudate persists and eventually undergoes fibrosis) in which fibrous tissue forms in the alveoli. The phase of resolution and/or remodeling following bacterial infections is commonly referred to as organizing pneumonia, both clinically and pathologically.

Cause

COP/BOOP may be triggered by infections from bacteria, viruses and parasites, drugs, or toxic fumes. It was identified in 1985, although its symptoms had been noted before but not recognised as a separate lung disease. The risk of BOOP is higher for people with inflammatory diseases like lupus, rheumatoid arthritis, and scleroderma.

Rituximab, is a chimeric monoclonal antibodyagainst the protein CD20, which is primarily found on the surface of B cells. Rituximab is used in the treatment of many lymphomas, leukemias, transplant rejection and some autoimmune disorders.

The antibody binds to the cluster of differentiation 20 (CD20). CD20 is widely expressed on B cells, from early pre-B cells to later in differentiation, but it is absent on terminally differentiated plasma cells. CD20 does not shed, modulate or internalise. Although the function of CD20 is unknown, it may play a role in Ca2+ influx across plasma membranes, maintaining intracellular Ca2+ concentration and allowing activation of B cells.

The exact mode of action of rituximab is unclear, but the following effects have been found.

The Fc portion of rituximab mediates antibodydependent cellular cytotoxicity (ADCC) and complement-dependent cytotoxicity (CDC).

Rituximab has a general regulatory effect on the cell cycle.

It increases MHC II and adhesion molecules LFA-1 and LFA-3 (lymphocyte function-associated antigen).

It elicits shedding of CD23.

It downregulates the rB cell receptor.

It induces apoptosis of CD20+ cells.

Rituximab may infrequently cause serious (sometimes fatal) side effects including severe breathing problems (e.g., hypoxia, pulmonary infiltrates, acute respiratory distress syndrome) or heart problems (e.g., heart attack, irregular heartbeats, low blood pressure). These effects are more likely if you already have heart or lung problems. Your doctor will carefully watch you during treatment and may stop or slow down your treatment if you have any signs of a reaction. If these serious side effects occur, it will usually be within 30 minutes to 2 hours of receiving this drug. The risk is also higher during your first treatment. However, severe side effects may occur several weeks to months after your last treatment, so it is very important to keep all your follow-up appointments. Seek immediate medical attention if you have trouble breathing (e.g., cough, wheezing), itching, swelling (especially of the throat/lips), dizziness, fast/slow/irregular heartbeat, or chest pain.

Rarely, serious (sometimes fatal) skin reactions (e.g., Stevens-Johnson syndrome) have occurred in people taking this medication.. These reactions can occur weeks to months after treatment has ended.

Rarely, a serious (sometimes fatal) Progressive Multifocal Leukoencephalopathy-PML can occur in people taking this medication .

CONCLUSION:

The focus of this presentation is to create awareness about some of the rare, serious complications of rituximab therapy which have a significant morbidity. In our patient CMV retinitis was a complication due to rituximab therapy.

REFERENCES:

1. "bronchiolitis obliterans with organizing pneumonia" at Dorland's Medical Dictionary

2. White, Eric J. Stern, Charles S. (1999). Chest radiology companion. Philadelphia: Lippincott Williams & Wilkins. pp. 76. ISBN 9780397517329. http://books.google.com/ books?id=keNyAl8AArUC&pg=PA76&dq=%22noninfectious+pn

3. Epler GR. (2011). "Bronchiolitis obliterans organizing pneumonia, 25 years: a variety of causes, but what are the treatment options?". Expert Rev Respir Med. 3: 353-61. PMID url=http://www.ncbi.nlm.nih.gov/ pubmed?term=21702658 21702658 url=http://www.ncbi.nlm.nih.gov/ pubmed?term=21702658.

4. Alasaly K, Muller N, Ostrow DN, Champion P, FitzGerald JM (July 1995). "Cryptogenic organizing pneumonia. A report of 25 cases and a review of the literature". Medicine (Baltimore) 74 (4): 201–11. doi:10.1097/ 00005792-199507000-00004. PMID 7623655. http://meta.wkhealth.com/pt/pt-core/ template-journal/lwwgateway/media/ landingpage.htm?issn=0025-7974&volume=74&issue=48

5. Geddes DM (August 1991). "BOOP and COP". Thorax 46 (8): 545–7. doi:10.1136/ thx.46.8.545. PMC 463266. PMID 1926020. http://www.pubmedcentral.nih.gov/ articlerender.fcgi?tool=pmcentrez&artid=463266.

6. Cotran, Ramzi S.; Kumar, Vinay; Fausto, Nelson; Nelso Fausto; Robbins, Stanley L.; Abbas, Abul K. (2005). Robbins and Cotran pathologic basis of disease. St. Louis, Mo: Elsevier Saunders. pp. 731. ISBN 0-7216-0187-1.

7. Oymak FS, Demirbaş HM, Mavili E, et al. (2005). "Bronchiolitis obliterans organizing pneumonia. Clinical and roentgenological features in 26 cases". Respiration 72 (3): 254–62. doi:10.1159/000085366. PMID 15942294. http://content.karger.com/produktedb/ produkte.asp?typ=fulltext&file=RES2005072003254

Mononucleosis-Like Drug Rash: An Interesting Case Presentation

Reshma T. Vishnani, Ram H. Malkani, Afsha A. Topal, H. G. Desai

J Fam Med Primary Care 2014;3:74-6.

Abstract

Dapsone hypersensitivity syndrome (DHS) is a rare adverse effect of the commonly prescribed drug dapsone. We present a case of a 35-year-old male who was referred to us from the gastroenterologist with complaints of rash, nausea, vomiting, and jaundice for 2 days with a provisional differential diagnosis of infectious mononucleosis or viral exanthema. On enquiry patient gave history of taking dapsone a week prior for refractory urticaria. After thorough investigations we diagnosed him with DHS. This syndrome occurs in a relatively small proportion of patients, but it is associated with considerable morbidity and mortality. The reason for presenting this case is to remind physicians of the unpredictability and potential severity of this reaction which makes it a major concern in clinical practice.

Introduction

Dapsone is a potent anti-inflammatory and antiparasitic compound with a variety of adverse effects, including hemolytic anemia, methemoglobinemia, hepatic involvement (hepatocellular or cholestatic disease, or both), cutaneous involvement (exanthematous eruption, Steven-Johnson syndrome, or toxic epidermal necrolysis), agranulocytosis, nephritis, pneumonitis, hypothyroidism, and the potentially fatal DHS.[1,2] DHS is a known but rare idiosyncratic multiorgan syndrome which was first reported in as early as 1950 by Lowe and was termed as dapsone syndrome by Allday and Barnes in 1951.[1] The incidence of DHS ranges from 0.5 to 3%.[3,4] It typically presents with a triad of fever, skin eruption, and internal organ (lung, liver, neurological, and other system) involvement, occurring several weeks to as late as 6 months after the initial administration of drug.

We present an interesting case of a 35-year-old male patient with DHS in whom the clinical presentation mimicked an infectious mononucleosis-like viral exanthema.

Case Report

A 35-year-old male was referred to us from the gastroenterologist for minimally itchy red rash all over the body along with swelling over the face for 2 days. He also had moderate continuous fever, sore throat, weakness, jaundice, nausea, and vomiting for 1 day. The patient was icteric, had hepatosplenomegaly and generalized lymphadenopathy (bilateral cervical, preauricular, submandibular, retroauricular, axillary and inguinal). Cutaneousexamination revealed generalized erythematous maculopaplular rash with acral and facial edema. On further enquiry, we found that the patient had been on treatment for refractory urticaria with dapsone in a dose of 100 mg/day;

this medication was started a week before the appearance of symptoms. In view of his history and clinical features, a provisional diagnosis of DHS, infectious mononucleosis, and leukemia were considered. Pertinent laboratory investigations revealed a hemoglobin of 10.9 gm/dl, an elevated total white cell count of 16,270/mm3 with 10% eosinophils, along with elevated levels of serum bilirubin (total: 6 mg/dl; direct: 3.6 mg/dl) and liver enzymes [aspartate transaminase (AST): 495; alanine transaminase (ALT): 768; gamma-glutamyltransferase (GGT): 179; alkaline phosphatase (ALP): 247]. Urine examination showed presence of bile salts, bile pigments, and granular casts. Heterophile antibody test done immediately, and repeated at 1 and 2 weeks were persistently negative, thus ruling out infectious mononucleosis. Patient did not have glucose-6-phosphate dehydrogenase deficiency (G6PD). Computerized tomography (CT) scan (chest and abdomen) showed multiple enlarged nonnecrotic lymph nodes in the neck, axilla, and inguinal regions; right pleural effusion with basal atelectasis; and mild hepatosplenomegaly. Skin biopsy showed mild spongiosis, focal parakeratosis and interface changes with moderately dense, superficial perivascular infiltrate of lymphocytes, histiocytes, and occasion eosinophils. Occasional necrotic keratinocytes were also seen, consistent with maculopapular drug eruption. No evidence of leukemic cells infiltration in the dermis or subcutaneous tissue. In view of the clinical and laboratory findings, a final diagnosis of DHS was made. Dapsone was discontinued and the patient was started on tablet prednisolone 40 mg/day along with supportive therapy; the dose of prednisolone was tapered slowly over a period of 6 weeks. The patient responded well to therapy; 10 days following the start of therapy his rash had considerably reduced and fever subsided, and over a period of 4 weeks his serology values were within normal limits.

Discussion

Dapsone is a widely used drug because of its antibiotic and anti-inflammatory effects, which is mainly related to its interference with neutrophil chemotactic migration and adherence.[3] Dapsone, after absorption from the gastrointestinal tract, is metabolized in the liver and excreted by the kidneys.[4,5] It has a long elimination half-life (about 24-36 h). Thus, the adverse reactions may appear after a long metabolite period; in our case, the reaction was seen after 1 week.[5,6] Though, the exact immune mechanism causing DHS is not clear, some mechanisms proposed are: DHS might be a combination of type I, type IV, and perhaps type III Gel and Coombs hypersensitivity reactions[7,8] or it could be a modified graft versus host disease mediated by activated T-lymphocytes.[7,8] Prussick and Shear have suggested that there is some evidence suggesting that the metabolic differences in the production and detoxification of reactive metabolites are an important factor in sulfonamide hypersensitivity reactions.[2] Richardus and Smith have outlined the following criteria for diagnosis of DHS: (a) Symptoms manifesting within 8 weeks of starting therapy and resolving after withdrawal of the drug; (b) symptoms not attributable to any other drug used simultaneously; (c) symptoms not attributable to lepra reaction; (d) no other disease liable to cause similar symptoms is diagnosed, and e) two of the following signs and symptoms are present: Fever, skin eruption, lymphadenopathy, liver pathology (hepatomegaly, jaundice, and/or abnormal liver function tests (LFTs)).[9] These criteria were met in our patient. Though unlike other drug hypersensitivity syndromes, eosinophilia is usually absent in DHS.[10] Our patient did show eosinophilia. Thus, our case of DHS may potentially be considered a variant of DRESS syndrome (drug reaction with eosinophilia and systemic symptoms). Furthermore, Therapy slow acetylators may be associated with an increased risk of development of this syndrome. Prompt withdrawal of dapsone, initiation of systemic glucocorticoids (1 mg/kg/day prednisolone tapered over 5-6 weeks),[2] supportive measures and minimal use of other drugs are essential in the management of DHS. For patients with dapsone-induced hemolysis, vitamin E supplementation might be beneficial while in patients with methemoglobinemia coadministration of cimetidine can have an ameliorative effect.[5,8] These were not required in our case. Rechallenge with dapsone can be performed but is not recommended due to potential hazards associated with it. An important issue to remember in the management is that patients with DHS are at a higher risk of development of hypothyroidism after 3 months, suggesting the need to repeat thyroid function tests at 3 monthly intervals, our patient was tested for the same and his result was within normal limits. The etiology attributed seems linked to the presence of autoantibodies, including antimicrosomal antibodies.[11] This hypersensitivity reaction appears in patients who are generally unable to detoxify reactive metabolites produced by thyroid peroxidase.[11] For genetic factors have been implicated in the pathogenesis of DHS, we made the relatives aware of this syndrome and their enhanced risk of developing similar adverse reaction should they take dapsone.

Conclusion

The focus of this presentation is to create awareness and vigilance towards the well-known but rare complication of the widely used drug dapsone (even in non-leprosy use), which closely mimics infectious mononucleosis-like syndrome and has significant morbidity and mortality associated with it.

Acknowledgement

We would like to acknowledge Dr. Maninder Singh Setia for editorial help with this article.

References

1. Aldday EJ, Barnes J. Toxic effects of diaminodiphenylsulphone in treatment of leprosy. Lancet 1951;2:205-6.

2. Prussick R, Shear NH. Dapsone hypersensitivity syndrome. J Am Acad Dermatol 1996;35:346-9.

3. Zhu YI, Stiller MJ. Dapsone and sulfones in dermatology: Overview and update. J Am Acad Dermatol 2001;45:420-34.

4. Sago J, Hall III RP. Dapsone. Dermatol Ther 2002;15:340-515.

5. Sener O, Doganci L, Safali M, Besirbellioglu B, Bulucu F, Pahsa A. Severe dapsone hypersensitivity syndrome. J Investig Allergol Clin Immunol 2006;16:268-70.

6. Zuiderna J, Hilbers-Modderman ES, Merkus FW. Clinical pharmacokinetics of dapsone. Clin Pharmacokinet 1986;11:299-315.

7. Knowles SR, Shapiro LE, Shear NH. Reactive metabolites and adverse drug reactions: Clinical considerations. Clin Rev Allergy Immunol 2003;24:229-38.

8. Kosseifi SG, Guha B, Nassour DN, Chi DS, Krishnaswamy. The Dapsone Hypersensitivity syndrome revisited: A potentially fatal multisystem disorder with prominent hepatopulmonary manifestations. J Occup Med Toxol 2006;1:9.

9. Richardus JH, Smith TC. Increased incidence in leprosy of hypersensitivity reactions to dapsone

after introduction of multidrug therapy. Lepr Rev 1989;60:267-73.

10. Kano Y, Shiohara T. The Variable clinical picture of drug-induced hypersensitivity syndrome/drug rash with eosinophilia and systemic symptoms in relation to the eliciting drug. Immunol Allergy Clin North Am 2009;29:481-501.

11. Gupta A, Eggo MC, Uetrecht JP, Cribb AE, Daneman D, Rieder MJ, et al. Drug-induced hypothyroidism: The thyroid as a target organ in hypersensitivity reactions to anticonvulsants and sulfonamides. Clin Pharmacol Ther 1992;51:56-67.

Review Articles

Oral Retinoids in Dermatology

Ram Malkani, Ajay Kumar, D.C. Patel

Bulletin of the Jaslok Hospital & Research Centre Vol XIV No. 2 Oct 1989 p.37

Oral retinoids are the natural or synthetic analogues of Vitamin A acid. These represent one of the major dermatologic achievements in recent years, next only to the corticosteroids. The concept of dermatologic therapy has undergone a revolutionary change with their spectacular success in a number of chronic dermatoses for which the treatment till now had been either emperical or totally unsatisfactory. The drug has been found useful in the management of congenital disorders of keratinisation such as icthyoses, Darier's disease, Pityriasis rubra pilaris, Keratoderma palmare et plantare and porokeratoses. It has also been very valuable in several other disease like Psoriasis, nodulocystic acne, erosive mucosal lichen planus, Keratoacanthoma, Epidermodysplasia Verruciformis etc.

HISTORICAL

Vitamin A, the parent compound of retinoids, was first discovered in 1909 as an essential fat soluble vitamin from egg yolk. Despite its widespread use this drug has not proved of much success in skin disorders. Three major forms of vitamin A, viz., vitamin A aldehyde (retinal), vitamin A alcohol (retinol) and vitamin A acid (retinoic acid or tretinoin), represent its bioligical activity in the body. Tretinoin, the forerunner of modern oral retinoids, was first synthesized in 1946, and because of systemic toxicity, its use is restricted to topical application only in some skin disorders. Further screening efforts have led to the discovery of three clinically important retinoids, isotretinoin or 13 cisretinoic acid (Ro 4-3780), etreinate (Ro 10-9359) and arotinoid (Ro 13-6298). At present we have used only the former two therapeutically. The latest, arotinoid, is a third generation synthetic oral aromatic retinoid and is under experimental clinical evaluation. It is presumed to be the most effective and least toxic retinoid tested so far.

Isotretinoin (13-cisretinoic acid), the first generation oral retinoid is available commercially for the treatment of nodulocystic acne in the USA under the trade name Accutane. Etretinate (Ro 10-9359), the second generation retinoid is available as Tigason, used in the treatment of disorders of Keratinisation.

MODE OF ACTION OF ORAL RETINOIDS

They have a broad spectrum activity, such as, antiinflammatory, antikeratinising, antineoplastic, hormonomimetic and immunomodulatory effects.

They promote synthesis of extracellular glycosaminoglycans, which are important for the cohesive property of epidermal cells, accounting for their efficacy in bullous disorders.

They exert cytostatic effect, due to their inhibitory effect on ornithine decarboxylase activity and hence promote tumour prevention. The anti-inflammatory activity of these drugs is obvious from their clinical effect on severe inflammatory nodulocystic acne and the early disappearance of neutrophils in the lesions of Psoriasis.

PHARMACOLOGY OF ORAL RETINOIDS

Isotrenoin and Etretinate are administered orally in the dose of 0.5 to 2 mg/kg/day in two divided doses. These are readily absorbed from the gut and undergo extensive enterohepatic cycling before entering into the systemic circulation. Peak blood levels with isotretinoin, etretinate occur in 2 and 4 hrs. respectively. Its metabolic products are excreted in the bile and urine. The drug is stored in the body tissues to the toxic proportions during long term therapy mainly in the liver and to a lesser extent in the skin. Traces of etretinate could be detected in the body even 110 days after cessation of therapy. Unlike etretinate, isotretinoin is not much stored in the body. Both the retinoids are transported to the skin by binding to the plasma proteins, especially the albumin and lipoproteins.

TOXICOLOGY OF ORAL RETINOIDS

Systemic side effects with oral retinoids are much less serious in comparison to vitamin A. Both isotretinoin and etretinate exhibit similar adverse effects although their relative frequency and severity differs. The more frequently side effects are, cheilitis, desquamation of palms, soles and central face, dryness of the nose, mouth, ocoular irritation, transient thinning of hair, paronychia, skin rashes such as urticaria, petechiae, photosensitivity, hypo or hyper pigmentation and exhuberant granulation tissue formation over the healing lesions of acne. In addition there may be mild gastrointestinal disturbances, headache, irritability and loss of weight. Children on etretinate therapy have been noted to have skeletal anormalities such as calcification of the spinal ligaments, hyperostosis of the vertebrae frequently referred to as diffuse idiopathic skeletal hyperostosis (DISH syndrome). Similar changes have been noted in the epiphyses of long bones resulting in growth abnormalities.

Laboratory abnormalities on long term retinoid therepy include, dose dependent and reversible elevation of liver enzymes, mainly SGOT, SGPT and alkaline phosphatase. There is elevation of serum lipids especially triglycerides.

More serious but less common side effects which need cessation of retinoid therapy include pseudomotor cerebri (benign intracranial hypertension), corneal opacities, inflammatory bowel disease and teratologic abnormalities (hydrocephaly, microcephaly and microophthalmia). No definite evidence of mutagenicity is available in humans.

CLINICAL INDICATIONS OF ORAL RETINOIDS

Oral retinoids have been found useful in the management of disorders hitherto unresponsive to conventional therapy.

a) Congenital disorders of keratinisation:

Several studies have confirmed the effectiveness of oral retinoids in almost all types of icthyoses including the lamellar, x-linked and epidermolytic hyperkeratoses for which the presently available treatment is disappointing. Etretinate (Tigason) was found to be superior to isotretinoin (Accutane) in disorders of keratinisation. Initially a dose of 1-2 mg/kg/ds is needed to produce clinical resolution, followed by a long term maintenance therapy to avoid relapse. Surprisingly, inspite of the good clinical improvement, the histopathological abnormalities persist.

Gratifying results have been obtained in other congenital keratotic disorders such as Darier's disease, Pityriasis rubra pilaris, Erythrokeratoderma variabilis, all types of Porokeratoses, Pachyonichia congenita and verrucous epidermal nevus. The exact mechanism as to how the defective keratinisation is taken care of, is not known. It is believed, that these drugs inhibit or regulate the proliferation and differentiation of the keratinocytes.

b) Psoriasis: Etretinate (Tigason), has been found useful in the management of recalcitrant Psoriasis, generalised Pustular Psoriasis, psoriatic erythroderma and arthropathy.

c) Nodulocystic acne:Isotretinoin (Accutane) is extremely useful in severe uncontrollable inflammatory acne that fail to respond to conventional therapy. The effectiveness of isotretinoin in acne appears to be due to effect on the physiology of sebaceous gland resulting in a decrease in the sebum secretion rate and ductal hyperkeratinisation. The exact reason for the lack of beneficial effect in acne with etreinate is not clear.

The drug is administered in the dose of 0.5 to 1.5 mg/kg/day for a period of atleast 3 to 4 months. A second course of the drug in a few patients with residual lesions cleared the acne with no further evidence of relapses during the period of two years under observation.

d) In tumour prevention: Oral retinoids in combination with BCG afford protection against some premalignant and malignant conditions such as basal cell epithelioma, multiple solar keratoses, epidermadysplasia verruciformis, keratoacanthoma, T cell lymphoma, Mycosis fungoides and malignant Melanoma. The antineoplastic effect of oral retinoids appears to be due to the inhibition of ornithine decarboxylase induction which is an essential prerequisite for the initiation of complex events concerned in carcinogenesis.

e) Miscellaneous disorders: The oral retinoids have been successfully used in other chronic dermatoses like, rosacea, gram negative folliculitis, mucosal and disseminated lichen planus, multiple plantar warts, Reiter's disease, subcorneal pustular dermatosis, chronic bullous disorders, scleroderma, LSA, DLE, Kyrle's disease and sarcoidosis.

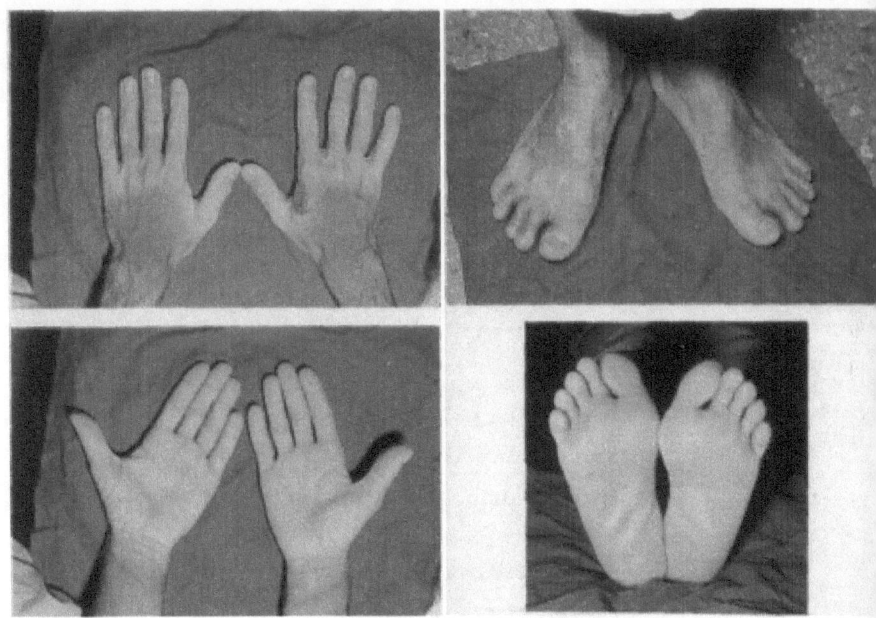

A case of Keratoderma palmare etplantare — after ten days of 1 mglkglday of oral Tigason therapy, showing softening of the skin of palms, soles and selectiv desquamations on the dorsal aspect.

CONTRAINDICATIONS TO ORAL RETINOID THERAPY

In view of their potential teratogenecity, these drugs should be avoided in pregnancy. Patients with obesity, alcoholism and abnormality of the lipid metabolism should avoid them. Similarly, these drugs should not be given to patients suffering from tumour cerebri, corneal opacities, inflammatory bowel disease and hyperostosis of the bones.

PRECAUTIONS DURING ORAL RETINOID THERAPY

Vitamin A should not be given concomitantly to avoid addition of the effects. The efficacy of oral retinoid is altered if given with other drugs like betablockers, chloroquine, aspirin and high doses of tetracycline. Laboratory studies comprising LFT, serum lipid profiles, pregnancy tests in females should be undertaken before treatment and during follow-up.

REFERENCES

1. Orfanos C.E. et al: Retinoids—Advances inBasic Research and Therapy,Springer—Verlag Berlin Heidelberg New York, 1981.

2. Orfanos C.E.:Oral retinoids—Presentstatus, Brit J Dermatol, 1980; 103: 473-481.

3. Jones D.H.: Retinoids for skin disorders,Practitioner, 1984; 228: 1043-1048.

4. Marks R: Synthetic retinoids in: Recent Advances in Dermatology,No.6,Editors,Rook A and Maibach H.I.: ChurchillLivinstone, Edinburgh, 1983; p 237-264.

5. Pochi P.E.: Oral retinoids in Dermatology(Special report), Arch Dermatol, 1982; 118:57-61.

6. Marks R, Finlay A and Holt P.J.A.: Severedisorders of keratinisation— Effects oftreatment with Tigason (etretinate), Brit. J.Dermatol, 1980; 104: 667-673.

7. Peck G.L. et al: Prolonged remissions ofcysticand conglobate acnewith 13-cis-retinoic acid, N Eng J Med,1979; 300:329-333.

8. Jones H. et al: 13-cis-retinoic acid and acne,Lancet, 1980; 2: 1048-1049.

9. Moriarty M. et al: Etretinate in treatmentof actinic keratoses, Lancet, 1982;1:364-365.

10. HaydeyR.R.etal:TreatmentofKeratoacanthomas with oral 13-cis-retinoicacid, N Eng J Med, 1980; 303: 560-564.

11. Reddy B.S.N.: Oral retinoids in Dermatology, Indian J Dermatol Venereol Leprol,1986; 52: 15-19.

IgE

Ram Malkani, Ajay Kumar

Bulletin of the Jaslok Hospital & Research Centre Vol XIV No.4 April 1990 p.15

Reagenic antibodies are characterised by their ability to sensitise human skin. These are confined to the IgE class of antibodies, which were added to the already existing IgA, IgM, IgG and IgD antibodies after they were discovered independently by two groups of investigators. Ishizaka and associates in 1966 reported the presence of these immunoglobulins as a unique class of antibodies, which were carriers of reagenic activity and were named IgE by Ishizaka. Johannson and Berrich discovered a myeloma protein IgND which could not be categorised among the then known classes of immunoglobulin and which was found to block the Pransnitz-Kustner (P.K.) passive skin sensitivation reaction[4,5] Ig ND was subsequently shown to be the same as IgE and the World Health organisation has adopted the name IgE in 1968[5]. Coombs et al[7] reported the detection of IgE specific antibody to castrobean allergen by the red-cell linked antigen-antibody reaction. Serum IgE concentrations must be measured by sensitive assay procedure, the mean serum level, in healthy adults is 250 nanogram (ng) per milliliter. Gleich and associates reported a mean IgE level of 160 ng/ml in non-allergic persons.

The serum IgE levels in various diseases have been summarised by Johanson et al. The levels are high in patients with atopic diathesis i.e., extrinsic asthama, hay fever and atopic dermatitis. The levels progressively increase from birth to adulthood in children with atopic diseases. High levels are also found in Wiskott-Aldrich's Syndrome in parasitic diseases such as ascariasis, trichinosis intestinal capillariasis and visceral larva migrans, and in apparently healthy Ethiopian children, which may have been as a result of ascariasis or other helminthic infections. They are also raised in a variety of non allergic conditions. Normal serum levels of IgE have been reported in a variety of skin conditions including acne, alopecia areata, scleroderma, and vitiligo. Kringer and co workers found that IgE levels were normal in numeral eczema and icthyosis. Winkelman and Geich have noted a chronic acral dermatitis in patients who had no features of the atopic diathesis but did have extremely high levels of IgE.

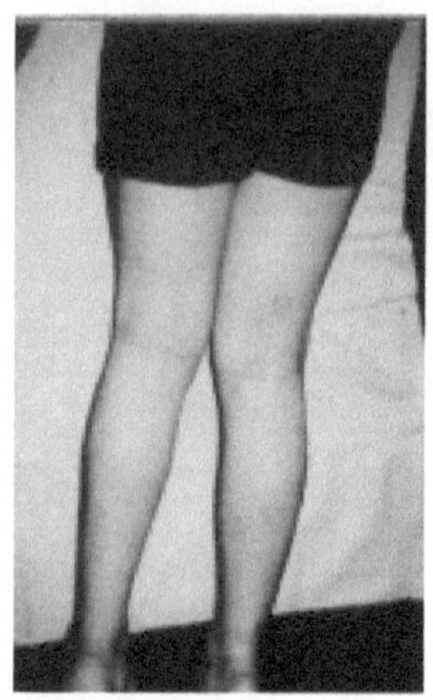

Fig. 1. Atopic dermatitis with papular lesion in popliteal fossa in a child

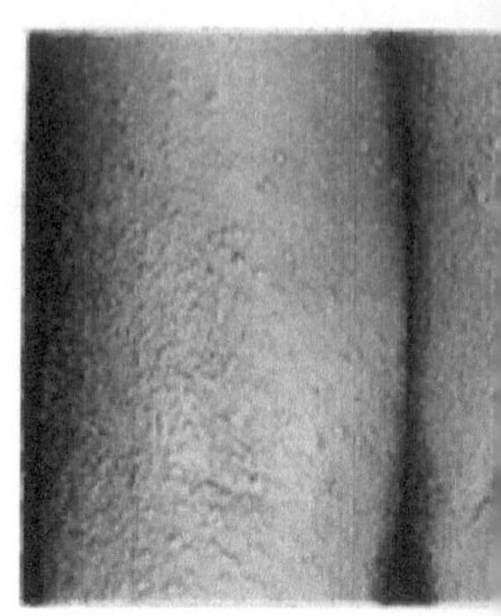

Fig. 2. Papules with excoriati

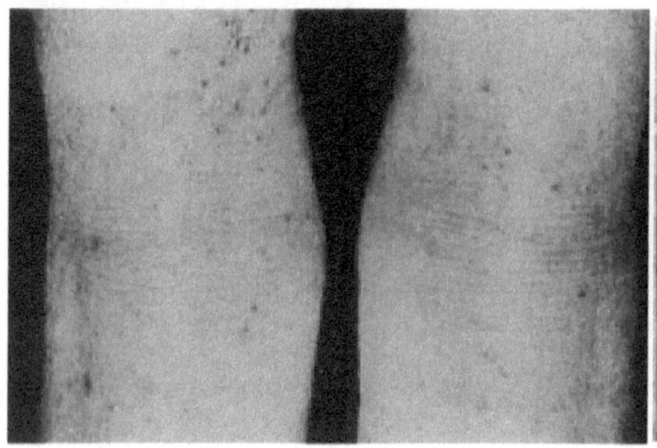

Fig. 3. Excoriated papules in cubital fossa

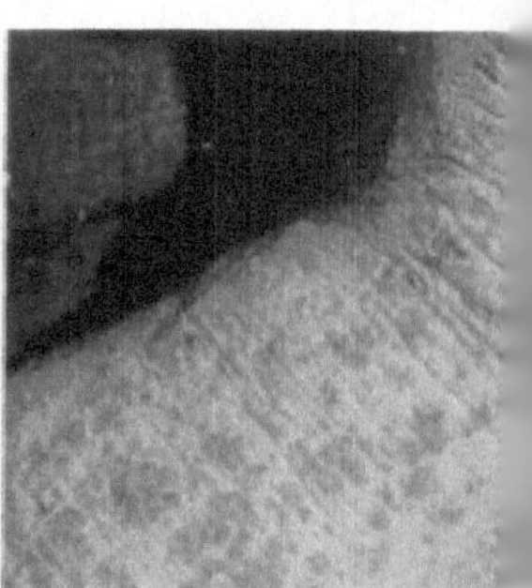

Fig 4 Atopic dermatitis with

The term atopy, since its first application by Coca and Coke, has been widely used to describe a human hypersensitivity state characterised by an enhanced capacity to form reagins in response to a variety of antigens. This hypersensitivity can be demonstrated by immediate erythemawheal type skin reactions in atopic individuals, and by the ability to transfer this hypersensitivity by Pransnitz Kustner (PK) test. The usual clinical manifestations are allergic rhinitis and asthma. The term atopic dermatitis was subsequently carried by Sulzberge and refers to a form of eczematous dermatitis which appears closely related to this hypersensitivity state. More than 70% of patients with this type of dermatitis have either a past or family history of asthma or allergic rhinitis and show many a constitutional and biologic features of the atopic diathesis. However it is far from certain that there is any pathogenetic relationship between an enchanced capacity to form reagenic antibodies and atopic dermatitis.

The injection of non antibody rabbit IgG into guineapig skin followed by an injection of antirabbit IgG gives an immediate wheal and flare reaction and is called the reverse passive cutaneous anaphylaxis (PCA) reaction. Ishizaka et al demonstrated an anologous situation in humans by an injection of rabbit or guinea-pig anti IgE serum into human skin and termed the phenomenon the reversed Pransnitz Kustner (PK) reaction. A normal reaction is a wheal and flare seen in 15 minutes at the site of injection. They postulated the mechanism to be a reaction between cell-fixed IgE and the injected anti-IgE with release of vasodilator metabolites. Individual sensitivity of IgE differs. Patients with defects in immunoglobulin synthesis fail to react to anti IgE except in very high doses

Although IgE levels are increased in atopic dermatitis, there is controversy as to whether these levels are related to the extent or severity of disease. Juhlin et al had reported that they were unable to find a correlation between IgE levels and the severity of atopic dermatitis although IgE levels did return to normal in patients free of dermatitis for a year or more. On the contrary Ogawa and Co-workers and

Gurevitch and his associates reported that IgE levels did corelate with severity of the dermatitis, if severity was defined on the basis of a number of areas of involvement.

Table 1 : IgE level in Corelation with disease activity

No.	Clinical appearance of Atopic Dermatitis (Normal Range 0-180) lU/ml.	IgE level
I.	Papular lesions on cubital fossae and wrist.	875
2.	Oozing and crusting over neck and cubital fossae	1050
3.	Lichenification over the cubital and popliteal fossae	650
4.	Extensive oozing and crusting over wide areas	1000
5.	Hand eczema with oozing	230
6.	Excoriated papules over the neck and hands	700
7.	Papules and oozing over the neck, popliteal fossa and leg.	440
8.	oozing and crusting over the face, neck, behind the ears.	970

Table : 2 : IgE levels in non atopic dermatoses

No.	Dermatoses	IgE level
1.	Vitiligo	170
2.	Psoriasis	105
3.	Acne vulgaris	5
4.	Allergic contact dermatitis	155
5.	Herpes simplex	40
6.	ENL	230
7.	Lichen planus	60
8.	Alopecia areata	45

Table : 3 : IgE levels not in correlation with presence of disease

No.	Clinical Presentation	IgE level (lU/ml)
1	Pitryasis alba	135
2	Hand eczema	80
3	Generalised itching and crusting, more in fluxures	170
4	Papules over neck and wrist with oozing	65
5	Lichenified lesions over popliteal and cubital fassae.	180

Review of IgE levels:

Serum IgE levels were estimated in a number of patients with manifestation of atopic dermatitis and other Cutaneous disorders. The observations are noted in tabular form. Table 1 indicates the IgE levels of atopic dermatitis, patients whose IgE levels correlated with the activity of the disease. Table 2 indicates the IgE levels in various dermatoses with their clinical presentation. Table 3 shows the IgE levels in patients with atopic disease where the IgE levels were not in correlation with disease activity.

Serum IgE levels though not diagnostic of the presence of atopic dermatitis, were found to be in correlation with the area of involvement of the lesions. This was in confirmity with the observations in the reviewed literature.

REFERENCES

1. Ishizaka K.,Ishizaka T, Hornbrook MM:
Physiocochemical properties of human reagenic

antibody. Presence of unique immunoglobulins as
carrier of reagenic activity. J. Immunol 97 :75-85
1966.

2. Ishizaka K: Human reagenic antibodies Ann
Rev. Mod 21:187-200 1970.

3. Johanson SCO, Bennich H: Immunological
studies of anatypical myeloma immunoglobulin.
Immunology 13:381-394, 1967.

4. Johansson SCO, Bennich H, Wide L: A new
class of immunoglobulin in human serum.
Immunology 14:265, 272, 1968.

5. Stanworth DR et al: Specific inhibition of the
Pramnitz Kustner Reaction by an Atypical
Human Myeloma Protein, Lancet 2:
330-332;1967.

6. Bennich HH, et al: Immunoglobulin E: A new
class of human immunoglobulin. Bull WHO
38:151 1968.

7. Coombs RRA et al: Detection of IgE (Ig ND)
Specific antibody (probably Reagin) to
castor-Bean Allergen by the Red-cell Linked

Antigen-Antibody Reaction, Lancet 1:115-1118 1968.

8. JoKanson SGO: Serum IgND levels in Healthy children and Adults. Int Arch Allerg 34:1-8;1968.

9. Johansson SGO: Bennich H, Berg T et al: Some factors influencing the serum IgE levels in atopic diseases. Clin Exp. Immun 6:43-47, 1970.

10. Raised levels of a new immunoglobulin class (IgND) in asthma, Lancet 2: 951-953 1963.

11. Berg T, and Johansson SGO: IgE levels in children with atopic disease: A clinical study. Arch Allerg.

12. Berglund, G, et al: Wiskott-Alderich Syndrome. A study of 6 cases with determinations of the immunoglobulins A I) G M and ND, Acta Paed Scand 57:89-97 1968.

13. Johansson SGO., Mellbin T., and Vahlquis B:Immunoglobin levels in Ethiopian preschool children with special reference to High concentrations of immunoglobulin E (IgND) Lancel 1:118, 1121 1968.

14. Johansson SGO, Bemich HH, Berg T: The clinical significance of IgEt Prog clin Immunol, 1:157-181, 1972.

15. Krueger GG et al: IgE levels in numnuralar eczema and icthyosis. Arch Dermatol 107: 56-58, 1973.

16. Winketmann RK, Gleich GJ: Chronic acral dermatitis. Association with extreme elevation of IgE, JAMA, 225:378-381, 1973.

17. Coca AF, Cooke RA: on the classification of the phenomenon of hypersensitivilies. J Immunol 8:163-182, 1923.

18. Ishizaka T, Ishizaka K, Johansson SGO, et al:Histamine release from human leucocytes by antigamma-E antibodies. J Immun 6:43-47,1970.

Induction of contact dermatitis as a therapeutic measure in Alopecia Areata and Warts

Ram Malkani, Ajay Kumar

Bulletin of the Jaslok Hospital & Research Centre Vol XIV No. 4 April 1990 p.47.

Intentional induction of Allergic contact dermatitis (ACD) by the application of potent contact allergens has been effectively used in the treatment of cases of alopecia areata (AA) which are otherwise difficult to treat, and in recalcitrant warts.

ALOPECIA AREATA AND AUTOIMMUNITY:

The etiology and pathophysiology of alopecia areata are still unclear. Defects in immunoregulation leading to autoimmunity have been proposed but not clearly proved. Alopecia is associated with several autoimmune disease including Addison's, thyroditis, ulcerative collitis and idiopathic hypoparathyroidism. Although no antibody to follicular tissue has been demonstrated, autoantibodies to a number of tissues have been found. Histopathologically the key findings is a predominantly lymphocytic infiltrate around the hair bulbs. In addition hair loss may be reversed by local or systemic steroids especially in the early stages.

CELL MEDIATED IN ALOPECIA AREATA:

Abnormalities of both humoral and cell mediated immune system have been described in alopecia areata. The histology of alopecia areata is certainly consistent with an aberrant T cell response.

The possible reason being first, that the hair follicle unit itself has undergone some antigenic change, which incites a normal response by the patient's immune system. Second, some serum factor may be missing, that, permits the patient's T cells to recognise 'self antigens'. This would explain the multiple autoantibodies observed in many of these individuals. Peribulbar round cell infiltrate reflects a CMI response to some hair associated antigen.

CONTACT ALLERGY AS A THERAPEUTIC TOOL IN ALOPECIA AREATA:

No curative treatment is currently available for alopecia areata, though a number of modalities are available which have resulted in hair regrowth. They include topical and systemic steriods, topical irritants, minoxidil and PUVA. The most interesting observation is the therapeutic effect of induced hypersensitivity reaction to a variety of sensitizers with topical application of potent contact allergens such as (DNCB)(3,1) squaric acid dibutyl ester (SADBE)(2,4) and diphencyprone.(6,12) The goal is to produce mild contact dermatitis. It requires that the skin of the subject be exposed to a toxic dose of the chemical during the induction phase and to a subtoxic dose two weeks later to elicit the immunological response.

The procedure entails topical application by a cotton wool bud on first visit to induce sensitisation. The patient is observed two weeks later to see whether sensitisation has developed in the form of mild eczema. The application is repeated till sensitisation occurs. Once the patient is sensitised, treatments are performed at weekly intervals. The concentrations are adjusted as per the patient's reactivity, so as to maintain erythema and pruritus for 24 to 36 hours. Time taken for the procedure entails application of the contactant initially to produce sensitisation. A 2% solution of DNCB in acetone is applied to a 2 sq. cm area on the arm or a region of the wart involvement and covered for 24 hrs. After 7 days 0.1% DNCB in quaphor is applied to the warts and occlusion applied overnight.

In a study carried out on 14 patients with recalcitrant warts, 9 patients had complete clearing. The mean duration of the warts was 1.4 years. A one year follow up showed no recurrence. There was no scarring or pigment alteration observed.

The mechanism of action is obscure. The effect is not due to irritation, since warts have been seen to disappear without direct contact with the agent. Most of the lesions disappeared without a clinically observable local inflammatory reaction. The intensity of immune reaction to the hapten did not seem to correlate with the ratio of resolution.

Regrowth varies from 5 to 18 weeks. Treatment is to be maintained as long as the disposition for alopecia areata exists. The frequency of application later on may be reduced to 2 to 3 weeks intervals.

The success of contact allergens in the treatment of alopecia areata further suggests the role of autoimmunity in its pathogenesis as their mode of action appears to be immunoregulatory rather than simply irritant . It has been postulated that the response to contact allergens induce non specific T suppresser cells into upper dermis which inhibits the lymphocytes associated with hair follicle damage (8). Although the non specific immunoregulatory activity exerted by the supressor cells that accumulate at the site of alopecia areata during the development of allergic contact dermatitis is too weak to suppress the response to contact allergens, it is sufficiently strong to inhibit the immune reaction to the hypothetical hair-associated antigen, responsible for alopecia areata.

SIDE EFFECTS AND LIMITATIONS:

The resulting contact eczema ranges from minimal itching to a severe reaction with blistering and weeping. There may also be local adenopathy and urticaria. Local side effects are dose related and reversible.

Dinitrochlorobenzene has been found to be mutagenic in Ames test. In light of this it has to be used with caution. SADBE and diphencyprone are safer.

Treatment with contact allergens does not appear to offer much for patients with long standing extensive hair loss, and in those with immunologic disturbances with auto antibodies.

CONTACT ALLERGY AS A THERAPEUTIC TOOL IN WARTS:

Delayed hypersensitivity or CMI is considered to be important in wart involution. Intentional induction of a CMI response appears to be a valuable tool in the treatment of warts. The treatment is relatively painless, nontraumatic and the mild itching and dermatitis was found acceptable to patients with resistant warts.

REFERENCES

1. Friedman P S: Alopecia areala and autoimmunity, BR J. Dermatol. 198];105:153.

2. Haple R: Contact allergy as a therapeutic toolfor alopecia areata- Application of squaric aciddibutyl ester, Dermatologica 161:289,1978.

3. Happle R.Buchner. V.Kalveram KL et al: Dinitrochlorobenzene for alopecia areata. Arch Dermatol 114:1629,1978.

4. Happle R. Buchner. V. Kalveram KL et al: Con tact allergy as a therapeutic toolfor alopecia areata: application of squaric acid dibutylester: Arch dcrmatol Res. 1979 264: 101-2.

5. Happle R. Echternach K:Induction of hair growth in alopecia areala with DNCB, Lancet 1977: ii 1002-1003.

6. Happle R. Hansen, Wcisner. Menzel L: Diphen cyprone in the treatment of alopeia areala, Acla Dermal vencrol (skotch) 1983, 63 : 49-52.

7. Haeza Petal:Immunological studicsin patients with alopecia areata. Int. Arch. Allergy. Appl. Immunol 1979, 212-18.

8. Milchell AJ el al: Alopecia areala-Palhogcncsis and Irealmenl. J Am. Acad Dcrmalol 1984: 5 : 763-75.

9. Ferret C et al: In silu demonslralion of T cells in alopecia areata. Arch. Dermalol. Res. 1982: 273 : 155-8.

10. Sauder D N el al in: Alopecia areala: an in-heriled auloimmunc disease in Hair, Irace ele-menls and human illness. Ediled by AC Brown, RG Gounse. New York, Prager 1989, P.343.

11. SchenlE Aelal: Aulo anlibodiesin alopecia and vililigo in Hair, trace elements and human ill ness, Edited by AC Brown, RG Gounse New York, Pager 1980 p. 334

12. Susan Macdonald Hull, Novis J F: Diphen cyprone in the treatmenl of long slanding alopecia areala. BR J dermalol: 119: 367, 1988.

13. Swanson NA, Mitchell AJ el al: Topical treat mentof alopeciaareatawithdinilro chlorobenizcne. Arch dermalol 1978: 114 : 1030.

Essential fatty acids and the skin

Ram H. Malkani, Belinda Vaz

Bulletin of the Jaslok Hospital & Research Centre Vol XVI No. 2 October 1991 p.44

The history of dermatology is littered with the corpses of discarded dietary hypotheses, some of which still stir when prodded. The idea that some types of cutaneous inflammation can be diminished by oral fatty acid supplements has recently been exhumed and resuscitated. It seems likely that fatty acids may be involved in cutaneous pathophysiology in atleast 3 different ways.

1. A direct structural role in maintaining the integrity of the cell membranes.

2. Modification of the metabolic pathway of the eicosanoids (prostaglandins, leukotrienes and thromboxanes)

3. Amplification of cell signals which govern basic processes such as cell division and secretion .

Nomenclature of essential fatty acids

Two fatty acids, linoleic and alphalinolenic acid, are essential for mammalian life. Linoleic acid is a polyunsaturated fatty acid and forms a precursor for the formation of the other polyunsaturated fatty acids, linolenic and alphalinolenic acid.(1) Linoleic and alphalinolenic acid are desaturated at the omega 6 and omega 3 positions respectively, i.e., they have their first double bonds at 6 and 3 carbon atoms along the fatty acid chain, starting from the methyl end of the molecule. These two fatty acids and their metabolites are called the omega 6 and omega 3 series of fatty acids respectively(2).

EFA

Omega -3 = marine source

Omega 6 = plant

Non EFA = animal fats

Sources and requirements of EFA

All food fats contain atleast small amounts of both alpha linoleic and linolenic acid(3). The omega 6 acids (eg. linoleic acid) come from plant sources mainly. Safflower, soy and corn oils are rich in linoleic acid. The evening primrose seed oil is a rich source of linoleic and gammalinolenic acid. Human breast milk also contains substantial quantities of gamma linolenic acid (5) The omega 3 series of fatty acids come mainly from marine sources

The recommended intake of linoleic acid to cover the metabolic need is 1 to 2% of total caloric intake for adults and 3% of calories for infants.

Metabolism of EFA

Essential fatty acids are stored in the phospholipids in the cell membranes and also act as precursors of prostaglandins. They are liberated from the cell membranes by enzymes such as phospholipase and converted by a further series of enzymes to metabolites such as arachidonic acid and eicosopentaenoic acid which eventually produce the eicosanoids (see fig. 2). These are vitally important in the production of inflammation and the regulation of cell division. Glucocorticoids inhibit the release of EFA from cell membrane by the action of lipocortin and this is one way in which steroids suppress inflammation (see fig. 3)(1).

RAM MALKANI

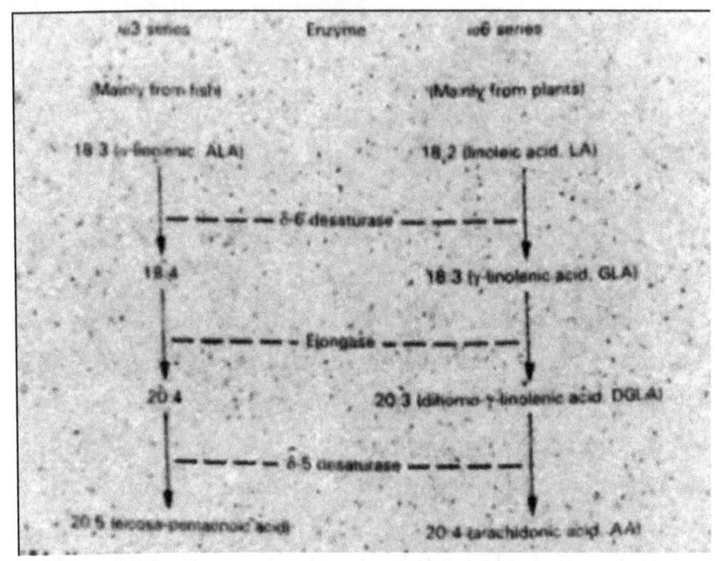

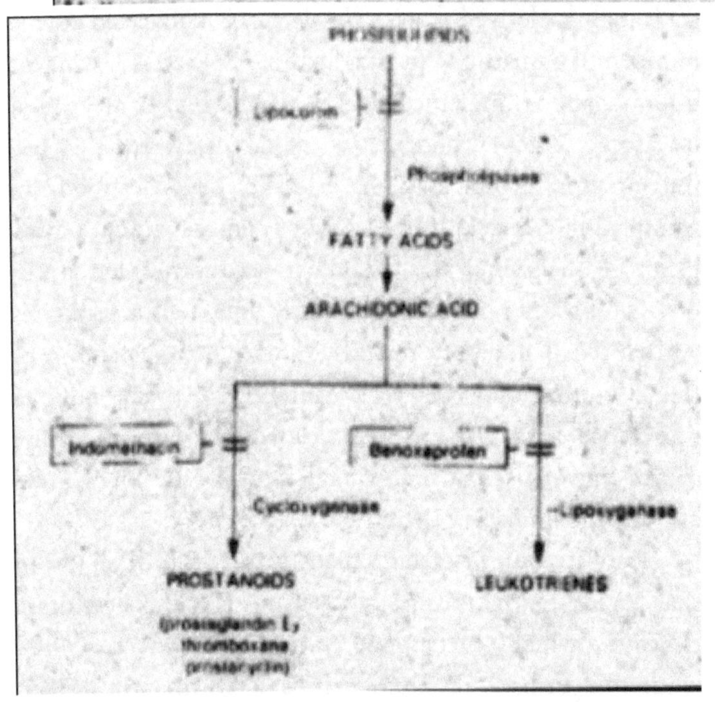

ω3 series
Enzyme
ω6 series
(Mainly from fish)
(Mainly from plants)
18:3 (α-linolenic, ALA)
18:2 (linoleic acid, LA)
δ-6 desaturase
18:4
18:3 (γ-linolenic acid, GLA)
Elongase
20:4
20:3 (dihomo-γ-linolenic acid, DGLA)
δ-5 desaturase
20:5 (eicosa-pentaenoic acid)
20:4 (arachidonic acid, AA)

PHOSPHOLIPIDS
Lipocortin
Phospholipases
FATTY ACIDS
ARACHIDONIC ACID
Indomethacin
Benoxaprofen
Cyclooxygenase
Lipoxygenase
PROSTANOIDS
LEUKOTRIENES
(prostaglandin E,
thromboxane,
prostacyclin)

Nonsteroidal anti-inflamatory agents such as indomethacin inhibit the cyclooxygenase pathway; benoxaprofen inhibits both the lipoxygenase and the cyclooxygenase pathways.

EFA of the omega 3 and omega 6 series are metabolised by a series of elongase and desaturase enzymes to form arachidonic acid and eicosapentaenoic acids, respectively (see fig. 2) These fatty acid substrates together with other dietary fatty acids compete with each other so that the quantities of the eicosanoids produced depend on the diet, ie., different prostaglandins are produced according to whether the fatty acids consumed are predominantly from the omega 3, the omega 6 or the later series. Arachidonic acid, mainly derived from animal fats, is converted to the more inflammatory prostaglandin 2 series, whereas dihomogamma linolenic acid (DGLA) which is decreased in atopic eczema patients is metabolised to the less inflammatory prostaglandin 1 series. DGLA is derived from gamma linolenic acid (GLA) a major component of evening primrose oil. Guinea pigs fed on barage, another rich source of GLA, produce increased quantities of DGLA metabolites with anti inflammatory potential namely prostaglandins of the 1 series and 15 hydroxy-DGLA which inhibits lipoygenases. Eicosapentaenoic acid, derived from marine sources, gives rise to the prostaglandin 3 series, which are also less inflammatory than the 2 series.

The metabolism of fatty acids in the skin differs from that in most other tissues since skin lacks the desaturase enzymes which metabolize fatty acids. Because the epidermis turns over rapidly, it is likely that it has no substantial stores of these important metabolites, and it is dependent on a supply of these metabolites being produced in other organs such as the liver.

Essential fatty acid deficiency

Rats fed on a diet deficient in the two fatty acids, linoleic and alpha linolenic acids fail to thrive and acquire skin changes including redness, scaling and hyperkeratosis of the sebaceous follicles .

Similar changes occur in EFA deficient human beings but these changes can be corrected by the topical application of linoleic acid . Simple dietary deficiency is rare, but there have been many cases due to chylous ascities, intestinal resection or prolonged parenteral feeding. Various skin changes have been reported in these patients including dryness, scaliness and erosions in the intertriginous areas .

Essential fatty acids and the epidermal barrier

EFA deficient rats lose water through the skin because the epidermal permeability barrier is defective. This barrier which partly "water proofs" the skin, is in the lowest part of the stratum corneum, just above the granular layer. The integrity of the barrier effect depends on interlocking sheets of lipid which act as a kind of "mortar" around the corneum. (see fig. 4). These lipid lamellae are secreted from granules (also called odland bodies) in the granular layer and they contain a unique sphingolipid of which linoleic acid is a vital component, (see fig. 5). The waterproofing effect depends on the stereochemical configuration of this sphingolipid. In the

EFA-deficient rat the linoleate portion of the sphingolipid is replaced by oleate, which gives it a different and "leaky" configuration. Thus, a defect in the barrier function of the epidermis might account for the dry skin of eczema patients: The lamellar bodies are abnormal in the dry but non-eczematous skin of atopic patients and the concentrations of the linoleate rich acyl sphingolipid are reduced in the skin of atopic eczema patients.

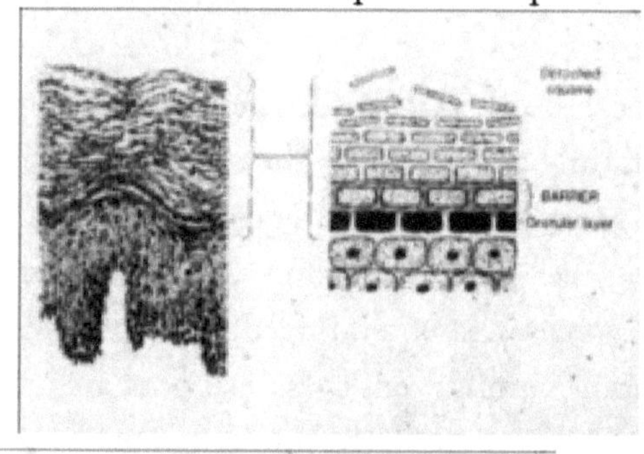

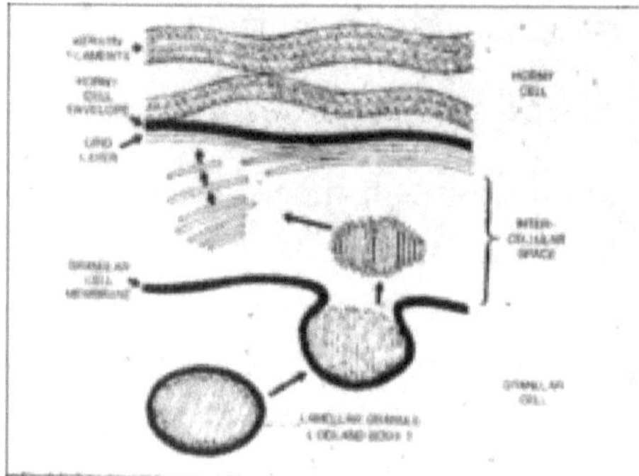

Essential fatty acids and psoriasis

Eskimos taking their traditional fishy diet have very little psoriasis, but it does tend to develop when they take a western diet with a higher intake of saturated fats.

Uncontrolled studies by Ziboh et al, Maurice et al, Alien et al and Kragballe et al(9) have suggested that dietary supplementation with fish oil with or without a low fat diet can improve psoriasis. In a controlled study, Bittiner et al(10) found a significant lessening of itching, erythema and scaling in patients with stable chronic psoriasis receiving 10 fish oil capsules daily, during the 8 week long study. Each capsule of 1 gm offish oil contains 180 mg of Eicosapentaenoic acid, 120 mg of docosahenxaenoic acid.

However Bjorneboe et al(11) in a double blind, 8 week long test using moderate doses of omega 3 fatty acids, found psoriatic lesions to be unresponsive and suggested further examination of both higher doses and longer period of treatment.

The possible mechanisms of action of EFA in psoriasis are:

1. The cellular content of free arachidonic acid in psoriatic lesions is increased 20 fold as compared to uninvolved epidermis.

Free arachidonic acid may be converted by specific enzymatic reactions to prostaglandins, leukotrienes and 12 hydroxyeicosatetraenoic acid (12HETE) (see fig. 6). These products are all mediators of inflammation. Increased levels of leukotriene B4 and 12-HETE have been observed in psoriatic epidermis, Leukotriene B4 formed from arachidonic acid is a very potent chemotaxin and Eicosapentaenoic acid is the precursor of the 3-series of prostaglandins and leukotriene B5. These eicosanoids are less inflammatory than those derived by conservation of arachidonic acid, and LTB5 is a less potent stimulator of keratinocyte proliferation than LTB4. Eicosanoid metabolism is largely dependent on the amount and types of fatty acid precursors in the diet, and in western diets n-6 fatty acids are most abundant. Arachidonic acid and eicosapentaenoic acid are cleared, elongated and desaturated by the same enzyme systems. When omega-3 fatty acids are supplied in the diet, competitive inhibition of omega 6 eicosanoid metabolism with formation of omega 3 eicosanoids may occur. Kragballe et al found that maximum LTB5/LTB4 ratios preceeded the maximum clinical improvement.

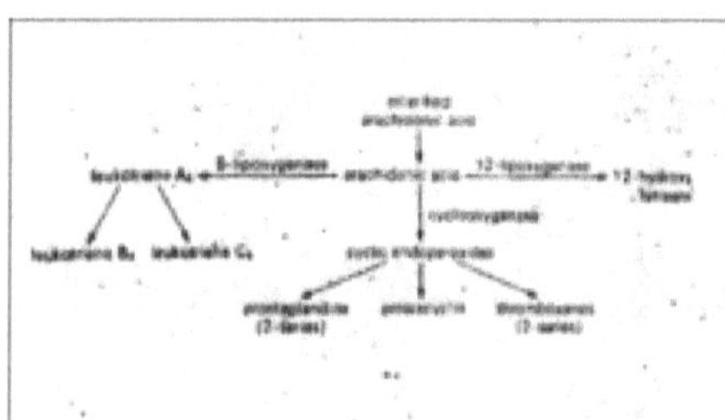

2. Dietary fats may be able to modify the cell signalling system. Many extracellular signals which stimulate a cell to perform a particular function such as division or secretion act by inducing phospholipid turnover in the cell membrane. After the cell receptor receives a

signal, a phospholipid component of the cell membrane is degraded to inositol triphosphate (IPS) and diacylglycerol (DAG). DAG then activates protein kinases, important enzymes which stimulate many cell functions by phosphorylating a range of cell proteins.

Many of the cells in the psoriatic plaque are overactive, including the keratinocytes, granulocytes, monocytes, T. cells, endothelial cells, fibroblasts, etc. IPS and DAG are increased in the psoriatic plaque. A defect in the transmembranous cell signalling system could explain some of these abnormalities seen in psoriasis, (see fig. 7)2.

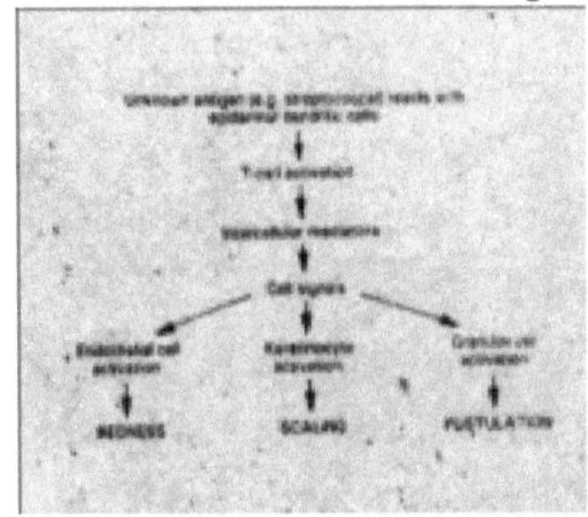

In view of the possible role of leukotrienes in the pathogenesis of psoriasis, more profound effects are likely in the inflammatory unstable variants such as erythrodermic and generalised pustular psoriasis. Treatment with eicosapentanoic acid (EPA) would have considerable advantage over the current therapies for these patients, such as methotrexate, etretinate and PUVA especially in women of childbearing age. The effectiveness of EPA could probably be improved by increasing dietary intake of oily fish and reducing that of foods with a high arachidonic acid content10. Kragballe et al recommended a diet low in fat as well. On the negative list of the administered diets were fats and oils, red meats, whole milk dairy products, baked goods, egg yolk, salad dressings and nuts. On the positive list of the administered diets were fish, poultry, fruits (except banana), vegetables (except avocado), grains, skim milk dairy products, carbonated beverages, coffee and tea.

A further possible advantage of the use of dietary fish oil supplements in psoriasis treated with etretinate is that fish oils decreases the hypertriglyceridaemia which is a common complication of this treatment.(2)

Essential fatty acids and atopic dermatitis

Several authors have confirmed that essential fatty acids of the omega 3 and the omega 6 series both produce significant clinical improvement in atopic eczema, particularly with regard to the severity of itching.

A double blind controlled crossover study conducted by Wright and Burton of the effect of various doses of oral evening primrose oil in 99 patients with atopic eczema showed that the preparation produced a significant clinical improvement when taken in high dosage.

Evening primrose oil in the form of 500 mg capsules, each containing 40 mg of gammalinolenic acid, has been recommended twice daily in adults and 2 to 4 capsules daily for children. Clinical improvement is usually noted after a few weeks, though some patients take 8 to 12 weeks to respond and some do not respond at all.

No serious adverse effects have been noted from this treatment, though occasional patients complain of nausea or belching. The capsules can safely be given during pregnancy and lactation.

The mechanism of action of essential fatty acids in atopic dermatitis could be as follows.

1. Linoleic acid and its derivative DGLA (see fig. 2.) are metabolized to the less inflammatory prostaglandins on the 1 series and block conservation of arachidonic acid to more inflammatory prostaglandin 2 compounds(2).

2. There is some evidence that prostaglandins are involved in the regulation of T lymphocytes. Some patients with atopic eczema have deficiencies of T lymphocyte functions and dietary essential fatty acid supplementation could alter the T-lymphocyte functions .

3. The dryness of the skin in eczema might be due to increased transepidermal water loss due to a defect in epidermal ceramides. Linoleic acid, an essential fatty acid, forms an integral part of the ceramides which are important in maintaining the permeability barrier of the epidermis.

Essential fatty acid therapy could be added to the therapeutic regimen of patients of atopic dermatitis who do not respond to conventional therapy.

Many patients who use oral evening primrose oil notice that their skin becomes smoother even if their eczema does not remit. Topical application of fish oil in atopic dematitis has proved helpful but not as effective as a fluorinated steroid cream.

Essential fatty acids and acne vulgaris

Acne patients have a low concentration of linoleic acid in their sebum and a relative essential fatty acid deficiency in the pilosebaceous epithelium may account for the characteristic follicular hyperkeratosis of acne. Acyl ceramides recovered from comedones contain much less linoleic acid than those from the normal epidermis. Downing found that oral essential fatty acid supplements have little or no effect in acne after 2 months treatment, but by 6 months about 90% of patients had improved.

Essential fatty acids and other dermatoses

A linoleic acid dimer used topically has protected against contact dermatitis to poison ivy. Essential fatty acids have also shown promise in carboxylase deficiency, acathosis nigricans associated with lipodystrophic diabetes and pruritus of biliary cirrhosis.

To conclude a new look at essential fatty acids has opened up exciting and promising new leads towards safer alternative therapeutic regimes in chronic dermatoses.

References

1. Burton J.L. 1989; Dietary fatty acids and inflammatory skin disease; Lancet: 27-31

2. Burton J.L. Essential fatty acids and the skin. Ed. R.H. Champion, p 129-145 ch. 9, vol.8., R.J. Pyc, Churchill Livingstone 1990

3. Suitor C.J.W., Crowlcy M.F., 1984, In nutrition-Principles and application in health promotion (2nd Edn) J.B. Lippincotl Company, Philadelphia pg. 36-37

4. Anderson 1., Dibble M.V., Turkki P.U., Mitchell H.S., Rynbergcn H.J., 1982, In Nutrition in health and disease (17th Edn) J.B. Lippincott Company, Philadelphia pg. 40-45.

5. Wright S., Burton J.L.,1982, Oral Evening Primrose-Seed Oil improves atopic eczema. lancet 11; 1120-1122.

6. Ziboh V.A., Cohen K.A., Ellis C.N., Miller C., Hamilton T.A., Kragballc K., Hydrick C.R., Voorhces J.J., 1986. Effects of dietary supplementation of fish oil on neutrophil and epidermil fatty acids. Arch Dcrmatol 122: 1277-1282.

7. Maurice P.O., Alien B.R.., Barkley A.S J., Cock-bill S.R., Stammers J., Bather P.C., 1987. The effects of dietary supplementation with fish oil in patients with psoriasis, Br. J. Dcrmatol 117: 599-606

8. Alien B.R., Maurice P.D.L., Goodfield M.W. ct al 1985. The effects on psoriasis of dietary sup-plementation with eicosapentaenoic acid (Abstract) 113: 777.

9. Kragballc K., Pogh K., 1989, A low fat diet supplemented with dietary fish oil (Max-EPA) results in improvement of psoriasis and in formation of leukotricnc B.5. Acto Derm Venereol (Stockh) 69: 23-28.

10. Brittncr S.B., Cartwright I., Tucker W.F.G., Bleehcn S.S., 1988, A double blind randomized placebo controlled trial of fish oil in psoriasis. Lancet i :378-380

11. Bjorneboe A., Smith A.K., Bjorneboe G.E., Thunc P.O., Drevon C.A., 1988, Effects of dietary supplementation with n-3 fatty acids on clinical manifestations of psoriasis. Br. J. Dcrmatol 118:77-83.

12. Rhodes E.L. 1984, Max EPA in the treatment of eczema. Br. J. Clin. Pr. (Suppl) 31.

Cetirizine in urticaria and atopic dermatitis

Ram H. Malkani

MEDIFACTS from Doctors for Doctors - an in house bulletin of Alkem Labs vol12;1994: p2

Introduction

Whenever a new drug is introduced the obvious question comes to the mind is "How is the new drug better than the presently available remedies ?"

Any switch in the prescription practice must have justification. Sometimes a switch would take place even if the new drug does not offer any advantages over the currently available drug. Like, we do prescribe a new drug to break the monotony, to see for ourselves the efficiency of the new drug or to satisfy our curiosity about the effect on the patient like conducting a self styled undocumented mini drug trial.

But one is forced to prescribe the new drug and change the prescription habit, if the new drug is definately superior to the presently available ones. As a clinician, the aims are always to try to give quick, long lasting relief to the patient's symptoms, to impress the patient with the therapist's sharp accumen, to show concern by giving relief to the patient, to make use of modern medicine, to get the satisfaction that one is updated & hence ahead. A good clinician must find time to go into the details of the new drug introduced and assess for himself the value of the new drug.

Cetirizine: The New Drug

Cetirizine dihydrochloride is a new second generation H1 antagonist antihistamine introduced. A H1 blocking agent and antihistamine is used in alleviating allergic conditions like allergic rhinitis & urticaria. Apart from the above allergic conditions, there is evidence that cetirizine is beneficial in asthma, atopic dermatitis and preventing pruritus from mosquito bites. A discussion of the pharmacology, therapeutic efficacy, the mechanism of action, of cetirizine in allergic processes, is undertaken in this communication.

Cetirizine and H1 Receptor Antogonism

Cetirizine, theprincipal metaboliteof hydroxyzine, is a member of a new therapeutic class of H1 antagonists. Cetirizine is a potent and highly selective antagonist at the peripheral H1 receptor site and it is characterised by greater selectivity for H1 receptors than that exhibited by other antihistamine agents. The disadvantages associated with the sedative properties of older antihistamines were overcome in the 1970-80's with the development of second generation nonsedating antihistamines eg. terfenadine, astemizole, loratadine and cetirizine. Adverse CNS events such as sedation, experienced with first generation H1 receptor antagonists are less likely to occur during Cetirizine therapy because of its reduced ability to cross the blood brain barrier. (Snowmen AM, Synder SH, Cetirizine action on neurotransmitter receptors. Journal of Allergy & clinical immunology 86: 1025-1028, 1990).

In 10 multicenter placebo controlled studies comprised of approximately 2000 patients, the mean incidence of sedation of cetirizine, 5 mg. was 12% versus 8% placebo and 17% of cetirizine, 10 mg. The incidence of sedation was less with Cetirizine than with hydroxyzine (36%), chlorpheniramine (23%) or diphenhydramine (30%).

In short Cetirizine has no significant anticholinergic or serotonergic effects. Cetirizine is possibly the most potent of the new generation of peripheral HI receptor antagonists, which have a low incidence of CNS adverse effects.

Like hydroxyzine, Cetirizine potently inhibits histamine induced wheal and flare reactions. In a skin model in which antihistamine potency is measured by wheal and flare inhibition after intradermal histamine injection, 10 mg. Cetirizine was found to be more potent than 10 mg. loratadine and 10 mg. astemizole.

Cetirizine has also shown greater potency than that of hydroxyzine and other antihistamines (e.g. mepyramine, clemastine and terfenadine) in antagonising the continuous effects of histamine in several animal models (De Vos C. Maleux MR, Baltes E. Gobert G). Inhibition of histamine skin wheal in four animal species. (Annals of Allergy 50 : 278-282, 1987). Cetirizine is characterised by rapid absorption after oral administration with maximum plasma concentrations, achieved within 1 hour of administration. Bioavailability is not significantly affected by the co-administration of food.

Cetirizine's low rate of hepatic metabolism makes it unique among the H1 antihistamines. Most H1 receptor antagonists are metabolised by the hepatic cytochrome system. Hence cetirizine may be an antihistamine of choice for patients with hepatic dysfunction. There is no interaction with hepatically metabolised drugs like theophylline, pseudoephedrine or cimetidine. It does not potentiate the effects of alcohol. It is eliminated through the renal route. It's prolonged duration of action permits once daily dosing.

Allergic Process

The allergic process is generally recognised to consist of 2 phases-immediate and late. The immediate response consists mainly of allergen-provoked, IgE mediated release of histamine and other chemical mediators of inflammation from mast cells. The main feature of the late-phase response is migration of inflammatory cells, particularly eosinophils, to the allergic site (Gibson et al. 1990; Gleich 1990; Kay 1979).

Immediate Allergic Response Mast Cell Degranulation:

Mast cells and basophils synthesise histamine, which is stored in secretory cytoplasmic granules. Mast cells degranulate when IgE molecules on their surface become crosslinked by a specific antigen or allergen, or when they come into contact with other non-IgE-mediated activators (Ryhal & Fletcher 1991).

Degranulation causes the release of preformed mediators such as histamine, and the synthesis and release of other chemical mediators such as platelet activating factor (PAF) and various products of arachidonic acid metabolism (eicosanoids) including prostagladins, leukotrienes and hydroxyeicosatetraenoic acids (HETEs). Macromolecular substances from the granule matrix are also released, such as tryptase, chymase, peroxidase and arylsulphatase B (Kaliner & Lemanske 1992) Additionally, degranulation initiates the transcription, synthesis and secretion of certain cytokines (nonspecific soluble mediators of the immune response) over a period of hours. These cytokines include the interleukins IL-3, IL-4, IL-5 and IL-6, together with tumour necrosis factor alpha (TNF - alpha), and granulocyte macrophage colony -stimulating factor (GM-CSF) (fig. 1).

Late-Phase Allergic Response Eosinophil Chemotaxis:

The inflammatory infiltrate seen during the late-phase allergic reaction is characterised by neutrophil, basophil, monocyte and, particularly, eosinophil infiltration of the allergic site. The response seen in allergic patients differs from that found in normal subjects.

Skin challenge with anti-lgE in normal subjects produced a cellular response involving mainly neutrophils and monocytes; in allergic subjects, significant accumulation of eosinophils occurred with a corresponding decrease in neutrophils (Rihoux et.al. 1990a). Similarly, eosinophil migration occurred in atopic individuals, but not in normal subjects, after intradermal injection of specific allergen, PAF or the synthetic chemotactic factor formyl - methionyl - leucyl - phenylalanine (FMLP); significant degranulation of eosinophils also occurred (Henocq & Vergaftig 1988).

The cellular response differed significantly from that in normal subjects, in whom neutrophil, but not eosinophil, infiltration was identified.

The mechanisms by which cells are attracted to the allergic site are not fully understood. A number of mediators released by mast cells are chemotactic for leucocyte and cause leucocyte migration to the site of inflammation. These mediators include PAF, leukotriene B4 (LTB4) and .some cytokines, and it is possible that mast of cells of allergic individuals produce an increased quantity of a specific eosinophilotactic mediator compared with mast cells in normal subjects (Gleich 1990b). Increased release of eicosanoids, including LTB4, from anti -IgE - challenged peripheral blood leucocytes has been demonstrated in patients with atopic dermatitis compared with normal individuals (Ruzicka & Ring 1987). However, factors other than chemotactic mediators are also implicated in the eosinophil accumulation seen in atopic patients.

Other Mechanisms of Eosinophil Accumulation

There appear to be 3 main mechanisms for the preferential accumulation of eosinophils: selective adhesion to vascular endothelium; preferential diapedesis of primed eosinophils; and cytokine -enhanced survival of eosinophils (Kay 1990).

Leucocyte adhesion to vascular endothelium occurs at an early stage in cellular infiltration and is dependent on cell adhesion molecules. These are leucocyte membrane proteins, which act as receptors and interact with structural counterparts on other cells to facilitate intercellular adhesion. Both eosinophils and neutrophils express 3 receptors of the leucocyte integrin family which are involved in cell adhesion. These receptor molecules lymphocyte - function - associated antigen-1 (LFA-1), complement receptor type 3 (CR3) and '150, 95-consist of 2 polypeptide chains. The alpha chains are distinct and comprise LFA-1-alpha (CDlla), CR3-alpha (CDllb) and 150, 95-alpha (CDllc), respectively while the beta chain (CD18) is common to all 3 receptor proteins (Kay 1990).

Cytokines are thought to play a significant role in eosinophil accumulation. Incubation with IL-5 increased the adherence of eosinophils, but not neutrophils, to cultured human vascular endothelial ells or plasma-coated glass, whereas IL-3 and iM-CSF enhanced both eosinophil and neutrophil adhesion. This selective action of IL-5 was at least tartly dependent on CD11/18 leucocyte integrins, in articular CR3, and to a lesser extent on LFA-1 Walsh et al. 1990). It is not clear whether increased adherence of eosinophils result from increased expression, or from some conformational change in be receptors (Kay 1990).

Other cell adhesion molecules include intercellular adhesion molecule-1 (ICAM-1 or CD54) and endothelial cell leucocyte adhesion molecule-1 (ELAM-1). CD54 plays a major role on pathological cell adhesion by interacting with its structural counterpart LFA-1. CD54 expression has been demonstrated on conjunctival epithelium in sensitised subjects following conjunctival allergen challenge. This expression together with a mild inflammatory cell infiltrate, may persist in patients chronically exposed to allergens such as dust mites, thus, a subclinical inflammatory state exists, known is minimal persistent inflammation, which increases susceptibility to acute exacerbations of allergic disease; non-allergic subjects do not exhibit his response (Canonica et al. 1992). It is therefore possible that increased expression of cell adhesion molecules in atopic individuals may contribute to eosinophil accumulation in the late-phase response.

The induction and upregulation of adhesion molecules on eosinophils and endothelial cells, by cytokines and other mediators, is of major importance in the pathogenesis of allergic disorders, indeed, mast cells are known to contain significant quantities of preformed and inducible TNF-alpha and IL-1 were found to induce endothelial ICAM-1 and ELAM-1, thereby increasing adhesion of eosinophils to endothelial cells (Hansel Walker 1992). IL-5 selectively primed eosinophils, but not neutrophils, for PAF - and LTB4 - induced locomotion, while IL-5, IL-3 and GM-CSF promoted differentiation and increased survival of eosinophils, while may partly account for eosinophil acumulation (Kay 1990; Losewicz a Davies 1991).

Degranulation of Eosinophils

Once at the allergic site, eosinophils degranulate and release a number of mediators including histaminase, PAF and leukotriene C4. Potent cytotoxic proteins are also released, such as eosinophil cationic protein (ECP), major basic protein (MBP), and eosinophil peroxidase (EPO). All 3 of these proteins can cause desquamation of the airways in asthma, and MBP and EPO can also induce further mast cell degranulation and release of histamine from basophils (fig. 2; Gleich 1990b). This could contribute to the chronicity of the disease.

Therapeutic Efficacy

Histamine is the oldest and most familiar substance among the mediators of the inflammatory response. At the cellular level, it is found largely in mast cells and basophils, when it is held in intra-cellular of granules.

Histamine released from mast cells during allergic reactions acts on specific histamine receptors. Some of the effects, e.g. Pruritus, bronchoconstriction and contraction of the smooth muscles of the gut, are mediated through the Ha receptors and are blocked by the classical antihistamines, while other effects, most notably gastric secretion, involved H2 receptors and will be blocked by H2 blockers. Still other effects, such as hypotension, resulting from vasodilation may be mediated by both H1 and H2 receptors.

Urticaria

Urticaria is characterised by raised, erythematous wheals involving the superficial part of the dermis. Episodes of urticaria persisting for 8 weeks or more are termed chronic, and although some forms of the condition are related to specific stimuli, in most cases, no underlying cause can be identified (Soter 1990).

Both subjective and objective improvement occurred in 28 patients with chronic idiopathic urticaria treated with cetirizine 10 mg. daily (Goh et al. 1991) and, in another study of 30 similar patients who had previously failed to respond to antihistamines, cetirizine caused significant reduction in wheals, erythema & pruritus (Quhlin and Arendt 1988).

Cetirizine is also effective in delayed pressure urticaria. Cetirizine was found to be more effective than terfenadine (Macher & Eichelberg 1989).

Cetirizine had a more rapid onset of action than astemizole. Cetirizine was associated with significant fewer wheals than astemizole during the first 2 weeks of a 4 week trial (Alomar et al 1990), and symptoms improved within 24 hours of Cetirizine, compared with 3 to 4 days of astemizole administration (Breneman et al. 1992).

Atopic Dermatitis

Atopic dermatitis affects upto 5% of the population. The condition has been defined by Rajka (1986) as a specific dermatitis in the abnormally reacting skin of the atopic, resulting in itch with sequelae as well as inflammation. Pruritus is the primary feature of atopic dermatitis and following morphological symptoms are secondary to this: prurigo — a discrete pruritic papule, lichenification plaques of thickened skin which result from scratching; and eczematous lesions - erythematous, papulous, scaling lesions.

Atopic dermatitis commonly affects anticubital and popliteal areas, and the face, hands and feet are also frequently affected (Rajka 1986).

Hanifin and Rajka, (1980) produced guidelines for the diagnosis of atopic dermatitis based on the presence of 3 major features out of the following important symptoms:

1. Pruritus

2. Typical morphology

3. Flexural lichenifications of linearity in adults. Facial and extensor involvement in infants and children.

4. Chronic or chronically relapsing dermatitis.

5. Personal or family history of atopy (asthma, allergic rhinitis, atopic dermatitis).

Histamine is thought to be involved in atopic dermatitis, particulars as raised levels of histamine have been demonstrated in plasma and skin during acute exacerbations of the condition. Antihistamines would therefore seem a logical treatment choice and first generation HI receptor antagonists have previously been used in this indication.

Pruritus in atopic dermatitis was significantly reduced by the 20 and 40 mg. dosages of cetirizine and the 40 mg. dosage also significantly reduced erythema, lichenification and area of involvement and total symptoms score (Hannucksela et al. 1992).

In a 4 week double blind multicentre study, cetirizine 10 mg. twice daily was compared with terfenadine 60 mg. twice daily in the treatment of 168 adult patients with atopic eczema. There was marked improvement in pruritus and in activity and extent of eczematous skin lesions, with both drugs. Therapeutic benefit, as assessed by its investigators and patients, was significantly greater with cetirizine than terfenadine (Behrendt & Ring 1990).

Anti Allergic Properties

Cetirizine 10 mg. daily reduced the cutaneous reactions induced by pollens or histamine and inhibited the migration of eosinophils to the allergic site (Charlesworth et al. 1989, Fadel et al. 1987, 1988, 1989).

Cetirizine pre-treatment, at the same dosage also inhibited anti-IgE-induced accumulation of eosinophils in 10 atopic subjects (Rihoux et al. 1990a). Such inhibition of eosinophil accumulation probably accounts for the clinical effects of cetirizine on the late phase allergic response (Charlesworth et al. 1989).

Following cutaneous allergen challenges, cetirizine inhibited late-phase, but not immediate, histamine release from mast cells but release of prostaglandin D2 was not. Thus cetirizine has no direct effect on mast cells (Michel et al.1988, 1989, 1990).

Cetirizine inhibits migration of eosinophils by a local action unrelated to H1 receptor antagonism or direct effects on circulating eosinophils (Martins et al. 1992).

IgE dependent activation of blood platelets, a mechanism which may contribute to the allergic reaction, was inhibited in vitro by therapeutic concentrations of Cetirizine (Joseph et al 1989). The drug may have a direct effect on platelet (Coyle et al 1991).

Mosquito Bites

The cutaneous response to mosquito bites varies from wheal & flare reactions and delayed papules to severe Arthrus type reactions, with even small lesions producing intense pruritus.

Cetirizine 10 mg. daily significantly reduced immediate wheal and flare responses in volunteers exposed to mosquitoes but had no significant effect on delayed symptoms (Reunala et al. 1991).

In another study both immediate wheal and flare and the delayed papules were significantly reduced by pretreatment with Cetirizine 10 mg. daily. Additionally pruritus was also markedly reduced (Reunala et al. 1992).

Contraindications & Precautions

Cetirizine is contraindicated in patients with a history of hypersensitivity to the drug.

In pregnancy and lactation Cetirizine should be avoided, though no adverse effects have been reported in animal studies.

Conclusions

Cetirizine is a piperazine derivative and a carboxylated metabolite of hydroxyzine. It is a long-acting peripheral histamine H1 receptor antagonist with a relative absence of adverse CNS effects Cetirizine is more potent than chlorpheniramine, clemastine, terfenadine, astemizole loratadine, ebastine, oxatomide and ketotifen in reducing histamine induced wheal & flare in volunteers or patients.

A novel feature of cetirizine is that it inhibits the recruitment of infiltrating inflammatory cells during the cutaneous allergic responses. This property is partially due to a direct effect on eosinophils. Such characteristics makes it useful in ameliorating the late phase allergic inflammatory changes which are intimately linked to the release of mediators from cells recruited to the immunologically stimulated sites and which may be responsible for the chronic nature of severe allergic problems.

References:

1. Alomar A. De La Cuaudra J. Fernandez J. Cetirizine vs. astemizole in the treatment of chronic idiopathic urticaria Journal of International Medical Research 18:358-365, 1990.

2. Behrendt H. Ring J. Histamine, antihistamines and atopic eczema. Clinical and Experimental Allergy 20 (Suppl. 4) 25-30, 1990.

3. Breneman D. Bergstresser P. Boggs P. et al. A multi-site comparative study of the efficacy and safety of cetirizine vs astemizole and placebo in the treatment of chronic .idiopathic urticaria. Abstr. 418. Journal of Allergy and Clinical Immunology 89:249, 1992.

4. Canonica GW. Ciprandi G. Bagnasco M. Allergic reaction and adhesion molecules

International Academy for Biomedical and Drug Research, Monte Carlo, November 1992, p.p. 51,53.

5. Charlesworth EN., Kagey-Sabotka A. Norman "PS. Lichtenstein LM. Effect of cetirizine on mast cell-mediator release and cellular traffic during the cutaneous late-phase reaction Journal of Allergy and Clinical Immunology, 83, 905-912, 1989.

6. Coyle AJ, Lefort J. Vargaftig BB. The effect of cetirizine on antigen - dependent leucopenia in the guinea-pig. British Journal of Pharmacology 103 : 1520-1524, 1991.

7. De Vos C. Maleux MR, Baltes E. Gobert G. Inhibition of histamine skin wheal in four animal species. Annals of Allergy 50: 278-282, 1987.

8. Fadel R. Herpin - Richard N. Rihoux JP. Henocq E. Inhibitory effect of cetirizine 2HCL on eosinophil migration in vivo Clinical Allergy 17: 373-379, 1987.

9. Fadel R. Herpin - Richard N. Rihoux JP. Henocq E. Effect of cetirizine on in vivo cutaneous leucocytes migration in allergic rhinitis. Journal of Allergy and Clinical Immunology 81: 178, 1988.

10. Fadel R. Herpin - Richard N. Rihoux JP. Henocq E. Inhibition by cetirizine 2HCL of antigen - induced eosinophil migration in allergic subjects Health Science Review 3. 11-13, 1989.

11. Fadel R. David B. Herpin - Richard N. et al. In vivo effects of cetirizine on cutaneous reactivity and eosinophil migration induced by platelet - activating factor (PAF - acether) in man. Journal of Allergy and Clinical immunology 86: 314-320. 1990.

12. Gibson PG, Delovich J. Girgis - Gabardo A et al. The inflammatory response in asthma exacerbation changes in circulating eosinophils, basophils and their progenitors. Clinical and Experimental Allergy 20: 661-668, 1990.

13. Gleich GJ. The eosinophil and bronchial asthma; current understanding Journal of Allergy and Clinical Immunology 85: 422-436. 1990a.

14. Gleich GJ. The role of eosinophils in allergic disease. Current concepts in the treatment of allergic disorders. Baltimore 28 March, 1990 pp. 6-7, Adis International 1990b.

15. Goh CL. Wong WK, Lim J. Cetirizine vs placebo in chronic idiopathic urticaria — a double blind randomised cross-over study.

Annals of the Academy of Medicine 20: 328-330,1991.

16. Hanifin JM. Rajka G. Diagnostic features of atopic dermatitis. Acta Dermatovenereologica (Suppl.) 92: 44-47, 1980.

17. Hannucksela M. Kalimo K. Lammintausta K. et. al. Dose ranging study; cetirizine in the treatment of atopic dermatitis in adults. Annals of Allergy 69, 1992.

18. Hansel TT, Walker C. The migration of eosinophil into the sputum of asthmatics the role of adhesion molecules. Clinical and Experimental Allergy 22 : 345-356, 1992.

19. Henocq E. Vargaftig BB. Skin eosinophllia in atopic patients. Journal of Allergy and Clinical immunology 81: 691-695, 1988.

20. Joseph M. Vorng H. Lassalle P. et al. In vitro activity of cetirizine on platelets. Health Science Review 3: 8-10, 1989.

21. Juhlin L. Arendt C. Treatment of chronic urticaria and cetirizine dihydrochloride a non-sedating antihistamine. British Journal of Dermatology 119: 67-72, 1988.

22. Kaliner M. Lemanske R. Rhinitis and asthma. Journal of the American Medical Association 268 : 2807-2829, 1992.

23. Kay AB. The role of the eosinophil. Journal of Allergy and Clinical Immunology 64 : 90-104, 1979.

24. Kay AB. Modulation of eosinophil function in vitro. Clinical and Experimental Allergy 20 (suppl. 4): 31-34, 1990.

25. Losewicz S. Davies RJ. Inflammatory cells in allergic rhinitis. Respiratory Medicine 85: 259-261. 1991.

26. Macher E. Eichelberg D. Terfenadine and cetirizine in chronic idiopathic urticaria; p. 91. Allergologie abstracts to the XIV congress of the European Academy of Allegology and Clinical Immunology, Berlin, 1989.

27. Martins MA. Pasquale CP. Silva PMR. et al. Interference of cetirizine with the late eosinophil accumulation induced by either PAF or compound 48/80. British Journal of Pharmacology 105: 176-180, 1992.

28. Michel L. De Vos C. Rihoux JP. et al. Inhibitory effect of oral cetirizine on in vivo antigen-induced histamine and PAF-acether

release and eosinophil recruitment in human skin. Journal of Allergy and Clinical Immunology 82 : 101-109, 1988.

29. Michel L. Jeanlouis F. Burtin C. et al. Measurement of cetirizine effects on protein diffusion, mediator release and eosinophil recruitment during in vivo anaphylactic cutaneous reactions. Health Science Review 3(1): 14-17, 1989.

30. Michel L. De Vos C. Dubertret L. Cetirizine effects on the cutaneous allergic reaction in humans. Annals of Allergy 65 : 512-516, 1990.

31. Rajka G. Natural history and clinical manifestations of atopic dermatitis. Clinical Reviews in Allergy 4 : 3-26, 1986.

32. Reunala T. Lappalainen P. Brummer Korvenkontio H. et al. Cutaneous reactivity to mosquito bites; effect of cetirizine and development of anti-mosquito antibodies. Clinical and Experimental Allergy 2 : 617-622, 1991.

33. Reunala T. Brummer-Korvenkontio H. Karppinen A. et al. Treatment of mosquito bites with cetirizine. Clinical and Experimental Allergy 22, 1992.

Keloids and Hypertrophic Scars A Therapeutic Enigma

Ajay Chaudhary, Ram Malkani

The Bombay Hospital Journal Vol. 39 No. 3 July 1997 p.548.

INTRODUCTION

The biochemical process of wound repair normally culminates in fine line scars as the only evidence of dermal injury. In certain individuals, however the repair process may go away and wounds may heal with large, raised collagenous scars known as keloids or hypertrophic scars. These abnormal scars are variations of a normal wound healing process. Keloids frequently persist at the site of injury, often recur after excision, and always overgrow the boundaries of the original wound. In contrast, hypertrophic scars, although often red and raised, remain within the confines of the original wound and tend to regress over an extended period.

AETIOLOGY

For unknown reasons, keloid and hypertrophic scars formation is unique to man. Despite numerous studies, there is no valid theory or explanation to indicate which factor(s) initiate keloid or hypertrophic scar formation. Proposed causes of abnormal scar formation have included foreign body reaction, bacterial infection, or the possibility that degraded or denatured collagen serves as a catalyst to scar hyperplasia. HLA types seems to be unrelated. However, family members are commonly afflicted. The role of immune system in abnormal scar formation is unclear. Initial studies that showed increased IgG and C1q complement component, immune lymphocyte characterisation failed to demonstrate cellular, systemic or local immunologic factors in keloid formation. Other possible causes of keloid formation include thyroid hormone alteration, ingrown hairs and excessive melanocyte stimulating hormone production. Again, none of the hypothesis have ever been validated.

TREATMENT

Several forms of treatment have been utilised for keloids and hypertrophic scars, with varying degrees of success. At an early stage the clinician should ascertain whether the patient's objective is to eradicate the esthetic and/or functional deformity, to prevent recurrence by surgery with adjuvant pharmacologic therapy or whether the objective is merely to ameliorate the physical discomfort and itching. Both the clinician and patient must accept the reality that neither pharmacological intervention nor surgical skill will ensure total cure or prevention.

RADIATION

Immature dividing fibroblasts are particularly vulnerable to the ionizing effects of radiation and are either killed or sterilized, preventing further multiplication of the treated cells. This effect is both permanent and additive. Irradiation is only effective in newly forming scars, in an individual who has a diathesis to keloid that cannot be managed with the use of steroids and pressure alone. Irradiation is not indicated in the treatment of scars in children or in any growing tissue. Furthermore it is inconvenient and is an added expense to the surgical procedure. Surgical excision alone rates for 55% to 100%. However, when results in recurrence patients are treated with irradiation following surgery, the overall control rate was found to be around 73%. 100 to 600 cGy doses for a total of 1000-1500 cGy over a period of 3 to 20 days is recommended starting from the 3rd postoperative day.

MECHANICAL PRESSURE

Mechanical pressure has been reported to inhibit hypertrophic scar formation. Larsson and colleagues have shown that pressure reorients collagen bundles parallel to the surface of skin. It has also been hypothesized that mechanical pressure altered the glycosaminoglycan content and blood vessel permeability of the healing wound. Others suggested that mechanical pressure increases tissue collagenase activity which in turn prevents excess collagen deposition. The exact mechanism of action of pressure is unknown; but it is thought that hypoxia may play a causative role in these effects.

The simplest way of applying pressure is to place a piece of foam rubber directly over the exact dimensions of the scar; then compress it with an elastic bandage. Alternatively, the patient can be measured for a custom fitted elastic garment that fits snugly over the contour of the scar involved. Although the skin must be cleaned from time to time, pressure cannot be relieved for more than 30 minutes.

The great advantage in the use of pressure in the treatment of abnormal scars is that large areas can be treated with this modality. There are definite disadvantages, however, that it must be maintained continuously for a minimum of 9 Months and premature release is frequently followed by recurrence of the lesion. Secondly it usually isolates the patient, with obvious psychological disadvantage. In addition, in warm weather, the use of such compression bandage is uncomfortable.

PHARMACOLOGICAL

a. Triamcinolone

Triamcinolone is a powerful anti-inflammatory agent. When injected into the edges of a newly made wound, it modifies the inflammatory response; whereas if injected into an established hypertrophic scar, it activates the endogenous collagenase. It is often not possible to instill much fluid into the scar at the time of first injection; thus a priming dose is required, whereby the material is injected directly under the skin. In about 3 weeks, the scar will begin to respond by becoming softer. Steroids can now be instilled in a greater quantity into the scar. A series of injections over a period of months may be required to achieve a soft, flat scar. All the complications such as atrophy of the normal tissue around and under the scar, telangiectasia, and depigmentation are caused by over dosage instillation of the drug into the normal tissue.

Dosage Schedule for Triamcinolone

Age of patient and size of lesion	Dosage
1 to 5 years	40 mg. (Max.)
6 to 10 years	80 mg. (Max.)
ADULT	
1-2 sq. cm. lesion	20-40 mg.
2-6 sq. cm.	40-80 mg.
6-10 sq cm. or larger	80-120 mg.

A maximum dose of 120 mg. should not be exceeded in an one month period.

b. Retinoic Acid

Retinoic acid is known to inhibit fibroblast proliferation. Retinoic acid also reduces the rate of synthesis of collagen. Topical retinoic acid in varying concentration can be used as priming agents in the treatment of keloids.

Retinoic acid when used in combination with topical steroid causes the keloids to become softer; thus facilitating the use of triamcinolone. However, use of retinoic acid is also associated with mild side effects like pruritus, burning sensation and erythema and secondary bacterial infections.

c. Vitamin E, Pentoxyphyline

Palmieri B in 1995 showed that use of Vitamin E in combination with silicon gives better results as compared to the use of silicon alone.

In vivo studies where fibroblasts were cultured and treated with 100-1000 ug/ml pentoxyphylline showed that pentoxyphylline caused inhibition of proliferation of human fibroblasts. It also caused inhibition of fibronectin

production. It had no effect on the collagenous
activity.

d. Amino-Propionitrile (BAPN), Penicillamine

These drugs prevent collagen cross linking and render
the collagen molecule more susceptible to enzymatic
degradation. At present, long term use of these systemic
drugs is clearly not the answer to the control of abnormal
scar because of its generalised side effects.

SURGERY

The use of sound surgical principles and atraumatic
technique is absolutely essential in the prevention and
treatment of abnormal scar. In addition, surgery is also
helpful in reducing the size of an established keloid,
rendering it more amenable to treatment by pressure,
steroids, or irradiation. The only occasion in which surgery
alone would be indicated is in reorienting the direction of
the scar if the direction is perpendicular to the line of relaxed
skin tension (Langer's line), or if the scar is the result of an
infection.

CRYOTHERAPY

Increasing knowledge in the field of cryobiology, together
with the development of sophisticated cryoprobes and
liquid gas jets has led to a great increase in the use of
cryotherapy.

Amongst, the wide spectrum of skin lesions which, have
been treated with freezing is keloids. The cryogenic agents

commonly available are liquid nitrogen (boiling point -196°C), nitrous oxide gas (-89.5°C) and solid carbon dioxide (-78.5°C).

However, liquid nitrogen is nowadays most commonly used. Liquid nitrogen is universally available and is cheap. It is unstable at room temperature. A one litre unsealed flask full of liquid nitrogen will last a full day and treat 50-60 patients. It can be used either by cotton wool swabs cooper discs or by cryoprobes.

The exact mechanism of action of cryosurgery in the treatment of keloids is unclear. Probably freezing the keloid cause the lesion to become oedematous and less dense during thawing. Repeated use of cryotherapy every 2-3 weeks is helpful in the treatment of keloid. Cryotherapy can be continued till complete cure is achieved. The success rate of use of cryotherapy alone was found to be around 45% and that of a combination of cryotherapy along with triamcinolone is found to be much higher at around 73%.

Transient pain, oedema, blister formation, paraesthesia, and hypopigmentation are some of the side effects seen with use of cryogenic agents.

LASERS

Lasers mainly the low energy type are recently been used in the management of keloids. Low energy laser therapy (LELT) is used on the principle of "Bioinhibition" i.e. there is inhibition of fibroblast proliferation and dissolution of collagen tissue. The energy density used varies from 9-12J and it takes 15 to 25 minutes per exposure per keloid and on the area/size of the keloid. After about 3-4 exposures, patient reports marked improvement in the severity of itching. The frequency of exposure is daily for at least the first 12 weeks. However, depending on the progress, the frequency can be changed to alternate days. The total duration of treatment is at least 8-10 week.

The keloid during the course of treatment becomes soft in consistency and at this point of time, intralesional steroids can be given easily to ensure complete cure of the disease. LELT being totally non-invasive carries no risk of infection.

SILICON GEL AND SILASTIC GEL SHEET

Silastic gel sheet (SGS) is a soft, semiocclusive scar cover made up of cross liked polydimethyl siloxane polymer. It was first reported to be an effective treatment for burn scars and contractures in 1982. The water vapour transmission rate of SGS is half as compared to that of skin. Thus SGS probably acts by affecting scar hydration; thereby reducing water vapour loss. This is postulated to decrease capillary activity thereby reducing collagen deposition and scar hypertrophy.

Silicon gel also acts by hydration of epidermis and by cellular effect of release of low molecular weight silicon fluid into the tissue.

The shiny surface of the sheet is placed in contact with the skin and is attached with a dermatologic surgical tape. Patient is asked to wear the gel sheet for 24 hours. The material is washed daily with soap and water solution and is replaced at 7-10 days later. The results are seen after at least 2 months of use.

Minor complications like superficial maceration, foul smell, pruritus and rash have been reported. However, the problem resolves when the gel sheet is removed temporarily or its duration of use is reduced to 12 hours/day.

COMBINATION

Morbid fibrosis resulting from extensive keloids is the only indication where a combination of all the modalities can be used. In such an individual, it may be necessary to reduce the bulk of keloid by a surgical excision, eliminate tension of the wound; inject the wound edges with triamcinolone, irradiate the wound or use cryotherapy and then apply pressure.

Although the biochemical and histological puzzles of abnormal scar formation are slowly being solved, question still remains regarding the clinical findings in abnormal scars e.g.

1. Why do certain individuals seem more likely to produce keloids and hypertrophic scars?

2. Why certain areas are more prone than other in the same individual?

3. Why do abnormal scars form after one type of injury but not after another type in the same person?

Thus, though newer therapeutic modalities are being made use of, answers to some of these questions still remain a mystery.

REFERENCES

1. McCarthy JC. "Plastic Surgery"; Edition. 1990;
732-46.

2. Mercer SG. Silicone gel in the treatment of
Keloid scars. Br J Plast Surg 1989; 42 : 83-87.

3. Goldschmidt, el al. Ionizing radiation therapy
in dermatology. J Am Acad Dermatol 1991; 30 :
177.

4. Zoufoulis CC, et al. Outcome of Cryosurgery
in Keloid and Hypertrophic scars - A prospective
consecutive trial of case series. Arch Dermatol
Sept 1993; 129(9): 1146-51.

5. Palmieri B, Gozzi G, Palmieri G. Int J
Dermatol July 1995; 34 (7): 506-9.

6. Korepanov V. Applications of LASERS in
Cosmetology. 1995.

Lasers in Dermatology

Maithili Shrikhande, Ram Malkani

Bulletin of The Jaslok Hospital And Research Centre Vol. XXV No. 2 2000 p 15

Laser technology in medicine is evolving at a rapid pace, allowing further advances in the treatment of dermatologic diseases as well as improvements in cosmetic procedures.

Laser is an acronym for Light Amplification by the Stimulated Emission of Radiation. Maiman produced the first working laser, which was a Ruby laser. Goldmann performed the first dermatological application of laser in 1963.

Laser is a light source, which consists of a beam of tightly bundled light. This beam comprises of activated photons, which are identical in phase, frequency and direction and are coherent too. The monochromatic wavelength of light emitted from a laser can be used in selecting specific chromophores as targets within skin. Lasers are named after the lasing medium used to produce light. This medium could be in a solid state, for e.g. Ruby or a liquid e.g. dye or a gas for e.g. Argon or Carbon Dioxide etc.

Different lasers that are used in dermatology are:

Carbon dioxide (10,600 nm); Erb: YAG (Erbium Yttrium Aluminium Garnet) (2640 nm); Nd: YAG (Neodymiun Yttrium Aluminium Garnet) (1064 nm); Frequency-doubled Nd: YAG (532 nm); Diode (810 nm); Alexandrite (755 nm); Ruby (694 nm); Argon and Copper vapour (575/585 nm); Pulsed tuneable dye (585 nm)

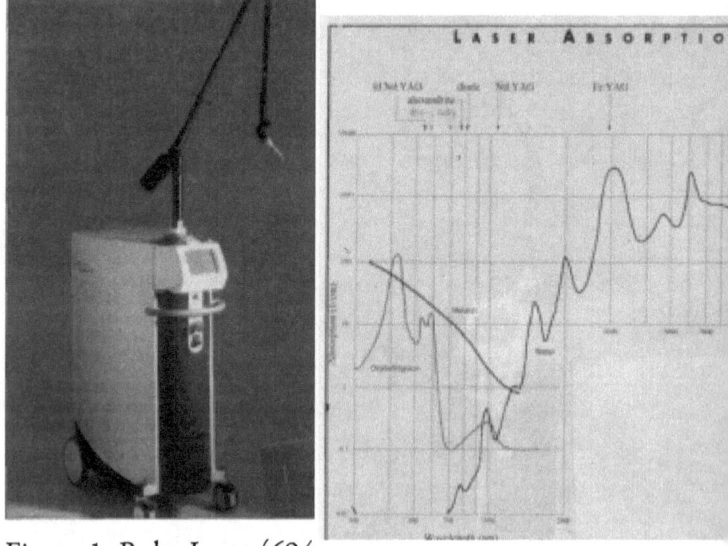

Figure 1: Ruby Laser (694 nm) machine for permanent hair removal

Figure 2: Various wavelengths with affinity for different chromophores

The mechanism of action of lasers is based on the principle of selective photothermolysis, i.e. the light energy is converted into heat energy upon tissue absorption and the heat generated brings about dessication, coagulation or vapourisation.

Various wavelengths have affinity for different chromophores (targets) within the skin. The green & yellow light lasers i.e. lasers with a wavelength of less than 600 nm e.g. Pulsed dye, Argon and Copper lasers and frequency doubled Nd: YAG lasers have an affinity for oxyhaemoglobin and hence can be used for cutaneous vascular lesions. The red and infrared light lasers like Ruby, Alexandrite, Diode and Nd: YAG lasers have an affinity for melanin and also for oxyhaemoglobin. These lasers can be used for pigmentary and vascular disorders and for hair removal. The long wavelength lasers like Carbon dioxide and Erb: YAG are used for skin resurfacing.

It is vital to understand some basic terms that are used routinely while discussing lasers.

Wavelength is the frequency of the monochromatic light. It is expressed in nanometres; larger the wavelength, deeper is the skin penetration. As explained earlier, certain wavelengths have affinity for certain chromophores within the skin.

Spot diameter is the diameter of the probe, through which the laser beam passes and enters the skin. Larger the spot size deeper is the penetration, but also more is the scattering of photons.

Pulse duration or pulse width is the time duration for which the laser energy is in contact with the target in the skin. It ranges from nanoseconds to microseconds to milliseconds.

The laser energy that is delivered is in Joules.

Fluence is energy density i.e. energy in Joules per cm

Cooling devices are an integral part of any laser system. There is a tendency for accumulation of laser energy near the skin surface for scattered media, resulting in unwanted epidermal heating which if not prevented could lead to either hypopigmentation or hyperpigmentation, blistering and crusting.

The types of cooling are:

1) Passive cooling with refrigerated ultrasound gel applied on the skin to be treated

2) Active cooling with water in glass window

3) Active cooling with water in sapphire window

4) Dynamic active cooling with cryogenic spray

There has been a great increase in the number of lasers and their applications in dermatology over recent years. It is useful to group them by their clinical applications, which are as follows.

1) Lasers for treatment of cutaneous vascular lesion (superficial lesions & leg vein telangiectasias)

2) Lasers for treatment of cutaneous pigmented lesions and tattoos

3) Skin resurfacing and ablative lasers

4) Lasers for hair removal

1) Lasers for treatment of cutaneous vascular lesion

The choice of laser to be used for vascular lesions depends on the diameter and the depth of the target vessel. Larger the diameter and deeper the target vessel, a laser with longer wavelength and also a longer pulsewidth is required for treatment.

a) Superficial vascular lesions:

• The target for treatment of superficial vascular lesions, for e.g. PWS or haemangiomas or telangiectasias is oxyhaemoglobin. The lasers with an affinity for these vessels need a shorter wavelength and shorter pulse duration i.e. a wavelength of less than 600 nm, which means green-yellow light lasers. The pulse duration is in nanoseconds and microseconds.

• The Pulsed tuneable dye laser with a wavelength of 585nm is safe for use in children, but has bruising as a side effect. The risk of scarring happens to be less than 1%, more so on the neck region.

• The other yellow and green light lasers are the argon pumped dye (577/585 nm),copper vapour and frequency doubled Nd:YAG (532 nm) laser.

The advantage of these lasers is the absence of bruising.

• Though primarily and widely used in the treatment of PWS, haemangiomas and telangiectasias, vascular lasers have been tried in warts, hypertrophic scarring and with doubtful benefits in striae and superficial rhytids.

b) Leg vein telangiectasias

• These vessels are larger and deeper and also less oxygenated. Therefore longer wavelengths and longer pulse duration's are required. Also higher atuence i.e. energy density is necessary and this warrants the need for good epidermal cooling system.

• The lasers used are the long pulsed dye (532 nm) with pulse duration of 1.5-4.0 milliseconds.

• The long pulsed Nd:YAG (1064 nm) or frequency doubled Nd:YAG (532 nm) with pulse width of 1-50 milliseconds are also used. Lasers having a wavelength of more than 600 nm for e.g. Alexandrite (755 nm) and Diode (810 nm), which also have an affinity for melanin can be used with longer pulse duration.

• There are a few, if at all, any controlled, long term studies to demonstrate the efficiency of lasers in treatment of leg veins and very often sclerotherapy remains the treatment of choice. Hence, in patients with a contraindication to sclerotherapy, or when the vessels are resistant to or are too small to cannulate or in needle phobic patients, lasers can be considered.

2) Lasers for the treatment of pigmented lesions and tattoos

• Because melanin absorbs over broad spectrum, a variety of lasers with different wavelengths can be used. Targetting of melanosomes within cells requires pulse durations in the domain of nanoseconds. Basically high energy, short pulses are necessary, which is achieved by the mechanism of Q-switching.

• The Q-switched ruby (694 nm) can treat lentigenes, freckles and blue-black with some green tatoos.

• Q-switched Nd:YAG (1064 nm) can treat dermal pigmented lesions like naevus of Ota because longer wave lengths penetrate deeper.

• For epidermal lesions like freckles and lentigo and red tatoo inks, the 532 nm frequency doubled Nd:YAG can be used.

- Q-switched Alexandrite can treat cafe-au-lait spots and green and blue-black inks.

3) Lasers in skin resurfacing

- They can be classified as ablative and nonablative lasers. The nonablative lasers e.g. Diode, NdrYAG, Flash Lamp Pulsed Dye and Intense pulsed light are under study.

- Amongst the ablative lasers, there are Carbon dioxide (CO2) and ERBIUM

- YAG lasers are with a longer wavelength of 10,600 and 2,940 nm respectively. They have affinity for water within the dermis. CC>2 has the advantage of haemostasis along with its resurfacing action. A CC-2 laser can be used in a focussed mode for haemostatic tissue cutting or in a defocussed, broad beam mode for skin resurfacing. The clinical improvement with CC>2 laser, although better than Erb:YAG, leads to more morbidity post- operatively. Erb:YAG has 10-15 times more affinity for water, offers shorter healing period but lacks haemostasis. Combining both lasers has proved beneficial.

4) Lasers for Hair removal

- The most rapidly evolving area in cutaneous laser surgery is lasers for hair removal. All these lasers target the follicular melanin.

- Best results are seen in fair skinned with dark hair, where the epidermal melanin would escape and the hair would be attacked.

- Repeated treatments are necessary for reduction in hair-growth.

- The laser treatment should be carried out when the hair are in the ANAGEN PHASE (growth-phase) of the hair cycle.

- Ruby laser (694 nm) has the highest affinity for melanin and thereby very effective, but one needs to be cautious with its use in dark skin.

- The other hair lasers are Alexandrite (755 nm) and Diode (810 nm), which allow more flexibility in treatment of darker skins also, the results with NdrYAG (1064 nm) have not been very encouraging so far.

- It is important to understand the concept of Thermal relaxation time (TRT) in hair removal. TRT is the time taken for a particular skin structure to come back to normal body temperature after exposure to the laser heat. For a laser to effectively epilate hair without attacking the epidermal melanin, the pulse width of the laser used should exceed the TRT of the epidermis but be less than that of the hair bulb.

Intense pulsed light

A number of broad band light sources have been marketed. These are not lasers, but flash lamps emitting non-coherent light. The operator has the option of selecting a particular wavelength range with the help of certain filters. Thus multiple treatment options are available i.e. the same machine could be used for vascular, pigmentary and / or hair disorder.

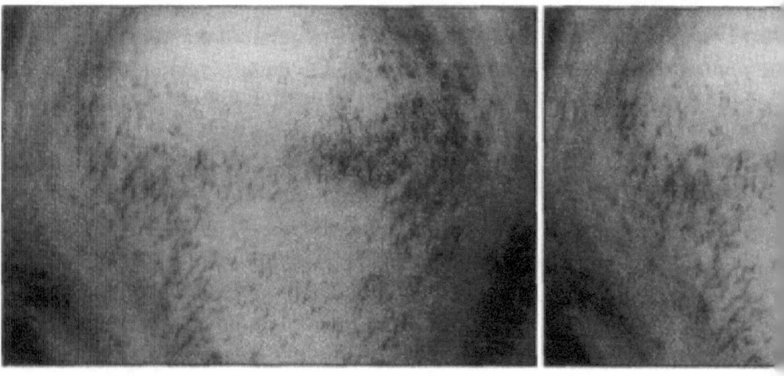

Figure 3a: A case of PCOD with Hirsuitism (Pretreatment)

Figure 3b: Posttre with Ruby Laser)

Lasers have a tremendous potential in dermatotherapeutics and the burgeoning are of laser treatment continues to expand. However, we must bear in mind that much of this rapid expansion is probably market-driven. More machines and more applications will undoubtedly appear in the coming years. It remains to be seen whether these promising advances stand the true test of time.

References

1) Sean W. Lanigan. Recent Developments in the use of Lasers in Dermatology, pp 25-29. In: Current Medical Literature"Dermatology (International Literature Review Service); Vol.5, No.2; 2000.

2) Hair restoration and Laser Hair Removal, pp 334-429. In: Dermatologic Clinics; Vol.17, No.2; April 1999.

3) Tina S. Alster. The Evolution of Laser-Assisted Hair Removal, pp 15-18. In: Cosmetic Dermatology; August 1999.

4) Lowe NJ et al. Nevus of Ota: Treatment with High Energy Fluences of the Q-Switched Ruby Laser, pp 997-1001. In: J Am Acad Dermatolo; Vol.29; 1993.

5) Ferguson JE et al. Evaluation of the Nd:YAG Laser for Treatment of Amateur and Profes sional Tattoos, pp 586-591. In: Br J Dermatol; Vol. 135; 1996.

6) Alster TS et al. Treatment of Facial Rhytides with a High-Energy Pulsed Carbon Dioxide La

ser, pp 791-794. In: Plast Reconstr Surg; Vol.98;
1996.

Psychogenic Pruritus - an overview

Farida Modi, Ram Malkani

Bulletin of The Jaslok Hospital And
Research Centre; Vol. XXV No. 3 2001
p14

Pruritus or itching can be simply defined as a cutaneous sensation that produces a desire to scratch.

Pruritus can be divided into three groups:

Group I: Pruritus of organic origin (in which group A refers to itching due to internal causes and group B to the various itchy dermatoses which have no primary emotional factors) e.g.: drug/food induced urticaria, scabies, contact dermatitis.

Group II: Pruritus of psychosomatic origin (those dermatoses where itching is related to primary emotional factors and there is presence of both primary skin lesions and emotional factors.) e.g.: urticaria, atopic eczema, etc.

Group III: Psychogenic pruritus (this is determined only by primary emotional factors and there is no primary cutaneous lesions)

Many dermatologists and psychiatrists as well, are unaware of the difference between the term psychosomatic and psychogenie. "Psychosomatic" is a disorder caused by the interaction of emotion and organic factors and "psychogenic" is a disorder caused by purely emotional factors. Hence, the term "psychogenic" is often applied erroneously to many dermatoses which are actually psychosomatic in origin.

Table 1: Organic causes of pruritus

- Hepatic disease
- Renal disease
- Infection
- Bacterial
- Parasitic
- HIV
- Food/drug allergy
- Diabetes
- Carcinoid
- Hyper/ hypothyroidism
- Polycythemia vera
- Malignancy
- Lymphoma
- Leukaemia
- Myeloma
- Atopy/ dermatographism
- Collagen vascular disease
- Xerosis

Thus psychogenic pruritus is defined in dermatology as a symptom caused by emotional factors, characterized by absence of primary skin lesions and occasionally by the presence of secondary skin lesions. Psychogenic pruritus thus becomes a diagnosis of exclusion where all organic causes and psychosomatic pruritus is excluded.

Psychological basis of pruritus is suggested by the fact that intensity parallels the emotional state, it is evoked by mention or thought and conversely distraction can make it disappear, it rarely prevents sleep.

Four major groups of psychological investigations have dealt with this problem.

The "ethologist" tends to ascribe scratching in animals, including man, to frustation and blocking of drive states.

The "psychoanalyst" tend to relate scratching behaviour to thwarted emotions arising from psychosexual complexities or to anxiety due to repressed, socially unacceptable drives.

The "behaviourists" have been interested in the scratch itch scratch cycle producing a habit pattern.

The "trait theorist" have attributed pruritus syndromes to constitutional predisposition, a hyper irritable autonomic nervous system, and to certain types of personality structure.

A study on the psychological profiles of such pruritus have shown the subjects to have a very strong feeling of self worth which is juxtaposed with a low objective feeling based on experience and judgement of others. This leads to individual's hostile behaviour towards his environment and assumes an aspect of "authentic intolerance". The personality of pruritus patient is that of constrained character but with egoistic character.

In some cases of senile pruritus, pruritus seems to be connected with common sociopsychological conditions like: emargination, isolation, sense of uselessness, frustration, depression resulting in diffuse or localised itching.The various psychological causes associated with psychogenic pruritus are anxiety disorders, depression disorders, obsessive disorders, personality disorders, psychosis and habit. Psychogenic Pruritus can present either as generalised pruritus or localised pruritus (pruritus ani or pruritus vulvae)

Generalised psychogenic pruritus:

In this type an early unsatisfactory mother child interactions in the background of many patients is believed to be significant. Guilt, anger, boredom, irritation and sexual arousal all predispose to itching.

Pruritus ani: Some investigators believe that compliance with or opposition to parental dictates regarding bowel training is the basis of character traits of many patients. Fixation at or regression to this anal stage of development leads to conflicts frequently involving sadistic impulses. Being intolerable, these impulses lead to defences like reaction formation, manifesting as gentleness and subservience toward authority. Scratching may become a manifestation of this aggression towards self. It may be both pleasurable and self punitive components. Defective heterosexual relationships are common in these patients and the fact that men are predominantly affected confirms the view that the anus is the site of expression of latent homosexuality. Patients are often depressed, feel 'dirty' with low self esteem and impaired sexual and family relationships.

Pruritus vulvae: Most patients have a long history of sexual frustration that frequently intensifies with the onset of pruritus. They may regress to masturbatory level of psychosexual development at times of intense frustation, but this leads to a self punitive feeling due to guilt. The pruritus vulvae thus strikes a balance between pleasure and pain.

Approach to the patient with psychogenic pruritus

The patients with psychogenic pruritus should be approached with the same objectively derived list of differential diagnoses and comprehensive treatment plan given to any other patient. Labels such as "psychogenic" frequently handicap the physicians ability to think critically and objectively about the causes of a symptom. It should be remembered that even crazy patients develop real organic illnesses and thus casual dismissal of complaints of these patients can result in oversights.

Evaluation and treatment options:

The therapy need not include lengthy psychotherapy sessions for meaningful therapeutic benefit to occur. The power of a strong doctor - patient alliance and emotional support from the physician cannot be overstated. This can be accomplished utilizing a "listen, ask and then tell" approach.

Most of the information regarding the personality and emotional state of the patient can be obtained from simply "listening" for a few minutes during which a patient typically describes the symptoms. Once some basic impression has been formed, the differential diagnosis can be refined by "asking" a few well focused questions. These questions are specifically designed to asses whether there is clinically significant anxiety, obsessive - compulsive disorder, depression or psychoses that need treatment. Finally, a few crucial things should be communicated to all patients with psychogenic pruritus. They need to be "told" and to feel that the intensity of their discomfort is genuinely understood, that their symptoms are taken seriously, and most important, that they will be helped to gain back "control".

Psychopharmacologic interventions:

The judicious use of psychopharmacologic agents can be effective in ameliorating symptoms of anxiety, depression, obsessive compulsive disorder, and psychoses that can be contributing to the patients pruritus - although an argument can be made that these agents may best be prescribed by a psychiatrist, it is within the scope of dermatology to use selected agents as part of a comprehensive treatment regimens perhaps more importantly, many patients in need of psychopharmacologic intervention refuse psychiatric referral and therefore will be denied this treatment if it is not provided by the dermatologist. Dermatologic patients can often be helped by lower dosing regimens than those used for psychiatric patient. The need for lower dosages may be a function of the antipruritic and sedating properties of many of these agents. Good results can often be achieved with the use of a sedating antihistaminic agent at night when pruritus is often most intense.

Table IV: If depression appears prominent, consider...

Drug	Starting dose	Antidepressant dose
Doxepin	25-50 mgq.h.s.	150 mg q.d.
Nortriptyline	50 - 75 mg q.h.s.	75 - 150 mg q.d.
Amitriptyline	25 - 50 mg q.h.s.	100- 300 mg q.d.
Fluoxetine	20 mg q. A.M.	20 - 40 mg q.d.
Sertraline	550 mgq. A.M.	50 - 100 mgq.d.

9. AM Each morning: q.d. - daily q.h.s. - each bedtime

Table V: If anxiety appears prominent, consider....

Drug	Dosage	Comment
Buspirone	5 mg t.i.d.	Increase 5 mg q. 2-3 days to 15 mg t.i.d. max.
Diphenhydramine	25-50 mg q. 6h.	Sedating, antipruritic
Hydroxyzine	25-50 mg q. 6h	Sedating, antipruritic
Doxepin	10-50 mg q.h.s.	Sedating, antipruritic
Clomipramine	25 mg q.d.	For Rx of obsessive-compulsive disorder: increase over 2 weeks to 100 mg q.d.
Alprazolam	0.25-0.5 mg t.i.d.	Addictive potential

Table VI: If delusional ideation appears prominent, consider....

Drug	Dosage	Comment
Pimozide	1-2 mg q.d.	Max. 4-6 mg q.d. Baseline and repeat EGG
Haloperidol	1-2 mg q.d.	4-8 mg q.d. if needed

Conclusion:

Pruritus is a frequent complaint seen in many patients. Rapid labelling of the complaint as psychogenic can be dangerous to the patient and a handicap of effective management. Appropriate evaluation to rule out an organic cause is necessary before the diagnosis of psychogenic pruritus can be made. Further more, an adequate and organized conceptualization of the cause of the symptom and a proper approach to treatment can be helpful in patient management. Finally, it should be recognized that psychologic factors including anxiety, depression, personality disorder and psychoses frequently underlie or accompany pruritus. In view of this, inter relation, judicious use of psychopharmacologic agents can be beneficial and at times essential in effective treatment of these patients.

References

1. Richard G. Fried. Evaluation and treatment of "psychogenic pruritus and self excoriation": A clinical review. J Am ACAD DERMATOL 1994; 30:993-999.

2. Engles DW. Skin disorders-Psychological fac tors affecting physical conditions Kaplan, ed. Textbook of psychiatry

3. A. Cotterill, L.G. Millard. Psychocutaneous disorder. In:Rook A, Wilkinson DS, Ebling FJG, et.al, eds. Textbook of dermatology. 6th ed. Ox

ford: Blackwell Scientific publications; 1998:2785-2814

5. Panconesi E. Psychosomatic dermatology. Clin Dermatol 1984; 2:94-179.

6. Gupta MA, Gupta AK, Haberman HF. Psychot- rophic drugs in dermatology. J Am Acad Derma tol 1986; 14:633-45.

Bifonazole: Focus on a Topical Azole

R. Malkani, S. Chaudhary

Bulletin of the Jaslok Hospital & Research Centre, Vol XXVII No.2 October 2002.

Introduction

Fungi are recognized as group of organisms differing from higher plants in structure, nutrition and reproduction. Dermatophytes, are superficial and do evoke a host of inflammatory response by their metabolic activities in the form of scaling, vesiculation, postulation and sometimes abscess formation.

The prevalence rates of undetected onychomycosis and tinea pedis with concomitant onychomycosis in the diabetic population were significantly higher compared to that in the non-diabetic group. The overall frequency of fungal infections among the diabetic population (59%) is almost double the frequency observed in non-diabetics (32%).

Classification based on Site of Infection

a) Superficial mycoses i.e. infection limited to the outermost layers of the skin and hair. They are usually cosmetic problems that are easily diagnosed and treated. These encompass four infections: two involving the skin (Pityriasis versicolor and Tinea nigra) and two involving the hair (Black piedra and White piedra).

b) Cutaneous mycoses i.e. infections that extend deeper into the epidermis as well as invasive hair and nail diseases. They are generally restricted to the keratinized layer. Dermatophytes cause most of these infections.

c) Subcutaneous mycoses i.e. infections involving the dermis, cutaneous tissues, muscle and fascia. These usually develop following trauma or skin injury. Often excision of the lesion is undertaken.

d) Systemic i.e. infections that originate primarily in the lung but may spread to many organ systems.

Chronology of Antifungal Drugs

At the beginning of this century drugs used for the treatment of superficial fungal infections had a non-specific action spectrum and minimal effectiveness. However, over the years, medical research has developed newer drugs to combat fungal infections.

Year First introduction (international)

1903 Potassium iodide was used to treat sporotrichosis

1951 Discovery of the first polyene antifungal antibiotic - Nystatin

1958 Use of Griseofulvin orally for superficial mycoses

1969 Clotrimazole and Miconazole

1974 Econazole

1977 Ketoconazole

1980 Itraconazole and Fluconazole

1984 Bifonazole (Bayer AG)

1990 Terbinafine

1994 Butanifine

Chemistry

Bifonazole is an imidazole derivative. 1-[alpha-(4-biphenyl)-benzyl]-imidazole and is stable in the acid and moderately alkaline range. Bifonazole displays pronounced lipophilic properties. This is important in respect of skin penetration and skin retention time because it gives Bifonazole good affinity for specific structures in the skin, e.g. keratin.

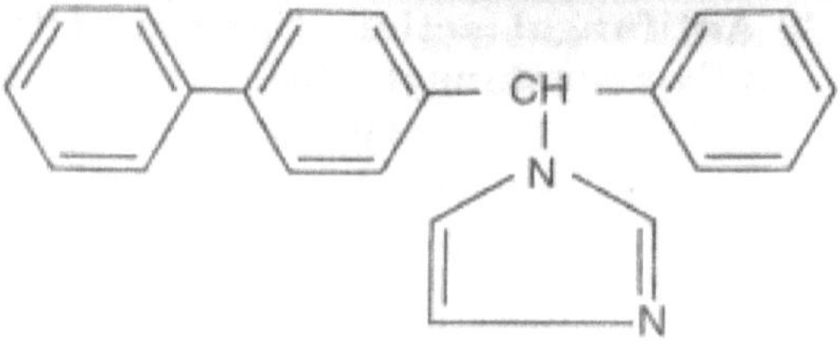

Fig. 1: Structural formula

Mechanism of action

a) Inhibition of ergosterol synthesis:

Bifonazole inhibits the synthesis of ergosterol, which is an essential constituent of the cell membrane of fungi. A lack of ergosterol leads to damage and death of the fungal cell.

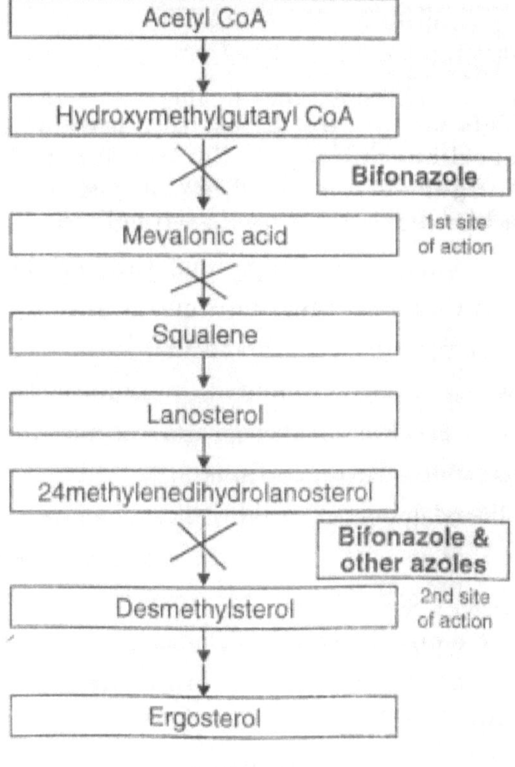

Cell Membrane

The biosynthesis of ergosterol, which passes through several different stages is inhibited by Bifonazole on two levelsunlike other "single-stage" imidazole derivatives and other broad-spectrum antifungals.

Action of Bifonazole is on two sites, reflecting in reduced synthesis of ergosterol. Bifonazole inhibits HMGCoA reductase which is the initial regulatory enzyme involved in ergosterol biosynthesis which is basically responsible for fungicidal activity.

b) Anti-inflammatory action: In clinical practice Bifonazole proves particularly effective in exudative forms of tinea. In addition, the itching of patients with dermatophytosis is rapidly relieved.

After application of Bifonazole or hydrocortisone treatment the intensity of erythema and urticaria were significantly reduced in comparison with the skin areas treated with the cream base or the untreated controls. The formation of weals (urticaria) and development of erythema were just as strongly inhibited by Bifonazole sa by hydrocortisone. Bifonazole has an anti-inflammatory effect similar to that of 1% hydrocortisone.

The clinical importance of this anti-inflammatory effect of Bifonazole can also be seen in the success achieved when treating rcsacea and, in particular, seborrhoeic dermatitis (i.e. skin conditions in which inflammatory reactions of the skin predominate). The effect against Pityrosporum ovale may also play a part in this success.

Early studies showed that Bifonazole intervenes directly in leukotriene metabolism. Leukotrienes were so named because part of them is formed primarily by leukocytes. Leukotrienes cause a sharp increase in permeability in the postcapillary venuoles of the skin and emigration of inflammatory cells into the pericapillary tissue. In experimental studies it was demonstrated that Bifonazole achieves partial or complete suppression of leukotriene formation in human granulocytes in a concentration dependent fashion.

It may be responsible to say that treatment of dermatophytoses with Bifonazole alone suppresses the signs and symptoms as quickly as initial treatment with a combined antifugal steroid cream.

Spectrum of Activity

Bifonazole has a broad spectrum of activity, with potent action on dermatophytes and moderate activity on yeasts and moulds.

In Vitro Activity

a) Inhibitory activity for fungi: Bifonazole is ideally suited for the treatment of fungal skin infections owing to its pronounced antimycotic efficacy.

Strain inhibitory activity

	% strains inhibited -Bifonazole 1-2 mg/L
Fungi	
Dermatophytes	
Tinea rubrum Tinea mentagrophytes Microsporum canis Epidermophyton floccosum	100%
Dimorphic fungi	
Blastomyces Histoplasma Coccidioides Paracoccidoides	100%
Moulds	
Aspergillus fumigatis Aspergillus niger	100%
Yeasts	
Candida spp. Torupsis spp. Other yeasts	50-83%

b) Antifungal action: Compared to other antifungals, Bifonazole has a pronounced primary fungicidal effect against dermatophytes, particularly Trichophyton species. Primary fungicidal action is killing of organisms by degeneration, which requires active metabolism of the organisms and occurs within a defined exposure time (e.g. 6-12 hrs.).

Secondary fungicidal activity

means the biologically induced death of organisms resulting from prolonged fungistasis — even when concentrations at the site of infection are sub-inhibitory.

Fungicidal against	Active substance concentrations	Exposure time
Trichophyton rubrum	5 mg/1	6 hours
Trichophyton mentagrophytes	< 5 mg/1	6 hours
Candida glabrata	5 mg/1	6 hours
Candida albicans	> 20 mg/1*	6 hours

* i.e. primary fungistatic action.

This means that Bifonazole provides excellent potency in the treatment of fungal skin infections, especially when dermatophytes are involved.

c) Activity at even low concentration: Sub-inhibitory means that an azole, at a concentration below the minimum inhibitory concentration (MIC), exerts a marked effect on the rate of growth and division of the fungi.

With Bifonazole this inhibitory effect at sub-inhibitory doses is particularly pronounced against dermatophytes. At sub-inhibitory concentrations which are below the MICs by a factor of 2 to 10, Bifonazole has a significant growth retarding effect of upto >- 90% against dermatophytes.

d) Antibacterial activity: In the case of gram-positive cocci (except enterococci), Bifonazole achieves MICs of between 4 and 16 mg/1; and against corynebacteria inhibitory concentrations of 0.5 to 2 mg/1 have been found. Corynebacteria are the organisms responsible for erythrasma, a mycosis-like bacterial infection which appears in the groin area. Corynebacteria are also found to cause super-infection in cases of interdigital fungal infection.

e) Resistance: Resistance means a lack of sensitivity of a pathogen to the antifungal used. In the case of primary resistance, this lack of sensitivity already exists before the antifungal is first administered. If the reduced sensitivity does not develop until the substance is taken, this is described as secondary resistance.

No variants of dermatophytes, yeasts and aspergilli with primary resistance to Bifonazole have yet been detected.

Pharmacokinetics

a) Skin penetration: Decreasing Bifonazole concentrations were found: from 1000 mcg/cms in the stratum papillare.

In virtually all skin layers there are Bifonazole concentrations which definitely reach the MICs of the fungi or are several times higher.

b) Skin retention time: The protective effect against infection was measured in hours from the time of pretreatment with cream to the onset of infection. The period measured is a clear gauge of how long the active substance is retained in the skin. It is revealed that Bifonazole Cream has a retention time of > 48 to > 72 hours.

Bifonazole was retained in the skin at least twice as long as the traditional azoles. The long retention time of Bifonazole at effective antifungal concentrations together with its fungicidal mode of action and good skin penetration form basis for single application of the topical treatment.

c) Absorption by fungi: Bifonazole is rapidly absorbed by the fungal cell. This results in high concentrations of active ingredient in the fungal cytoplasm. Maximum absorption is found after 10-30 minutes.

d) Absorption after topical application: It was found that a maximum of 0.6 to 0.8% of the topical dose was absorbed by healthy skin and between 2% and 4% by inflamed skin following application of Bifonazole Cream or Solution (concentrations are 5 times higher in the infected skin).

Indications

Bifonazole Cream contains 1% Bifonazole in a neutral cream base. It is useful for the mycoses of the skin and mucocutaneous parts due to dermatophytes, Candida species (specially in cases of candidal balanitis), Malassezia furfur, Aspergillus species and Corynebacterium spp.

The clinical and (mycological) cure rates after Bifonazole treatment were as follows at the follow-up examination:

	Clinical cure	Mycological cure
Candidosis	87.9%	84.5%
Tinea corporis / Tinea cruris	90.9%	91.6%
Tinea pedis	91.6%	91.3%
Tinea manus	86.9%	89.7%
Otomycosis	100%	100%
Pityriasis versicolor	91.1%	92.9%

Bifonazole used by more than 9,406 patients in multicentric trials reveal that the clinical and mycological cure rates of around 90% are achieved in cases of dermatophytosis, irrespective of the site of infection. These impressive results, especially in tinea pedis and tinea manus, well-known as obstinate mycoses, illustrate the outstanding clinical efficacy of Bifonazole.

Excellent treatment results were achieved with erythrasma and otomycosis, but the success rates were also around 90% for fungal skin infections. It is particularly impressive that there was no decrease in cure rates due to recurrence at the 2nd follow-up, showing that Bifonazole ensures lasting therapeutic success.

Clinical and mycological cure were achieved in over 90% of cases with Pityriasis versicolor, the recommended treatment period of only 14 days being adhered to in most cases. With this indication it may be possible to reduce the treatment time even further.

The mycological cure rates with candidal infections were 85% and clinical cure of 88% in cases of candidal balanitis, the common etiology of which is diabetes.

The cure rate for patients with otomycosis was 100% with Bifonazole Cream.

Dosage and administration

1) Frequency of administration: Bifonazole Cream, is used only once a day, preferably at night before retiring. They are applied thinly to the infected area of skin and rubbed in. Bifonazole is so effective that a small quantity (half finger tip unit) is enough to treat an area roughly the size of the palm of the hand.

2) Length of treatment: Bifonazole needs to be applied properly and for long enough to ensure lasting success. The treatment period will differ, depending on the causative organism, the extent and location of the infection.

Guidelines for treatment

Fungal infection			Duration	Other drugs
Tinea pedis,	Tinea	pedis interdigitals	3 weeks OD	4 weeks MA*
Tinea corporis,	Tinea	inguinalis, Tinea manus	2-3 weeks OD	4 weeks MA
Superficial candidosis			2-4 weeks OD	3 weeks MA
Pityriasis versicolor, Erythrasma			2 weeks OD	2 weeks MA

* Multiple application.

In seborrhoeic dermatitis and rosacea the treatment time depends on how the condition progresses in the individual case and usually runs into several weeks.

Compared with other antifungals, these are short treatment periods, and this helps to meet the patient's need.

Other Indications

• Seborrhoeic dermatitis / Rosacea: A

wide variety of treatment methods have been used to deal with seborrhoeic dermatitis and these have met with varying success. The substances used include sulphur and zinc compounds: They are effective against Pityrosporum ovale, they delay skin growth and suppress desquamation. The most commonly used are anti- inflammatory agents, such as hydrocortisone or even more potent corticosteroids. These are not effective against Pityrosporum ovale and only suppress the inflammatory reaction. The theory that seborrhoeic dermatitis is caused or sustained by Pityrosporum ovale is supported by the fact that antifungals have a very beneficial effect on the course of the condition. Topical application of azole such as Bifonazole, brings about a particularly marked improvement in the skin lesions, probably due to their effect on Pityrosporum ovale and other anti-inflammatory action.

There have been few reports on the use of Bifonazole in rosacea, where the patients applying Bifonazole Cream had marked improvement

	Clinical Cure	Mycological Cure
Erythrasma	100%	100%
Rosacea	65.1%	-
Seborrhoeic dermatitis	40%	Improvement 50%

Tolerability

It has been proved that Bifonazole is well tolerated and ADRs' are rare.

There has been no evidence of any primary allergising or sensitizing effects with Bifonazole. No phototoxic or photodynamic effects and no signs of systemic action after topical application have been established. Skin reactions, such as slight redness, burning, irritation and scaling, may occur especially in the presence of symptoms related to the clinical picture of predisposing local factors. However, they are rare and usually transient.

Only 3.7% of the 9406 patients assessed in clinical trials displayed any adverse reactions, mostly itching or burning

(1.8%) or skin reactions such as irritation, dryness or redness (1.7%). With these complaints it is often difficult to distinguish between a side effect of the treatment and a clinical manifestation of the fungal infection.

Features of Bifonazole

- Primary fungicidal action against dermatophytes, primary fungistatic action against yeasts, virulence of dermatophytes reduced by inhibition of keratinase.

- Good skin penetration.

- Prolonged retention time with therapeutically useful concentrations in the skin — from more than 48 hours to nearly 72 hours in the cream formulation (guinea pig studies).

- As a consequence of its long retention time in the skin. Bifonzole only needs to be applied once a day.

- Bifonazole has a rapid and prolonged action: the treatment period is shorter as a result of its fungicidal effect.

- Very well tolerated.

- Bifonazole combines potent antifungal action with simple application and excellent tolerability.

• Pleasant cosmetic properties: nongreasy, odourless, can be washed off and does not stain.

• An anti-inflammatory effect so that symptoms, in particular itching, subside very rapidly on Bifonazole treatment.

References

1. Drugs 38(2):204-225,199. International Journal of Clinical Practice, A Symposium Supplement on Bifonazole, 1998.

2. The Use of Antibiotics, Kucers, 5th ed., 1997, Pg.1460- 1464.

3. Antimycotic activity of Bifonazole in vitro and invivo, Arneimittel-Forscgybg/Drug Res.33 (I),No.4 (1983), Pg. 517-524..

4. Advances in topical antifungal therapy, R.J, Hay (Ed.), 1986, pg. 26-39. Japanese Journal of Medical Mycology, Vol.39, 11-16, 1998.

5. Clin. Ther. 13(1):126-146(1991). Drugs 1999, Jul. 58(1):179-202, Mykosen 30(10):482-'492

6. Evaluation of clinical efficacy and tolerance of Tazarotene 0.05% gel in the treatment of Acne vulgaris & Psoriasis-March 2003 to June 2003.

Epidemiological study of serum IgE levels in patients with atopic dermatitis.

Ram Malkani

To be published

Introduction

Atopy is defined as genetic disposition to develop an allergic reaction1 (as allergic rhinitis, asthma, or atopic dermatitis) and produce elevated levels of IgE upon exposure to an environmental antigen and especially one inhaled or ingested.

Atopic dermatitis is a chronically relapsing, inflammatory[1] and intensely pruritic skin disease.

IgE is a class of antibody which plays an important role in type I hypersensitivity, which manifests various allergic diseases, such as allergic asthma, allergic rhinitis, food allergy, and some types of chronic urticaria, atopic dermatitis and parasitic infestations.

Aims and objectives

To study the epidemiological profile of patients attending dermatology OPD and correlate their symptoms with total serum IgE levels.

---

1.   http://en.wikipedia.org/wiki/Inflammation

To analyze the presence of raised serum IgE levels in patients with intrinsic and extrinsic atopic dermatitis

Materials & methods

We included 24 patients with atopic dermatitis of all ages and both sexes attending dermatology OPD. Patients were analyzed with complete personal, family history Total serum IgE levels were done in all these patients. Patients on immunosuppressive agents were excluded.

Normal IgE levels

Age	Serum IgE (IU/ml)
4-11months	0-74
1yr	0-150
2yr	0-126
3yr	2.6-135
4yr	1.4-219
5-7yrs	1.6-158
7-10yrs	3.4-437
10-15yrs	3.7-260
Adults	0-180

Results

There were 24 patients in study population with 9 males and 15 females. Age group of the patients ranged from 11yrs to 65years with mean age being 44.65yrs. One of the patient was a known case of retroviral disease.

Duration of symptoms ranged from 3months to 6-7yrs for present episode with remissions and exacerbations in the past.

Most of the patients complained of generalized pruritus, itchy papular, eczematous lesions, lichenification over the flexures, recurrent eczemas including hand eczemas, allergy to artificial jewelry, and few having localized itcthing.

Total serum IgE levels were raised in 17 patients while 7 patients had normal serum IgE levels.

Table 1. Patients with intrinsic atopic dermatitis and normal IgE levels

Age (years)	Sex	S.IgE(IU/ml)	Age of onset(years)
55	F	13.26	45
65	F	21.68	37
56	M	32.03	52
20	F	73.73	19
25	F	55.57	23
55	F	30.72	48
56	F	263.2	55

Table 1 shows patients with intrinsic atopic dermatitis with higher age of onset (mean age-39.85yrs), female predominance(85%) as in previous studies, normal serum IgE levels and lack of history of atopyexcept in 1 patient.

Table 2. Patients with extrinsic atopic dermatitis and raised IgE levels.

Age(years)	Sex	S.IgE levels(IU/ml)	Age of onset(years)
62	M	2947	5
27	F	469	8
49	F	215.5	14
44	F	342.5	10
55	M	435.6	15
29	F	205.6	7
31	F	728	9
37	F	765.8	17
53	M	674	20
44	F	514	9
28	F	802	8
11	M	1364	7
57	M	4452.5	20
39	M	546.3	24
34	M	436.7	12
65	F	2647.5	19
33	M	33	8

Since the presenting symptoms of both intrinsic and extrinsic atopic dermatitis are indistinguishable, we divided our patients in the above two groups based on the following findings. Table 2 shows patients with extrinsic dermatitis having earlier age of onset(22.52yrs), nearly equal sex ratio(M-=8,F=9), personal or family history of atopy, raised total serum IgE levels and absence of icthyosis indicating filagrin gene mutations.

Discussion

Immunoglobulin E (IgE) is a class of antibody that has been found only in mammals. It exists as monomers consisting of two heavy chains (ε chain) and two light chains, with the ε chain.

Although IgE is typically the least abundant isotype - blood serum IgE levels in a normal ("non-atopic") individual are only 0.05% of the Ig concentration,(5) compared to 10 mg/ml for the IgGs - it is capable of triggering the most powerful inflammation reactions.

Atopic individuals can have up to 10 times the normal level of IgE in their blood (as in hyper-IgE syndrome). However, this may not be a requirement for symptoms to occur as has been seen in asthmatics with normal IgE levels in their blood - recent research has shown that IgE production can occur locally in the nasal mucosa.(6)

IgE that can specifically recognize an "allergen" with its high-affinity receptor FcεRI so that basophils and mast cells, become "primed" histamine, leukotrienes, and certain interleukins. These chemicals cause many of the symptoms we associate with such as airway constriction in asthma, local inflammation in eczema, increased mucus secretion in allergic rhinitis, and increased vascular permeability.

Atopic dermatitis (AD) is a chronic relapsing dermatitis which can be categorized into the extrinsic and intrinsic types.

The diagnostic Criteria for Atopic Dermatitis (AD) by Hanifin and Rajka(7) are as follows:-

Major criteria: Must have three or more of:

- Pruritus

- Typical morphology and distribution

- Flexural lichenification or linearity in adults

- Facial and extensor involvement in infants and children

- Chronic or chronically-relapsing dermatitis

- Personal or family history of atopy (asthma, allergic rhinitis, atopic dermatitis)

Minor criteria: Should have three or more of:

- Xerosis

- Ichthyosis, palmar hyperlinearity, or keratosis pilaris

- Immediate (type 1) skin-test reactivity

- Raised serum IgE

- Early age of onset

- Tendency toward cutaneous infections (especially S aureus and herpes simplex) or impaired cell-mediated immunity

- Tendency toward non-specific hand or foot dermatitis

- Nipple eczema

- Cheilitis

- Recurrent conjunctivitis

- Dennie-Morgan infraorbital fold

- Keratoconus

- Anterior subcapsular cataracts

- Orbital darkening

- Facial pallor or facial erythema

- Pityriasis alba

- Anterior neck folds

- Itch when sweating

- Intolerance to wool and lipid solvents

- Perifollicular accentuation

- Food intolerance

- Course influenced by environmental or emotional factors

- White dermographism or delayed blanch

Although the two forms are clinically indistinguishable based on the findings of the physical examination, there are numerous differences in other aspects. Extrinsic AD which is the classical type constituting 70% to 85% of the cases, intrinsic atopic dermatitis makes up the remaining 15% to 30% with a female predominance.

The onset of extrinsic AD typically is in early childhood while patients with intrinsic AD have a later onset. Other clinical features of intrinsic AD include milder severity, and Dennie-Morgan folds, but no ichthyosis vulgris or palmar hyperlinearity Finally, patients with intrinsic AD are characterized by an absence of other atopic disease, asthma, and allergic rhinitis (Schmid-Grendel meier et al., 2001).

The skin barrier is perturbed in the extrinsic, but not intrinsic type. Filaggrin gene mutations are not a feature of intrinsic AD.

Extrinsic or allergic AD shows high total serum IgE levels and the presence of specific IgE for environmental and food allergens, whereas intrinsic or non-allergic AD exhibits normal total IgE values and the absence of specific IgE. The intrinsic type is immunologically characterized by the lower expression of interleukin (IL) -4, IL-5, and IL-13, and the higher expression of interferon-gamma. It is suggested that intrinsic AD patients are not sensitized with protein allergens, which induce Th2 responses, but with other antigens, and metals, might be one of the candidates of such antigens.

References

1. Atopic dermatitis. In: Habif TP, ed. Clinical Dermatology. 5th ed. Philadelphia, Pa: Mosby Elsevier; 2009:chap 5.

2. Lewis-Jones S, Mugglestone MA; Guideline Development Group. Management of atopic eczema in children aged up to 12 years: summary of NICE guidance. BMJ. 2007;335:1263-1264.

3. Ascroft DM, Chen LC, Garside R, Stein K, Williams HC. Topical pimecrolimus for eczema. Cochrane Database Syst Rev. 2007 Oct 17;(4):CD005500.

4. Bath-Hextall FJ, Delamere FM, Williams HC. Dietary exclusions for established atopic eczema. Cochrane Database Syst Rev. 2008 Jan 23;(1):CD005203.

5. Liu FT[2], Goodarzi H[3], Chen HY[4].IgE, mast cells, and eosinophils in atopic dermatitis. Clin Rev Allergy Immunol.[5] 2011

---

2. http://www.ncbi.nlm.nih.gov/

pubmed?term=Liu%20FT%5BAuthor%5D&cauthor=true&cauthor_uid=21249468

3. http://www.ncbi.nlm.nih.gov/

pubmed?term=Goodarzi%20H%5BAuthor%5D&cauthor=true&cauthor_uid=21249468

Dec;41(3):298-310. doi: 10.1007/s12016-011-8252-4.

6. Stephen P. Stone, MD; Sigfrid A. Muller, MD; Gerald J. Gleich, MD. IgE Levels in Atopic Dermatitis.Arch Dermatol. 1973;108(6):806-811. doi:10.1001/archderm.1973.01620270032008.

7. Rothe MJ, Grant-Kels JM. Diagnostic criteria for atopic dermatitis. Lancet. 1996; 348: 769-770.

8. Rudikoff D, Lebwohl M. Atopic dermatitis. Lancet. 1998; 351: 1715-1721.

9. Simpson EL, Hanifin JM. Atopic dermatitis. Med Clin North Am. 2006 Jan;90(1):149-67.

---

4. http://www.ncbi.nlm.nih.gov/pubmed?term=Chen%20HY%5BAuthor%5D&cauthor=true&cauthor_uid=21249468

5. http://www.ncbi.nlm.nih.gov/pubmed/21249468

In the process of completion for publication

Serology A metanalysis ofthe results of CMV and HSV serology in Pregnancy

Manindersingh Setia, Ram Malkani

HIV A study of Anti Retroviral Resistance patterns in Treatment exposed and Treatment Naïve HIV infected patients

Principal Investigator, Raj Harjani, Ram Malkani, Manindersingh Setia

Generation next HIV free: New borns of HIV Sero discordantand Sero concordant couples

Delivering HIV negative babies – an experience of 11 couples

Raj Harjani, Ram Malkani